Obstetric Anesthesia Handbook

Fourth Edition

Obstetric Anesthesia Handbook

Fourth Edition

Sanjay Datta, MD, FFARCS (Eng)

Professor of Anesthesia
Brigham and Women's Hospital
Harvard Medical School
Boston, Massachusetts

With 72 Illustrations

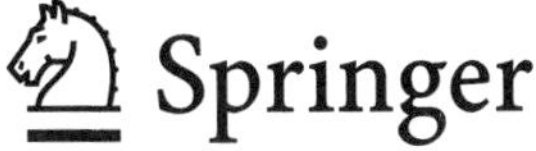

Sanjay Datta, MD, FFARCS (Eng)
Professor of Anesthesia
Brigham and Women's Hospital
Harvard Medical School
Boston, MA 02115
USA

Library of Congress Control Number: 2005926767

ISBN 0-387-26075-7
ISBN 978-0387-26075-4

Printed on acid-free paper.

Printed in the United States of America. (BS/MVY)

9 8 7 6 5 4 3 2 1

springeronline.com

Preface

Three previous editions of *Obstetric Anesthesia Handbook* have proven valuable in serving those interested in managing pregnant women, each edition has become popular among anesthesiology residents, fellows, staff, and also among obstetricians. This book has enjoyed strong international appeal and has been widely translated.

Obstetric anesthesia has undergone changes in its field, changes in the technique as well as in its specific pharmaceutical agents. Updating these fields has been the primary focus for the fourth edition. The text has been written to retain the cohesiveness of a single-author work; all efforts have been made to keep the text concise and to keep it in a true handbook format.

I sincerely hope the fourth edition will be as useful and as popular as previous editions. I thank Mrs. Elizabeth Kiernan, whose help has been immeasurable.

Sanjay Datta, MD

Contents

1
Maternal Physiological Changes During Pregnancy, Labor, and the Postpartum Period

▼

Parturients undergo remarkable changes during pregnancy, labor, and the immediate postpartum period that can directly affect anesthetic techniques; hence a broad knowledge of these changes is essential for proper management of these women.

Changes in Blood Volume

Maternal blood volume increases during pregnancy, and this involves an increase in plasma volume as well as in red cell and white cell volumes.[1] *The plasma volume increases by 40% to 50%, whereas the red cell volume goes up by only 15% to 20%, which causes a situation that is described as "physiological anemia of pregnancy"* (normal hemoglobin, 12 g/dL; hematocrit, 35).[2] Because of this apparent hemodilution, blood viscosity decreases by approximately 20%. The exact mechanism of this increase in plasma volume is unknown. However, several hormones such as renin-angiotensin-aldosterone, atrial natriuretic peptide, estrogen, and progesterone may be involved in this interesting phenomenon. Two current hypothesis attribute the increase to (1) an underfill state caused by initial vasodilation, which stimulates hormones such as renin, angiotensin, and aldosterone or (2) an overfill state characterized by an early increase in sodium retention (due to an increase in mineralcorticoids) that retains fluid, causing an increase in blood volume. Levels of clotting factors I, VII, VIII, IX, X, and XII, and the fibrinogen count are elevated during pregnancy as well. *At present the majority of observers report a statistically significant fall in platelet count as pregnancy progresses.*[3] A recent study that observed an increase in thrombopoietin with the advancement of the gestational age also confirmed this finding.[3a] Systemic fibrinolysis also may increase slightly.

Clinical Implications

The increased blood volume serves several important functions: (1) it takes care of the increased circulatory need of the enlarging uterus as well as the needs of the fetoplacental unit, (2) it fills the ever-increasing venous reservoir, (3) it protects the parturient from the bleeding at the time of delivery, and (4) parturients become hypercoaguable as the gestation progresses.

It takes about 8 weeks after delivery for the blood volume to return to normal.

Changes in the Cardiovascular System

An increase in cardiac output is one of the most important changes of pregnancy. *Cardiac output increases by 30% to 40% during pregnancy, and the maximum increase is attained around 24 weeks' gestation.*[4] The increase in heart rate lags behind the increase in cardiac output initially and then ultimately rises by 10 to 15 beats per minute by 28 to 32 weeks' gestation. The increase in cardiac output initially depends mainly on the rise in stroke volume, and later the increase in heart rate also becomes an important factor. With Doppler and M-mode echocardiography technique, increases in end diastolic chamber size and total left ventricular wall thickness have been observed in recent years. Cardiac output can vary depending on the uterine size as well as on the maternal position at the time of measurement. The enlarged gravid uterus can cause aortocaval compression while the pregnant woman is in the supine position, and this will lead to reduced venous return and ultimately maternal hypotension. This effect will be exaggerated in parturients with polyhydramnios or multiple gestations.

Cardiac output increases further during labor and may show values 50% higher than prelabor values. In the immediate postpartum period, cardiac output increases maximally and can rise 80% above prelabor values and approximately 100% above nonpregnant measurements. The increase in stroke volume as well as in heart rate maintains the increased cardiac output.

Clinical Implications

An increased cardiac output might not be well tolerated by pregnant women with valvular heart disease (e.g., aortic or mitral stenosis) or coronary arterial disease. A *severe decompensation in myocardial function can develop at 24 weeks' gestation, during labor, and especially immediately after delivery.*

Cardiac output, heart rate, and stroke volume decrease to pre-labor values 24 to 72 hours postpartum and return to nonpregnant levels within 6 to 8 weeks after delivery.[5]

Even with this increase in cardiac output the systolic blood pressure does not change during pregnancy; however, the diastolic blood pressure drops by I to 15 mm Hg. There is a decrease in mean arterial pressure because of an associated decrease in systemic vascular resistance. Pregnancy hormones like estradiol-17β and progesterone are probably responsible for these vascular changes.[6] Prostacyclin as well as nitric oxide also may play an important role.

The down regulation of α and β receptors may also be an important factor. The heart is displaced to the left and upward during pregnancy because of the progressive elevation of the diaphragm by the gravid uterus. The electrocardiogram of normal parturients may include: (1) benign dysrhythmia, (2) reversal of ST, T, and Q waves, and (3) left axis deviation.

Aortocaval compression is one of the most important events during pregnancy, especially when the parturient lies supine. Hence left uterine displacement must always be maintained. This becomes more important following regional (spinal or epidural) analgesia or anesthesia. Volume expansion is always important. Recently, however, the importance of infusion of predeterminant volume has been challenged.[6a] Engorgement of the epidural venous plexus increases the risk of intravascular catheter placement in pregnant women; direct connection of the azygos system to the heart as well as brain also increases the risks of local anesthetic cardiovascular and central nervous system toxicity.

Changes in the Respiratory System

Changes in the respiratory parameters start as early as the fourth week of gestation. Minute ventilation is increased at term by about 50% above nonpregnant values. The increase in minute ventilation is mainly due to an increase in tidal volume (40%) and, to a lesser extent, to an increase in the respiratory rate (15%).[7] Alveolar ventilation is greatly increased as the tidal volume increases without any change in the anatomic dead space. At term the P_{CO_2} value is decreased (32 to 35 mm Hg). Increased progesterone concentrations during pregnancy decrease the threshold of the medullary respiratory center to carbon dioxide.[8]

Functional residual capacity, expiratory reserve volume, and residual volume are decreased at term. These changes are related to the cephalad displacement of the diaphragm by the large gravid uterus. Inspiratory capacity increases because of increase in tidal volume and inspiratory reserve volume. Vital capacity is unchanged. Even with the presence of elevation of the diaphragm the total lung capacity is slightly reduced because of the presence of an increase in chest circumference.

Besides these changes in respiratory parameters, there are some structural changes. The respiratory mucous membrane becomes vascular, edematous, and friable.

Clinical Implications

A decreased functional residual capacity as well as increased oxygen consumption can cause a rapid development of maternal hypoxemia. *Decreased functional residual capacity, increased minute ventilation, as well as a decreased minimal alveolar concentration (MAC) will make parturients more susceptible to inhalational anesthetics as compared with their nonpregnant counterparts.*

Because of the increased edema, vascularity, and friability of the mucous membrane, one should try to avoid nasal intubation in pregnant women, and smaller endotracheal tubes should be used for oral intubation.

During the first stage of labor, in the absence of pain relief, hyperventilation can decrease the maternal $PaCO_2$ to values as low as 18 mm Hg and, subsequently, produce fetal acidosis. In the second stage of labor, $PaCO_2$ increases to a certain extent and may stay around 25 mm Hg.[9] Maternal alkalosis associated with decreased $PaCO_2$ values due to hyperventilation as a result of labor pain causes fetal acidosis because of (1) decreased uteroplacental perfusion (with significant drop of maternal $PaCO_2$) and (2) shifting of the maternal oxygen dissociation curve to the left. Decreased FRC decreases the time for denitrogenation. However, because of decreased FRC and increased oxygen demand the parturients rapidly become hypoxic when apneic. All respiratory parameters return to nonpregnant values within 6 to 12 weeks postpartum.

Table 1-1. Changes in the Renal System

	Nonpregnant	Pregnant
BUN (mg/dl)	13 ± 3	8.7 ± 1.5
Creatinine (mg/dl)	0.67 ± 0.14	0.46 ± 0.13

Changes in the Renal System

The glomerular filtration rate is increased during pregnancy because of increased renal plasma flow.[10] A rise in the filtration rate decreases plasma blood urea nitrogen (BUN) and creatinine concentrations by about 40% to 50% (Table 1-1). Tubular reabsorption of sodium is increased. However, glucose and amino acids might not be absorbed as efficiently; hence glycosuria and aminoaciduria may develop in normal gestation.[11,12] The renal pelvis and ureters are dilated, and peristalsis is decreased.

Clinical Implications

Normal parturients' BUN (8 to 9 mg/dl) and creatinine (0.4 mg/dl) values are 40% less than in nonpregnant women. So nonpregnant values in parturients will suggest abnormal kidney function. Physiological diuresis during the postpartum period occurs between the second and fifth days. The glomerular filtration rate and BUN concentration slowly return to nonpregnant values by the sixth postpartum week.

Changes in the Gastrointestinal System

Gastrointestinal motility, food absorption, and lower esophageal sphincter pressure are decreased during pregnancy, probably due to an increased level of plasma progesterone.[13] Lower esophageal sphincter pressure is decreased during pregnancy, on the other hand intragastric pressure is increased during the last trimester. Heartburn during pregnancy is the result of reduced barrier pressure. The gastric emptying time of solid as well as liquid material is not changed during pregnancy. Because of decreased plasma gastrin concentration during pregnancy, there is reduction in the total acid content of the stomach. Gastric emptying time is significantly slower during labor and hence gastric volume is increased. Analgesic drugs will further increase the gastric emptying time. The enlarged gravid uterus divides the stomach into fundal and antral parts and also increases gastric pressure (Fig. 1-1).

Serum glutamic oxaloacetic transaminase, lactic dehydrogenase, and alkaline phosphatase levels are elevated

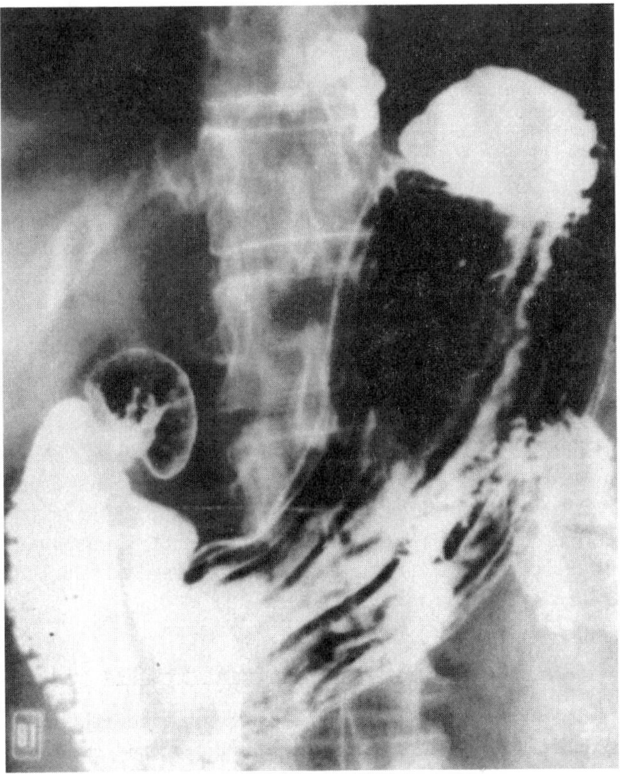

Figure 1-1. Fundal and antral sacs in parturients following a Barium meal. (From Holdsworth JD, et al. Fundal and autral sacs in parturients following a barium meal. Anaesthesia 1970; 35s641. Used with permission from Blackwell Publishing.)

during pregnancy and labor, and the sodium Bromsulphalein excretion test is also often abnormal in the majority of parturients. *Serum cholinesterase activity is reduced 24% before delivery and becomes lowest (33%) on the third postpartum day*[14] (Fig 1-2). *Even with this lower activity, normal dosing*

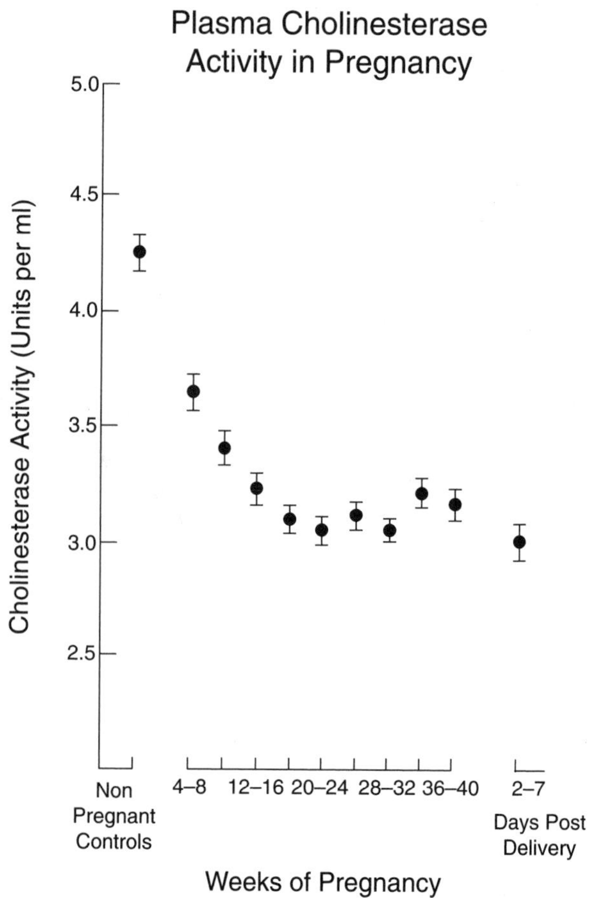

Figure 1-2. Plasma cholinesterase activity in pregnancy. (From Cohen SE: *Semin Anesthesia* 1982; 1:73. Used with permission from Elsevier.)

of succinylcholine for intubation (1 to 1.5 mg/kg) is not associated with prolonged neuromuscular blockade during pregnancy.

Gallbladder function and emptying are impaired during pregnancy, and there is evidence that parturients may be more prone to gallstone problems.

Clinical Implications

Pregnant women in labor should always be considered to have a full stomach irrespective of the time of their last meal. General anesthesia should be avoided when possible. The routine use of nonparticulate antacid is important before cesarean section and before induction of regional anesthesia, and one should allow for proper mixing of the antacid and stomach contents.

Although the mechanical effects of a gravid uterus on the stomach are resolved in a few days, the other gastrointestinal changes revert back to nonpregnant states within 6 weeks postpartum.

Changes in the Central and Peripheral Nervous Systems

The central and peripheral nervous systems undergo significant changes during pregnancy. The MAC is decreased by 25% to 40% (different inhalational anesthetics) during pregnancy.[15] Increased progesterone and endorphin concentrations during pregnancy have been implicated as a cause of this change. However, a few studies have shown that endorphin concentrations do not increase during pregnancy until the parturient is in active labor,[16] so endorphin might not be involved in the difference in MAC values. By injecting exogenous progesterone in oophorectomized rabbits, a decrease in MAC was observed when compared with control animals.[17]

A wider dermatomal spread of sensory anesthesia was observed in parturients following the use of epidural anesthesia as compared with their nonpregnant counterparts of the same age group.[18] This difference was explained on the

Table 1-2. Increased Sensitivity in Nerves From Pregnant Animals as Compared With Nonpregnant Ones*

Nerve Fibers (N = 6)	Pregnant Animals	Nonpregnant Animals†	P
A	11.2 ± 0.4	19.4 + 3.7	0.001
B	6.7 ± 2.8	17.9‡	0.03
C	12.1 ± 5.2	31.6‡	0.001

*From Datta S. Lambert H, Gregus J. et al. Anesth Analg 1983; 62:1070–1072.

†Time in minutes for a 50% block with 0.35 mM bupivacaine HCl in HEPES Liley's solution.

‡The statistical method employed does not yield a standard deviation here.

basis of a reduced epidural space volume caused by an engorged epidural venous plexus because of aortocaval compression by the large gravid uterus. However, a more recent report showed that this difference exists even during early pregnancy (8 to 12 weeks) when one might not expect any mechanical obstruction by the small gravid uterus and thus that other factors may be involved in this difference[19] The factors suggested are (1) compensated respiratory alkalosis of pregnancy, (2) reduced plasma and cerebrospinal fluid (CSF) protein levels during pregnancy, and (3) pregnancy hormones. An increased sensitivity of the pregnant nerve fiber to bupivacaine was observed in recent studies[20] (Table 1-2). This increased sensitivity was also observed in nerves from oophorectomized rabbits treated chronically with exogenous progesterone.[21] Interestingly, this phenomenon was not observed following acute exposure to progesterone.[22] More recently, enhanced sensitivity of the peripheral nerve to local anesthetic has been documented in humans.[23] It is possible that progesterone or one of its active metabolites is responsible for the observed increased sensitivity of the peripheral nervous system to anesthetics in parturients.

Clinical Implications

Even though the exact mechanism of the increased sensitivity of the central nervous system and peripheral nervous system to general and local anesthetics is not known, one must reduce the doses of anesthetics in pregnant women.

There is controversy regarding the time needed for these changes to revert back to their prepregnant state because of a lack of studies in this area. However, there is evidence that increased sensitivity to the local anesthetic used for epidural or spinal anesthesia can exist up to 36 hours postpartum.

Changes in the Musculoskeletal System

The hormone relaxin is responsible for both the generalized ligamentous relaxation and the softening of collagenous tissues.

Changes in the Dermatological System

Hyperpigmentation of certain parts of the body such as the face, neck, and midline of the abdomen is not uncommon during pregnancy. Melanocyte-stimulating hormone is responsible for this change.

Changes in Mammary Tissue

Enlargement of the breasts is an integral part of the physiological changes of pregnancy.

Changes in the Ocular System

Intraocular pressure has been shown to decrease during pregnancy; this is related to (1) increased progesterone levels, (2) the presence of relaxin, and (3) decreased production of aqueous humor due to increased secretion of human chorionic gonadotropin.[24]

Clinical Implications

Relaxation of ligaments and collagen tissue of the vertebral column is the main cause of lordosis during pregnancy.

Enlarged breasts, especially in parturients with short necks, may make intubation extremely difficult. A short-handled larygoscope as described by Datta and Briwa may be helpful in such cases.[25] Changes in intraocular pressure in parturients may produce visual disturbances as well as contact lens intolerance.

References

1. Lund CJ, Donovan JC: Blood volume during pregnancy. *Am J Obstet Gynecol* 1967; 98:393.
2. Ueland K: Maternal cardiovascular hemodynamics. VII. Intrapartum blood volume changes. *Am J Obstet Gynecol* 1976; 126:671.
3. Fay RA, et al: Platelets in pregnancy: Hyperdestruction in pregnancy. *Obstet Gynecol* 1983; 61:238.

3a. Frolich MA, Datta S, Corn SB: Thrombopoietin in normal pregnancy and preeclampsia. *Am J Obstet Gynecol* 1998; 179:100.

4. Mashini IS, et al: Serial noninvasive evaluation of cardiovascular hemodynamics during pregnancy. *Am J Obstet Gynecol* 1987; 156:1208.
5. Ueland K, et al: Maternal cardiovascular dynamics. III. Labor and delivery under local and caudal analgesia. *Am J Obstet Gynecol* 1969; 103:8.
6. Rosenfeld CR, et al: Effect of estradiol-17β on blood flow to reproductive and nonreproductive tissues in pregnant ewes. *Am J Obstet Gynecol* 1976; 124:618.

6a. Park GE, Hauch MA, Curlin F, Datta S, Bader A: The effects of varying volume preload before cesarean delivery on maternal hemodynamics and colloid osmotic pressure. *Anesth Analg* 1996; 83:299.

7. Prowse CM, Gaenster EA: Respiratory and acid-base changes during pregnancy. *Anesthesiology* 1965; 26:381.
8. Tyler JM: The effects of progesterone on the respiration of patients with emphysema and hypercapnea. *J Clin Invest* 1960; 39:34.
9. Reid DHS: Respiratory changes in labour. *Lancet* 1966; 1:784.
10. Digham WJ, et al: Renal function in human pregnancy. I. Changes in glomerular filtration rate and renal plasma flow. *Proc Soc Exp Biol Med* 1958; 97:512.
11. Christensen PJ, et al: Amino acids in blood plasma and urine during pregnancy. *Scand J Clin Lab Invest* 1957; 9:54.
12. Welsh GW, Sims EAH: The mechanism of renal glycosourea in pregnancy. *Diabetes* 1960; 9:363.

13. Lind LJ, et al: Lower esophageal sphincter pressures in pregnancy. *Can Med Assoc J* 1968; 98:571.
14. Cohen SE: Why is the pregnant patient different? *Semin Anesth* 1982: 1:73.
15. Palahniuk RJ, et al: Pregnancy decreases the requirement for inhaled anesthetic agent. *Anesthesiology* 1974; 41:82.
16. Steinbrook RA, et al: Dissociation of plasma and cerebrospinal fluid beta-endorphin-like immunoactivity levels during pregnancy and parturition. *Anesth Analg* 1982; 61:893.
17. Datta S, et al: Chronically administered progesterone decreases halothane requirements in rabbits *Anesth Analg* 1989; 68:46.
18. Bromage PR: Continuous lumbar epidural analgesia for obstetrics. *Can Med Assoc J* 1961; 85:1136.
19. Fagreus L, et al: Spread of epidural analgesia in early pregnancy. *Anesthesiology* 1983; 58:184.
20. Datta S, et al: Differential sensitivities of mammalian nerve fibers during pregnancy. *Anesth Analg* 1983; 62:1070.
21. Flanagan HL, et al: Effect of exogenously administered progesterone on susceptibility of rabbit vagus nerves to bupivacaine (abstract). *Anesthesiology* 1988; 69:676.
22. Bader AM, et al: Acute effect of progesterone on conduction blockade in the isolated rabbit nerve. *Anesth Analg* 1990; 71:545.
23. Butterworth JF, et al: Pregnancy increases median nerve susceptibility to lidocaine. *Anesthesiology* 1990; 72:962.
24. Weinreb RN, et al: Maternal ocular adaptations during pregnancy *Obstet Gynecol Surv* 1987; 42:471.
25. Datta S, Briwa J: Modified laryngoscope for endotracheal intubation of obese patients. *Anesth Analg* 1981; 60:120.

2
Local Anesthetic Pharmacology

▼

Local anesthetics are an integral part of obstetric anesthesia; hence an adequate knowledge of these chemical agents is absolutely essential.

Chemically, local anesthetics are classified into two groups: (1) amino esters and (2) amino amides (Fig 2-1).

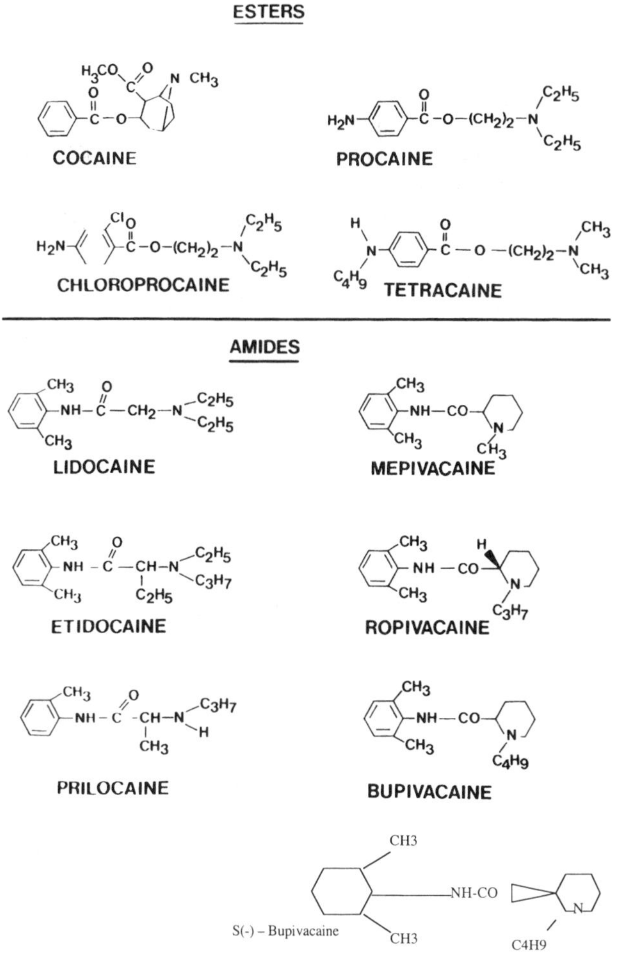

ESTERS

COCAINE

PROCAINE

CHLOROPROCAINE

TETRACAINE

AMIDES

LIDOCAINE

MEPIVACAINE

ETIDOCAINE

ROPIVACAINE

PRILOCAINE

BUPIVACAINE

S(-) – Bupivacaine

Figure 2-1. Local anesthetics. Esters and amides with chemical structures.

Amino esters are ester derivatives of para-aminobenzoic acid. These agents are metabolized by plasma cholinesterase, and the *first metabolic product is para-aminobenzoic acid, which is a known allergen. Hence allergic reactions to amino esters are not unusual* On the other hand, *amino amides* are associated with amide linkage, and these agents are metabolized by the liver; *thus allergic reactions to amides are extremely rare.* Two new amide local anesthetics recently approved by the Federal Drug Administration are ropivacaine and S-bupivacaine or levobupivacaine.[1] Interestingly, these agents are marketed as pure S forms.[1a]

Besides the chemical classification, another practical way to classify these agents is by their clinical properties:[2] (1) low potency with a short duration of action, e.g., procaine, 2-chloroprocaine; (2) intermediate potency with intermediate duration of action, e.g., lidocaine, mepivacaine, prilocaine; and (3) high potency with a long duration of action, e g., bupivacaine, tetracaine, etidocaine, ropivacaine and levobupivacaine. These differences in their activities can be explained to a certain extent by discussing both their physicochemical as well as their nonphysicochemical properties. Of the amide local anesthetics, prilocaine has the highest clearance rate.

Physicochemical Properties

Lipid Solubility

Lipid solubility influences the potency of the local anesthetic. The nerve membrane is a lipoprotein complex, and local anesthetics, which are highly lipid soluble, can pass through the membrane easily, thus requiring fewer molecules for conduction blockade. *Lidocaine and etidocaine possess similar pKa values; however, etidocaine is more potent than lidocaine because of its higher lipid solubility. As far as placental transfer is concerned, lipid solubility will enhance local anesthetic diffusion through the placental structures.*

Protein Binding

Protein binding influences the duration of action of local anesthetics. Local anesthetics produce nerve blockade by binding with the protein receptor located within the sodium channel of the nerve membrane. In vitro studies observing the neural blockade by different local anesthetics verify this notion. Procaine, an agent with minimal protein binding, will be washed out from the isolated nerve much more quickly than highly protein-bound local anesthetics such as etidocaine, bupivacaine, or tetracaine. Local anesthetic is bound to two principal sites in plasma: (1) a high-affinity, low-capacity α_1-acid glycoprotein and (2) low-affinity, high-capacity albumin. *Protein binding will inhibit placental transfer,* so etidocaine, because of its high-protein-binding property, will have less placental transfer.

pKa

pKa is the most important factor in determining the speed of onset of the local anesthetic agents. pKa is defined as the pH where 50% of the local anesthetic will remain in uncharged form and 50% will exist in charged form. Agents with pKa closest to the body's pH will have the fastest onset since a major amount of the local anesthetic will exist in uncharged form, the latter being primarily responsible for diffusion across the nerve membrane. Mepivacaine with a pKa of 7.6 has a faster onset than bupivacaine with a pKa of 8.1. Etidocaine, lidocaine, and prilocaine possess pKa values of 7.7, so at a normal tissue pH of 7.4, 35% of these agents will exist in base or uncharged form, whereas bupivacaine with a pKa of 8.1 will have only 15% in base form at a pH of 7.4. *However, one must remember that although the uncharged form is important for diffusion across the nerve membrane the charged form will be ultimately responsible for binding with protein receptors. Hence both forms of the local anesthetic are important for neural blockade. pKa also affects the placental transfer of the local anesthetic. Agents with low pKa values will transfer in larger amounts because of the greater amount of uncharged forms.* The umbilical vein/maternal vein (UV/MV) concentration ratio of a local anesthetic is inversely proportional to the pKa of the local anesthetic, e.g., mepivacaine with the lowest pKa (7.6) possesses the highest UV/MV ratio (0.8). *Although a lower UV/MV ratio has been recently implicated with higher tissue binding of the local anesthetic to neonatal tissue,*[3] *the clinical importance of this factor is not clear at the present time.*

Nonphysicochemical Properties

Tissue Diffusibility

Local anesthetics with high tissue diffusibility will have a faster onset of action. 2-Chloroprocaine, even with its high pKa (8.9), shows a rapid onset of action. Two factors have been suggested for this finding: (1) the high concentration of the drug used for clinical practice (because of the low toxicity) and (2) the high tissue diffusibility of this agent.

Inherent Vasoactive Property

Different degrees of vasodilation of the local anesthetic will modify its action (Fig 2-2). In in vitro nerve preparations, lido-

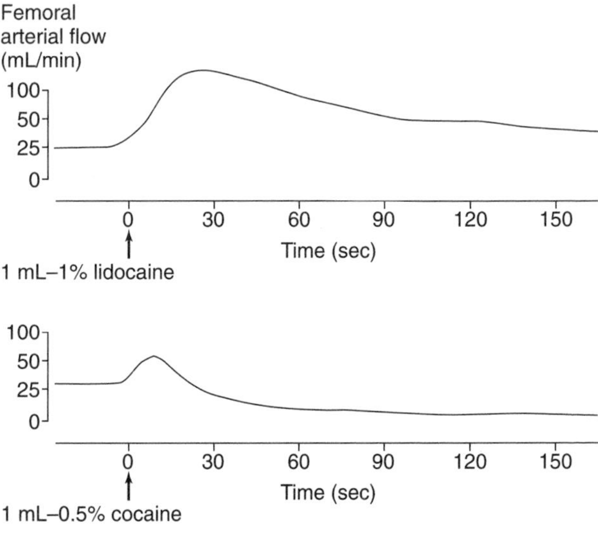

Figure 2-2. Effect of intraarterial injection of lidocaine and cocaine on femoral arterial blood flow in the dog. (Adapted from Covino BG, Vassallo HG: Mechanisms of action and clinical use. In *Local Anesthetics.* New York, Grune & Stratton, 1976.)

caine shows higher potency than mepivacaine in blocking the isolated nerve. However, in vivo studies, their relative potency has been observed to be similar. This might be related to the higher vasodilating property of lidocaine, in which case less drug will be available for neural blockade in the clinical situation. Besides these inherent properties, there are other factors that can modify the activity of the local anesthetic. Because of inherent vasoconstricting properties, the S-isomers including ropivacaine and S-bupivacaine, are associated with longer duration of infiltration block.

Other Factors Affecting Local Anesthetic Activity

Volume and Concentration

The total dose of the agents will ultimately dictate the onset, quality, and duration of the block. With increased doses of local anesthetic one can make the onset faster and the duration longer. In one study of obstetric population, it was shown that when the same volume is used, the onset, quality, and duration of the block improved by varying the concentration from 0.125% to 0.5% while using for epidural anesthesia.[4] Another interesting observation was discovered when 600 mg of prilocaine was used epidurally: no difference in onset, adequacy, or duration of block was observed by administering either 30 mL of a 2% solution or 20 mL of a 3% solution.[5] However, it is possible that one might observe a higher spread of the local anesthetic in the epidural space when a higher volume is used.

Addition of Vasoconstrictor Agents

Epinephrine is frequently used with local anesthetics to improve the quality and duration of analgesia. *Because of the vasoconstriction produced by epinephrine more local anesthetic will be available for neural blockade because of less absorption through vascular beds.* Besides epinephrine, norepinephrine and phenylephrine have also been used for prolonging the duration of blockade. Addition of epinephrine will also decrease the peak plasma concentrations of certain local anesthetics like mepivacaine and lidocaine. Because of inherent vasoconstriction with both ropivacaine and S-bupivacaine, the addition of epinephrine should not be necessary.

Site of Injection

The onset of action of a local anesthetic varies depending on the site of administration. Spinal and subcutaneous routes are associated with a more rapid onset, whereas epidural and brachial plexus blocks are associated with a slower onset of action.

Bicarbonation and Carbonation of Local Anesthetics

The addition of a bicarbonate solution to a local anesthetic has become very popular in recent years. It has been shown that the addition of bicarbonate to lidocaine, bupivacaine, and 2-chloroprocaine shortened the onset of action by 50%. The contents of the local anesthetic vials are maintained at a low pH (3.5 to 5) to increase the shelf life of these agents. The *addition of bicarbonate will increase the pH of these solutions and ultimately the percentage of uncharged forms, which is important for diffusion through the nerve membrane.*[6] However, when used with bupivacaine, one has to be very careful because of the chance of precipitation when the pH goes above 7.[7]

The mixing of carbon dioxide (CO_2) with a local anesthetic is also associated with a faster onset. However, the mechanism is different. *CO_2 rapidly diffuses through the nerve membrane and decreases the axoplasmic pH. This will increase the intracellular concentration of charged forms of local anesthetics, which is important for receptor binding and ultimate neural blockade.* [8]

Mixtures of Local Anesthetics

Combinations of local anesthetics have been used both to shorten the onset of action as well as to improve the quality of the block. A combination of 1% tetracaine and 10% procaine in equal volume was associated with superior sensory anesthesia when compared with hyperbaric tetracaine (5% dextrose) alone.[9] *Another interesting combination that evolved from taking advantage of the rapid onset as well as the longer duration of action was the mixture of 2-chloroprocaine and bupivacaine. However, the use of 2-chloroprocaine shortened the duration of bupivacaine's action. The mechanism of this interesting phenomenon is not known but may be related to inhibition of the binding of bupivacaine to membrane receptor sites in the presence of 2-chloroprocaine or its metabolite chloraminobenzoic acid.*[10]

Pregnancy

Pregnancy can alter the effect of local anesthetics in different ways. Smaller amounts of local anesthetic have been shown to be needed for both spinal and epidural anesthesia in parturients as compared with nonpregnant women in the same age group."[11,12] The onset of blockade is also faster with the use of spinal, epidural, and peripheral nerve blocks.[13] The mechanism for this phenomenon is not known; however, progesterone, an important pregnancy hormone, may be one of the responsible factors.[14–16]

Temperature

Warming the local anesthetic to a temperature of 100° F has been shown to reduce the onset of epidural anesthesia blockade. A decreased pKa due to increased temperature is probably the mechanism.[17]

Central Nervous System (CNS) and Cardiovascular System (CVS) Toxicity of Local Anesthetics

Compared with the central nervous system, the cardiovascular system is more resistant to local anesthetic toxicity.

CNS Toxicity

The clinical features will depend on the blood concentrations of the local anesthetics. In lower concentrations, the patient may complain of (1) tinnitus, (2) light-headedness, (3) metallic taste, and (4) circumoral numbness. With higher concentrations, convulsions and unconsciousness followed by respiratory arrest may ensue. *If a large bolus dose of local anesthetic is accidentally injected intravenously the parturient may manifest convulsions as the first sign. This may also occur if the pregnant woman receives large doses of diazepam or midazolam as premedication.* A direct correlation has been observed between the potency of local anesthetic and CNS toxicity. *The higher the potency of the local anesthetic the lower the amount necessary to produce CNS toxicity. Increased $PaCO_2$ as well as low pH will decrease the convulsive threshold and vice versa.* Hypercarbia will produce cerebral vasodilation and will increase the local anesthetic uptake. This will also decrease the intracellular pH and increase the charged form of local anesthetic. Acidosis will also decrease the protein-binding capacity of the local anesthetic and will increase the free local anesthetic concentrations.

CVS Toxicity

Local anesthetics will inhibit the sodium channels and will decrease the maximum rate of depolarization of Purkinje's fibers and ventricular muscles. Local anesthetic will also decrease the duration of both the action potential and the effective refractory period. More potent local anesthetics like bupivacaine, tetracaine, and etidocaine will produce significantly more cardiac depression than less potent agents like lidocaine, mepivacaine, or prilocaine. The ratio of cardiovascular collapse CC/CNS toxicity has been demonstrated to be 7 : 1 for lidocaine, whereas it was 3 : 7 and 4 : 4 for bupivacaine and etidocaine, respectively. Finally, increased CVS toxicity to bupivacaine and cocaine has been shown during pregnancy.

Two new amide local anesthetics have recently been introduced.[19,19a] These are S-isomer of propyl chained amide local anesthetic ropivacaine and S-isomer of butyl chained amide local anesthetic levo-bupivacaine.

Ropivacaine is a long-acting local anesthetic. Isolated nerve preparations with different concentrations of ropivacaine have shown that it possesses a significant differential nerve blockade activity.[20] The blockade of C-fibers is very similar to bupivacaine; however, A fiber blockade is significantly less with ropivacaine. Preliminary studies in orthopedic patients have shown that in a dose-dependent manner, ropivacaine, compared to bupivacaine, is associated with a similar degree of sensory anesthesia, however, less intensity of motor block. This property will be beneficial for the obstetric population. Human volunteers as well as animal studies showed that ropivacaine is associated with less central nervous system as well as cardiovascular system toxicity compared to bupivacaine. 0.5% ropivacaine was compared to 0.5% bupivacaine for cesarean section anesthesia. While they provided similar sensory anesthesia, motor blockade occurred, with slower onset and shorter duration in parturients who received ropivacaine. Relative analgesic potencies of epidural bupivacaine and ropivacaine was determined by their respective minimum local analgesic concentrations (MLAC) in laboring women. Analgesic potency was found to be 40% less in ropivacaine compared to bupivacaine.[20a] 0.0625% bupivacaine with fentanyl and 0.1% ropivacaine with fentanyl were compared for labor analgesia. There were no significant differences in sensory analgesia or motor block. These findings suggest that bupivacaine may be more potent compared to ropivacaine. Using 0.125% bupivacaine and ropivacaine with fentanyl in a laboring women a similar sensory anesthesia was observed, however, a significantly less motor block was found in case of ropivacaine. In another study, 0.08% bupivacaine plus fentanyl was compared to 0.08% bupivacaine plus fentanyl for ambulatory labor epidural analgesia.[20b] Spontaneous micturition was observed in 65% of the bupivacaine group, whereas 100% of the ropivacaine group. Ambulation was effective in 75% of the bupivacaine group compared to 100% of the ropivacaine. The incidence of forceps delivery was significantly higher in the bupivacaine group. However, a meta analysis comparing ropivacaine with bupivacaine for labor analgesia concluded that there was no statistical significant difference as far as the obstetrical and neonatal outcome was concerned.[20c]

Levobupivacaine is also a long-acting amide local anesthetic. One study in rats observed a shorter duration of motor block in case of levobupivacaine compared to bupivacaine. In a volunteer study, the duration of motor block using 0.25% of levobupivacaine was shorter compared to 0.25% of bupivacaine; 0.5% of levobupivacaine was compared to 0.5% bupivacaine for cesarean section anesthesia. Sensory anesthesia and motor block were similar in both groups. Minimum local analgesic concentrations (MLAC) of epidural levobupivacaine and bupivacaine were compared for labor analgesia. The potency of the two drugs were similar. So far the motor block is concerned potency of levobupivacaine is significantly less than bupivacaine in laboring women.[21] 0.125% of bupivacaine with sufentanil was compared to 0.125% of levobupivacaine with sufentanil for combined spinal epidural analgesia in laboring women. Duration of analgesia was similar, however, incidences of motor block were significantly less in cases of levobupivacaine. Although levobupivacaine has the similar anesthetic potency as bupivacaine it has been found to posses less cardiovascular and central nervous system toxicity in animal models as well as human volunteers.[22] The following interesting properties were observed in the two newer local anesthetics:

1. A greater degree of sensero motor differentiation (sensory > motor) compared with bupivacaine.
2. Lesser cardiac and central nervous system toxic properties.
3. Inherent vasoconstricting property may exclude the use of epinephrine.

References

1. McClure JH: Ropivacaine. *Br J Anaesth* 1996; 76:300.

1a. Nath S, Johansson G, Haggmark S, Reizs: Cardiotoxicity of ropivacaine—a new amide local anaesthetic agent. *Acta Anaesthesiol Scand* 1989; 33:93.)

2. Covino BG, Vassallo HG: Mechanisms of action and clinical use. In *Local Anesthetics.* New York, Grune & Stratton, 1976.

3. Finster M: Toxicity of local anesthetics in the fetus and the newborn. *Bull N Y Acad Med* 1976; 52:222.
4. Littlewood DG, Buckley P, Covino BG, et al: Comparative study of various local anesthetic solutions in extradural block in labour. *Br J Anaesth* 1979; 51:47.
5. Crawford OB: Comparative evaluation in peridural anesthesia of lidocaine, mepivacaine and L-67, a new local anesthetic agent. *Anesthesiology* 1964; 25:321.
6. DiFazio CA, Carron H, Gosslight KR, et al: Comparison pH-adjusted lidocaine solutions for epidural anesthesia. *Anesth Analg* 1986; 65:760.
7. Peterfreund RA, Datta S, Ostheimer GW: pH adjustment of local anesthetic solutions with sodium bicarbonate: Laboratory evaluation of alkalinization and precipitation. *Regional Anesth* 1989; 1:265.
8. Catchlove RFH: The influence of CO_2 and pH on local anesthetic action. *J Pharmacol Exp Ther* 1972; 181:291.
9. Chantigian RC, Datta S, Berger GA, et al: Anesthesia for cesarean delivery using spinal anesthesia: Tetracaine versus tetracaine and procaine. *Reg Anaesth* 1984; 9:195.
10. Corke BC, Carlson CG, Dettbarn WD: The influence of 2-chloroprocaine on the subsequent analgesic potency of bupivacaine. *Anesthesiology* 1984; 60:25.
11. Fargraeus L, Urban BJ, Bromage PR: Spread of epidural analgesia in early pregnancy. *Anesthesiology* 1983; 58:184.
12. Datta S, Hurley RJ, Naulty JS, et al: Plasma and cerebrospinal fluid progesterone concentrations in pregnant and nonpregnant women. *Anesth Analg* 1986; 65:950.
13. Datta S, Lambert DH, Gregus J, et al: Differential sensitivities of mammalian nerve fibers during pregnancy. *Anesth Analg* 1983; 62:1070.
14. Flanagan HL, Datta S, Lambert DH, et al: Effect of pregnancy on bupivacaine-induced conduction blockade in the isolated rabbit vagus nerve. *Anesth Analg* 1987; 66:123.
15. Flanagan HL, Datta S, Moller RA, et al: Effect of exogenously administered progesterone on susceptibility of rabbit vagus nerves to bupivacaine (abstract). *Anesthesiology* 1988; 69:676.
16. Bader AM, Datta S, Moller RA, et al: Effect of acute progesterone treatment on bupivacaine-induced conduction blockade in the isolated rabbit vagus nerve. *Anesth Analg* 1990; 71:545.
17. Mehta PM, Theriot E, Mehrotra D: A simple technique to make bupivacaine a rapid-acting epidural anesthetic. *Reg Anaesth* 1987; 123:135.

17a. Owen MD, Thomas JA, Smith T, et al: Ropivacaine 0.075% and bupivacaine 0.075% with fentanyl 2 mcg/ml are equivalent for labor epidural analgesia. *Anesth Analg* 2002; 94:179.
18. Datta S: *Pharmacology of Local Anesthetic Agents.* American Society of Anesthesiologists, Philadelphia, JB Lippincott, 1993; 21:241.
19. Capogna G, Celleno D, Fusco P, et al: Relative potencies of bupivacaine and ropivacaine for analgesia in labour. *Br J. Anaesth* 1999; 82:371.
20. Bader AM, Datta S, Flanagan HL, et al: Comparison of bupivacaine and ropivacaine induced conduction blockade in the isolated rabbit vagus nerve. *Anesth Analg* 1989; 68:724.
20a. Polley LS, Columb MO, Naughton NN: Relative analgesic potencies of ropivacaine and bupivacaine for epidural analgesia in labor. Implications for therapeutic indexes. *Anesthesiology* 1999; 90:9444.
20b. Campbell DC, Rhonda Z, Crone LL: Ambulatory labor epidural analgesia: Bupivacaine versus ropivacaine. *Anesth Analg* 2000; 90:1384.
20c. Halperin SH, Walsh V: Epidural Ropivacaine versus bupivacaine for labor: A meta-analysis. *Anesth Analg* 2003; 93:1473.
21. Lacassie HJ, Columb MO: The relative motor blocking potencies of bupivacaine and levobupivacaine in labor. *Anesth Analg* 2003; 98:1509.
22. Gristwood RW, Greaves L: Levobupivacaine: A new safer long acting local anesthetic agent. *Expert Opin Invest Drug* 1999; 8:861.

3
Perinatal Pharmacology

Perinatal pharmacology involves the three most important participants in pregnancy: the mother, the placenta, and the fetus (Fig 3-1). There are only a few drugs (heparin, protamine) used in parturients that cannot traverse the placenta and go to the fetal side. Therefore, most of the drugs used in pregnant

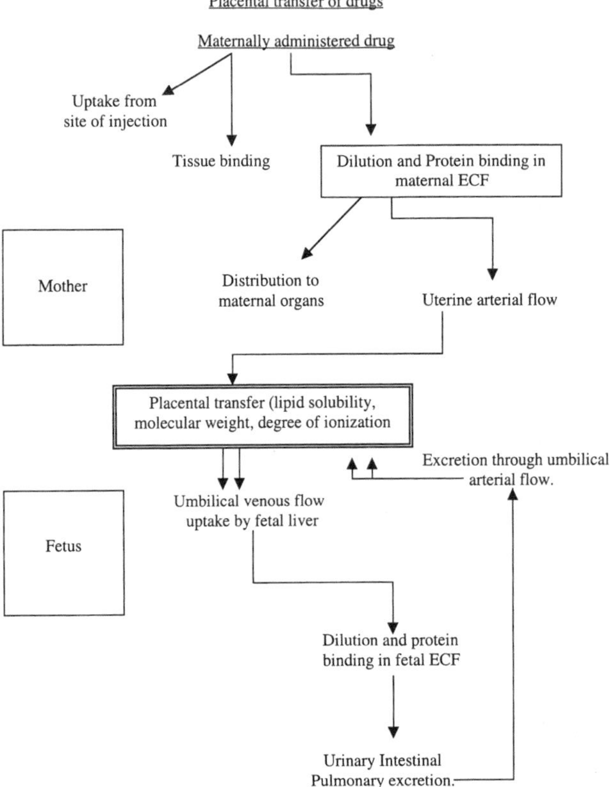

Figure 3-1. Drug disposition in the mother, placenta, and fetus.

women will affect the fetus to a certain extent; hence perinatal pharmacology should be an important part of obstetric anesthesia.

Maternal drug administration can affect the fetus mainly in two ways: (1) having a direct fetal effect and (2) indirectly involving the uteroplacental circulation. This chapter will discuss the three main participants.

Mother

The maternal plasma concentration of any agent will depend upon the site of administration as well as the amount of agent administered. In the case of local anesthetics, *the highest to lowest maternal plasma concentration will be achieved by the following route of administration: intravenous > paracervical > caudal epidural > lumbar epidural > intramuscular > subarachnoid block.* Once the drug reaches the maternal circulation, the maternal plasma concentration will depend upon several important factors: (1) the volume of distribution and elimination and (2) changes in the cardiovascular system due to pregnancy.

Increased Plasma Volume

An increase in plasma volume as well as total body water during pregnancy increases the volume of distribution mainly of lipid-soluble drugs. This increased volume of distribution can also increase clearance of the drugs. This increase in volume of distribution has an important clinical implication. Bupivacaine and fentanyl concentrations were measured from the mother's vein as well as an umbilical vein from parturients with long duration of labor. Free bupivacaine and fentanyl concentrations in both mother and baby were extremely small. Highly lipid-soluble drugs like bupivacaine and fentanyl are associated with rapid distribution as well as uptake by the maternal tissue. Hence a very small amount of the drug appears in the neonate.[1a] In non-pregnant women, the maximum and minimum concentrations of drugs will be higher than those observed at 10 to 40 weeks of gestation.[1]

Increased Blood Volume

Increased maternal blood volume as well as cardiac output will increase uteroplacental blood flow. The exact impact of these hemodynamic changes in placental transfer of drugs to the fetus is not clearly understood. However, an interesting concept has been suggested related to uterine contraction and the placental transfer of drugs. Placental transfer of drugs is especially reduced when they are injected intravenously into the mother at the beginning of the uterine contraction because of stoppage of placental circulation; *tissue redistribution of the drugs in the meantime will lower the maternal plasma concentration before re-establishment of the placental circulation.*

Free Drug Concentration

The free drug concentration in the uterine artery that will ultimately reach the placenta will depend on several important factors: (1) the addition of epinephrine, (2) maternal metabolism and elimination of drugs, (3) maternal protein binding, and (4) the maternal pH and pKa of the drugs.

Addition of Epinephrine

Epinephrine has been shown to reduce the peak maternal plasma concentration of lidocaine and mepivacaine.[2] However, epinephrine has an insignificant effect on peak concentrations of bupivacaine and etidocaine.

Maternal Metabolism and Elimination of the Drug

Ester drugs like 2-chloroprocaine, succinylcholine, and trimethaphan are destroyed by cholinesterase; hence the maternal plasma half-life of these drugs is very short, and thus less drug will ultimately reach the fetus. On the other hand, normeperidine, a metabolite of meperidine, is twice as toxic as the parent compound and interestingly only half as analgesic. This metabolite will ultimately reach the fetus.[3,4] These studies observed that infants born more than 4 hours after maternal medication have more time to accumulate normeperidine in their tissues, because of maternal metabolism of meperidine; however, infants born within 1 hour of maternal medication have less time for nomeperidine to accumulate and, neonatal depression can be due to direct action of meperidine.

Maternal Protein Binding

Plasma protein binding may be important for placental transfer. Local anesthetics like bupivacaine and etidocaine with significantly higher plasma protein-binding capacity than lidocaine and mepivacaine will have less placental transfer and lower fetal concentrations. *The umbilical vein and maternal vein (UV/MV) concentration ratio has been shown to be lower in the case of bupivacaine and etidocaine as compared with lidocaine and mepivacaine.* On the other hand, in a study in animals this lower UV/MV ratio has been explained by the higher fetal tissue uptake of bupivacaine and etidocaine because of their high lipid solubility.[5]

Maternal pH and Drug pKa

Drugs with a pKa close to the body's pH of 7.4 will remain in higher amount in nonionized form in maternal blood, and this will be associated with higher placental transfer. Mepivacaine with a pKa of 7.6 will cross the placenta in higher amounts when compared with bupivacaine with a pKa of 8.1. The two new local anesthetics, ropivacaine and levobupivacaine, are like the present form of bupivacaine because of their similar pKa.

Placental Transfer of Drugs

Placental transfer of drugs will depend on several important factors: (1) the area of transfer and the diffusion distance, (2) the molecular weight and spatial configuration of the drugs, (3) the pKa of the drugs, (4) the protein binding and lipid solubility of the drugs, (5) drug interaction, and (6) the metabolism of the drugs. Hence, placental transfer of drugs can be described by the diffusion equation

$$Q/t = \frac{KA(C_m - C_f)}{D}$$

where Q/t is the quantity of the drugs transferred in a unit of time; K is a diffusion constant; A is the total area of the placenta; C_m and C_f are the maternal and fetal concentration of free drugs, respectively; and D is the distance across the placenta.

Area of Transfer and Diffusion Distance

The rate of drug transfer will depend upon the area of transfer. The maternal part of the placenta contains 180 to 320 spiral arteries. The functional unit of the placenta is the "placentone", which is supplied by a single spiral artery. Reduced placental perfusion will decrease the blood flow through the "placentone" and will affect drug transfer. The distance of diffusion is also important. Pre-eclampsia, which is associated with placental abnormality, can increase the diffusion distance.

Molecular Weight and Spatial Configuration of Drugs

Drugs between 100 and 500 daltons (Da) will freely cross the placenta. Drugs above 500 Da will cross with difficulty, and drugs above 1,000 Da will not cross the placenta. Most of the clinically useful drugs will cross the placenta because of their low molecular weight. However, *heparin, and protamine cannot cross the placenta because of their large molecular weight.*

pKa of Drugs

Only the un-ionized form of drugs can cross the placenta; hence *drugs with a pKa closer to the maternal pH of 7.4 will be able to cross the placenta in a high amount.*

Protein Binding and Lipid Solubility of Drugs

Drugs bound to plasma protein cross a biological membrane like the placenta with great difficulty. Hence drugs such as bupivacaine, with its higher protein-binding capacity, will have less placental transfer. On the other hand, a higher total plasma concentration of any drug (administered in a large amount) will remain in unbound form and will cross the placenta in a higher amount. Lipid solubility eases the transfer of drugs through the placenta. *Highly lipid-soluble drugs, such as barbiturates, can reach the fetus in large amounts after easy placental transfer.*

Drug Interaction

Different drugs do possess different affinity for plasma protein-binding or tissue-binding sites. *Diazepam is a highly protein-bound drug. Diazepam given intravenously after local anesthetic administration will compete with protein binding and will thus increase the free local anesthetic concentration.*[6] Hence, multiple drugs administered at the same time to the mother may affect placental transfer and ultimately fetal drug concentration.

Metabolism of Drugs

The placenta can manufacture and excrete specific enzymes that will destroy maternally administered prednisone; hence it will not cross the placenta.

Fetus

Fetal uptake, distribution, and metabolism and elimination will ultimately be responsible for the fetal drug concentration and its effect on the fetus. Once drugs reach the fetus, several important factors will determine the free umbilical artery concentration of drugs.

Uptake

Fetal uptake of drugs will depend on protein binding, lipid solubility, and the pKa of the drugs. Because of lesser amount of total protein in the fetus, plasma protein-binding capacity in the fetus is less than in the mother; hence a higher amount of free drug will be available in plasma. Highly lipid-soluble drugs like bupivacaine and etidocaine have been shown to be absorbed by the fetal tissues in a significant amount and thus reduce the fetal plasma concentration.[5] Finally, the fetal pH is important for determining the proportion of ionized and un-ionized forms of the drug. Normal fetal pH varies between 7.32 and 7.38, whereas maternal pH varies between 7.38 and 7.42. In a normal situation, maternal fetal transfer of the drug will depend significantly on the concentration gradient. If the fetus is acidotic (pH > 7.20), then un-ionized drugs from the mother will reach the fetus and ultimately will be dissociated to ionized form. The *ionized form of drugs will get trapped in the fetus since they will be unable to cross the placenta. This phenomenon has been described as "ion trapping."*[7]

Distribution

Because of the uniqueness of the fetal circulation (Fig 3-2), there is a significant difference between umbilical vein and umbilical artery concentrations of drugs. The umbilical artery concentration is a true reflection of the fetal brain concentration.

Fetal Liver

The umbilical vein blood from the placenta either reaches the liver or flows through the ductus venosus. The left lobe of the liver is transfused by the umbilical vein blood, whereas the right lobe is perfused by portal vein blood. Thiopental administered intravenously to the mother is taken up by the fetal liver in a significant amount.[8] Thus the fetal liver helps in extracting substantial amounts of drug entering the fetus and thereby helps in protecting the fetal brain. This high uptake has also been observed with halothane, lidocaine, and cyclamate.

Progressive Dilution of Umbilical Vein in Blood Concentration

Umbilical vein blood going through either the fetal liver or the ductus venosus will ultimately be diluted by the blood received from the inferior extremity or gastrointestinal tract. This diluted umbilical vein blood will be shunted through the foramen ovale of the heart and ultimately to the fetal brain.

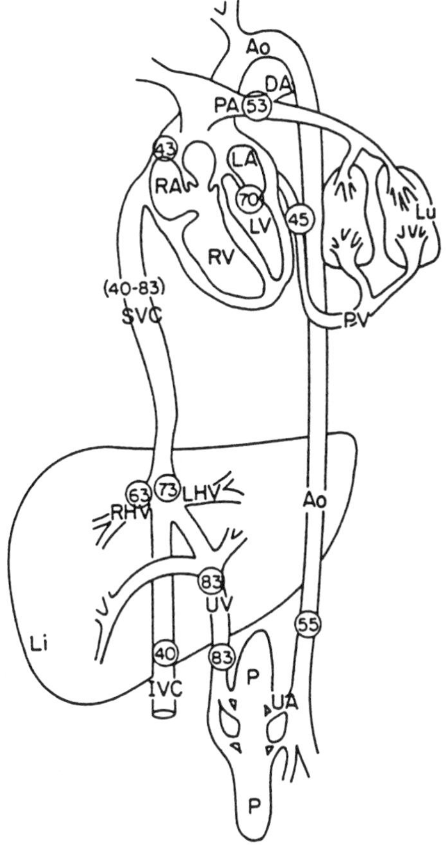

Figure 3–2. Fetal circulation (numbers indicate percent saturation). IVC = inferior vena cava; P = placenta; Li = liver; RHV, LHV = right and left hepatic veins; SVC = superior vena cava; RA, LA = right and left atria; DA = ductus arteriosus; PA = pulmonary artery; Ao = aorta; Lu = lung; DV = ductus venosus; PV = pulmonary vein; UV = umbilical vein; UA = umbilical artery. (From Martin R. Prepartum and Intrapartum fetal monitoring. In Datta S (ed): Anesthesthetic and Obstetric Management of High-Risk Pregnancy, 3rd ed. New York, Springer, 2004.)

Extensive Right-to-Left Shunt of the Fetal Circulation

About 57% of fetal cardiac output returns to the placenta without perfusing fetal tissues. This is related to extensive shunting of the fetal circulation via the foramen ovale of the heart as well as the ductus arteriosus. This mechanism leads to diminished exposure of the fetal brain to circulating drugs.

The three major reasons that thiopental, maternally administered in therapeutic doses (4 to 6 mg/kg), will result in an awake and screaming baby despite the mother being asleep are (1) *extraction by the fetal liver,* (2) *progressive dilution of umbilical vein blood concentrations, and* (3) *a large right-to-left cardiac shunt in the fetus.*

Metabolism and Elimination

Although hepatic enzyme activity in the fetus is usually less than that in the adult, the human fetus can take care of the drugs administered to the mother in therapeutic doses. The human fetal liver stores a significant amount of cytochrome P-450 and reduced nicotinamide-adenine dinucleotide phosphate (NADPH) cytochrome c reductase even at the 14th week of gestation. Hence premature fetuses can metabolize maternally administered local anesthetics. 2-Chloroprocaine was found to be metabolized by the human premature fetus without any problem.[9] On the other hand, mepivacaine's metabolism is incomplete, and the majority of this drug is excreted by the kidney in an unchanged form.[10]

In summary, the majority of maternally administered drugs will cross the placenta and reach the fetus, but because of the unique fetal circulation, only a small amount of the drugs will reach the fetal brain and myocardium and cause fetal depression. Apgar scores, acid-base values, and neurobehavior tests have been used to observe drug effects on the fetus.

References

1. Mattison DR: Physiologic variation in pharmacokinetics during pregnancy. In Fabro S, Scialli AR (eds): *Drug and Chemical Action in Pregnancy*. New York, Marcell Dekker Inc, 1986.

2. Covino BG, Vasallo HG: *Local Anesthetics: Mechanisms of Action and Clinical Use.* New York, Grune & Stratton, 1976, p 100.
3. Kuhnert BR, Kuhnert PM, Tu AL, et al: Meperidine and normeperidine levels following meperidine administration during labor: 1. Mother. *Am J Obstet Gynecol* 1979; 133:904.
4. Kuhnert BR, Kuhnert PM, Tu AL, et al: Meperidine and normeperidine levels following meperidine administration during labor. II. Fetus and neonate. *Am J Obstet Gynecol* 1979; 133:909.
5. Morishima HO, Finster M, Pedersen H, et al: Placental transfer and tissue distribution of etidocaine and lidocaine in guinea pigs (abstract). Presented at the Annual Meeting of the American Society of Anesthesiologists, Chicago, 1975, p 83
6. Denson DD, Myers JA, Thompson GA, et al: The influence of diazepam on the serum protein binding of bupivacaine at normal and acidic pH. *Anesth Analg* 1984; 63:980.
7. Biehl D, Shnider SM, Levinson G, et al: Placental transfer of lidocaine: Effects of fetal acidosis. *Anesthesiology* 1978; 48:409.
8. Finster M, Morishima HO, Mark LC, et al: Tissue thiopental concentrations in the fetus and newborn. *Anesthesiology* 1972; 36:155.
9. Kuhnert BR, Kuhnert PM, Reese AL, et al: Maternal and neonatal elimination of CABA after epidural anesthesia with 2-chloroprocaine during parturition. *Anesth Analg* 1983; 62:1089.
10. Brown WU, Bell GC, Lurie AO, et al: Newborn blood levels of lidocaine and mepivacaine in the first postnatal day following maternal epidural anesthesia. *Anesthesiology* 1975; 42:698.

4
Drug Interactions and Obstetric Anesthesia

Drugs Used for Maternal and Fetal Indications

Newer pharmacological agents are being used more frequently for the treatment of maternal and fetal pathological states. Obstetric anesthesiologists should be aware of the interactions of maternally administered drugs with anesthetic agents and techniques.

Drugs Used for Maternal Indications

Antibiotics

Rarely, parturients may receive antibiotics for various disease processes. *Most of the antibiotics will prolong the effect of nondepolarizing muscle relaxants, but prolongation of depolarizing muscle relaxants has also been observed* (Table 4-1).[1] The mechanism of this phenomenon is unknown. Antagonism of this action by neostigmine and pyridostigmine is found to be unpredictable; however, neuromuscular blockade from antibiotics could be reversed predictably by 4-aminopyridine.[2] *Interestingly, the neuromuscular blocking action of the local anesthetic lidocaine is found to be exaggerated in the presence of neuromuscular blocking drugs and aminoglycoside antibiotics.*[3]

Antiepileptic Drugs

Parturients may be taking antiepileptic drugs when they arrive in the hospital for labor and delivery. The common antiepileptic drugs at the present time include phenytoin, phenobarbital, benzodiazepines, and valproic acid. *The pharmacokinetics of most of the antiepileptic drugs are altered during pregnancy. Parturients need higher amounts of antiepileptic drugs because of increased volume of distribution; hence measurement of the plasma concentration is important.* Most of these drugs are metabolized in the liver and thus can interfere with the biotransformation of other drugs. The duration of action of the drugs, which are mainly metabolized by the liver, can be prolonged in parturients who are receiving antiepileptic drugs. *These drugs also cross the placenta and can thus*

Table 4–1. Interaction of Antibiotics, Muscle Relaxants, Neostigmine, and Calcium

	Neuromuscular Block From Antibiotic Alone Antagonized by		Increase in Neuromuscular Block of		Neuromuscular Block From Antibiotic and *d*-Tubocurarine Antagonized by	
	Neostigmine	**Calcium**	***d*-Tubocurarine**	**Succinylcholine**	**Neostigmine**	**Calcium**
Neomycin	Sometimes	Sometimes	Yes	Yes	Usually	Usually
Streptomycin	Sometimes	Sometimes	Yes	Yes	Usually	Usually
Gentamicin	Sometimes	Yes[†]	Yes	[‡]	Sometimes	Yes[†]
Kanamycin	Sometimes	Sometimes	Yes	Yes	Sometimes	Sometimes
Paromomycin	Yes[†]	Yes[†]	Yes	[‡]	Yes[†]	Yes[†]
Viomycin	Yes[†]	Yes[†]	Yes	[‡]	Yes[†]	Yes[†]
Polymyxin A	No	No	Yes	[‡]	No	No
Polymyxin B	No[§]	No	Yes	Yes	No[§]	No
Colistin	No	Sometimes	Yes	Yes	No	Sometimes
Tetracycline	No	[‡]	Yes	No	Partially	Partially
Lincomycin	Partially	Partially	Yes	[‡]	Partially	Partially
Clindamycin	Partially	Partially	Yes	[‡]	Partially	Partially

From Smith NT, Corbascio AN (eds): Drug Interactions in Anesthesia. Philadelphia, Lea & Febiger, 1986. Used by permission.

[†] In spite of this, difficulty with antagonizing the block from these antibiotics is still likely to occur.

[‡] Not studied.

[§] Block augmented by neostigmine.

interfere with the synthesis of vitamin K-dependent clotting factors in the fetal liver. Hence, careful observation of the neonate is absolutely essential. Regional anesthesia should be the anesthetic technique of choice because there is evidence that a local anesthetic like lidocaine can be an effective anticonvulsant in therapeutic doses.[4] *If general anesthesia is indicated, the use of enflurane should be avoided because of its epileptogenic property.*[5]

Enzyme Induction

Enzyme induction is an adaptive response associated with accumulation of specific mRNAs and increased expression of the associated enzyme system. *Oxidative metabolism is catalyzed by the P450 enzyme system.* P450 enzymes have been grouped into three families: CYP_1, CYP_2, and CYP_3. Several medications selectively induce specific families of the P450 enzyme system. Rifampicin decreased concentration of midazolam; its elimination half-life was also reduced.[6]

Sympathomimetic Drugs

Pregnant women may use both sympathetic nervous system agonist and antagonist drugs for either therapeutic or recreational reasons. *Sympathetic nervous system antagonists* are used for the treatment of hypertension; α-Methyldopa, reserpine, and guanethidine have been used in parturients. *Depletion of norepinephrine is possible*[6a] *in such a situation, and indirect-acting agonists like ephedrine may be ineffective following hypotension.* Direct-acting agonists like phenylephrine may be indicated in such a situation. Besides these antagonist agents, β-receptor antagonist drugs like propranolol can be used for therapeutic reasons. *If the parturient is taking propranolol, medications that increase airway resistance, such as large doses of morphine or prostaglandin F_{2a} (PCF_{2a}) (Prostin), should be used cautiously.* Calcium channel blockers with negative inotropic effects can exaggerate the depressant effect of propranolol. *Propranolol will cross the placenta and can cause fetal bradycardia and hypoglycemia.* Autonomic ganglionic blocking drugs like trimethaphan camsylate (Arfonad) are used occasionally to treat hypertension. Because this drug is destroyed by cholinesterase, which is also responsible for the metabolism of succinylcholine, a prolonged neuromuscular block has been described following the use of Arfonad and succinylcholine.[7] A few words of caution must be mentioned in using beta blockers such as esmolol. *Severe fetal bradycardia has been described when esmolol was given to the mother.* The proposed mechanisms include (1) large placental transfer and (2) more beta-specific medications have unrestricted alpha constriction of the uterine blood vessels.

Sympathetic Nervous System Agonist Drugs

Two drugs in this group that are used recreationally are worth mentioning:

1. *Amphetamine* is a central nervous system (CNS) stimulant. A new smoked form, "ice," that produces a "high" of long duration is popular in Hawaii and on the West Coast of the United States. The minimum alveolar concentration is increased in parturients who are addicted to amphetamines. Higher doses of narcotics and inhalational anesthetics may be needed for general anesthesia.[8] Vasopressors, both direct and indirect acting, should be used carefully for the treatment of hypotension.
2. *Cocaine* is one of the commonly used recreational agents at the present time. *It blocks the presynaptic uptake of norepinephrine, serotonin, and dopamine.* Chronic use will decrease α_2-adrenergic- and presynaptic cholinergic mediated norepinephrine release.[9] Cocaine is metabolized by cholinesterase and can affect the metabolism of 2-chloroprocaine. Ketamine or excessive catecholamines can cause severe hypertension and myocardial infarction. Tachycardia following cocaine use should be treated with labetalol because pure β-adrenergic agents will have unopposed α-adrenergic activity with associated hypertension.[10] Calcium channel blockers will also have unopposed action. Decreased pseudocholinesterase levels may prolong the duration of action of succinylcholine.

Antiasthmatic Drugs

Xanthine Derivatives

Xanthine derivatives such as theophylline and aminophylline may be associated with different drug interactions. Cimetidine has been observed to slow down the elimination of theophylline.[11] If general anesthesia is indicated, ketamine should be used carefully because the combination of *ketamine and aminophylline can cause significant lowering of the seizure threshold.*[12] *Methylxanthines are associated with the release of endogenous catecholamines; hence halothane can induce dysrhythmias. This problem can be exaggerated if the parturient receives ephedrine*[13] *or epinephrine at the same time.* Theophylline can antagonize a nondepolarizing muscle-relaxant block.[14] The mechanism is unknown. Pancuronium should be used cautiously because of the possibility of supraventricular tachycardia.[15]

Sympathomimetic Drugs

See the later section "Sympathomimetic Amines."

Corticosteroids

Corticosteroids have been observed to alter the disposition of theophylline. The intravenous administration of large doses of corticosteroids was associated with a twofold increase in serum levels of theophylline in patients who were receiving a theophylline infusion.[16]

Histamine H_2 Receptor Blockers

The use of H_2 receptor blockers has become a common practice before cesarean section. Both cimetidine and ranitidine have been used as premedicant agents. *Cimetidine binds to the hepatic microsomal cytochrome P-450 system. Cimetidine as well as ranitidine significantly decrease hepatic blood flow and thus can decrease hepatic clearance of various drugs. Chronic cimetidine use will decrease clearance as well as the metabolism of drugs like theophylline, benzodiazepines, morphine, lidocaine, and propranolol.* [17-20] Ranitidine does not bind with cytochrome P-450 and is more potent than cimetidine; hence drug interactions with ranitidine are extremely rare.

Psychotropic Agents

A broad range of antipsychotic drugs are available at the present time, and these drugs may be associated with multiple complex drug interactions. Three commonly used groups of drugs include phenothiazine, and butyrophenones. Antipsychotic drugs are associated with elevation of serum prolactin levels and blocking of dopaminergic receptors.[21]

Phenothiazine, Thioxanthenes, and Butyrophenones

Narcotic Analgesics. Most of the antipsychotic drugs will enhance the effect of narcotic analgesics. This might have additive and/or synergistic effects.[22] One has to reduce the dose of narcotics if the patient is taking antipsychotic drugs.

Central Nervous System Depressants. Antipsychotic drugs also exert an increased effect on sedative and hypnotic drugs. A study showed that chlorpromazine reduced the thiopental requirement as well as prolonged postoperative recovery following thiopental use.[23]

Sympathomimetic Drugs. Antipsychotic drugs can block the pressor effects of norepinephrine and other α-adrenergic agonist drugs.[24] Hence, higher doses of vasopressors may be necessary to treat hypotension in these cases. Selective α-adrenergic-blocking effects of these drugs may exaggerate the effects of drugs with β-agonist activity (propranolol).[25]

Anticholinergic Drugs. Some antipsychotic drugs like chlorpromazine and thioridazine do exert active anticholinergic effects: hence one has to be careful while administering anticholinergic premedications.[26]

Inhalation Anesthetics. Because of the higher incidence of hypotension when inhalational anesthetics are used in women taking antipsychotic drugs, one has to be careful when using general anesthesia in this population.

Regional Anesthesia. A higher incidence of hypotension has been described in women receiving chlorpromazine. Proper volume replacement and active treatment of hypotension are important.[27] Direct-acting α-agonists like phenylephrine (NeoSynephrine) may be necessary for the treatment of hypotension.

Other popular psychotropic drugs outside the three main groups (phenothiazine, thioxanthenes, and butyrophenones) are tricyclic antidepressants monoamine oxidase inhibitors (MAOIs), lithium, and serotonin reuptake inhibitors (SSRIs).

Tricyclic Antidepressants

This group of drugs has become very popular recently for the treatment of severe depression. Their mechanisms of action include blocking the uptake of norepinephrine, serotonin, or dopamine into presynaptic nerve endings, thus increasing central and peripheral adrenergic tone. Tricyclic antidepressants also possess a strong anticholinergic effect. Drug interactions with tricyclic antidepressants are complex, and the obstetric anesthesiologist must be aware of the problems. *Tricyclic antidepressants heighten the pressor response of direct-acting vasoactive drugs such as norepinephrine, epinephrine, or Neo-Synephrine.*[28] *Hence, local anesthetic solution containing epinephrine should be used very carefully. Ephedrine may not be effective for treating hypotension in this group of women following regional anesthesia. NeoSynephrine, in small doses, may be necessary in such a situation.* Tricyclic antidepressants will also exaggerate the response of anticholinergics and narcotics as well as other sedative and hypnotic drugs (Table 4-2).

Monoamine Oxidase Inhibitors

These drugs work by inhibiting the enzyme monoamine oxidase. Monoamine oxidase is responsible for the oxidative deamination of serotonin, norepinephrine, and dopamine (Table 4-3); thus their metabolism is disturbed by this group of drugs (MAOIs). These drugs can also inhibit other hepatic microsomal enzymes. Three important drug interactions to consider for parturients receiving MAOI agents are sympathetic amine interactions, narcotic analgesic interactions, and muscle-relaxant interactions.

Sympathomimetic Amines. *Indirect-acting sympathomimetic drugs such as amphetamine, methamphetamine, mephentermine, metaraminol, and ephedrine can release excessive amounts of catecholamine and can be associated with severe hypertension in parturients receiving MAOI agents.*[29] Direct-acting sympathomimetic amines have fewer problems,[28] *so in women receiving MAOI agents, a very small amount of a direct-acting vasopressor may be the drug of choice to treat hypotension following regional anesthesia.*

Narcotic Analgesics. Meperidine's interaction with MAOI agents is complex and can precipitate a hypertensive crisis. Severe respiratory depression, hypotension, and coma have also been described.[30,31] *The mechanisms are not completely clear; however, the hypertensive crisis may be explained by the presence of elevated brain serotonin concentrations in the presence of an MAOI and meperidine because of the inhibition of enzyme metabolism by MAOI agents.* Because meperidine is still one of the most common analgesics used for obstetric cases, one has to be very careful if the population is receiving an MAOI. Metoclopramide has been observed to potentiate opiate analgesia. The administration of metoclopramide was associated with a

Table 4–2. Some Interactions Between Tricyclic Antidepressants and Drugs Used in Anesthesia

Tricyclic Antidepressants	Interaction
Narcotics	↑Analgesia ↑Respiratory depression
Barbiturates	↑Sleep time
Anticholinergics	↑Central acitvity ↑Peripheral activity
Sympathomimetics	↑Effect of direct-acting agents

From Janowsky EC, Craig Risch S, Janowsky DS: Psychotropic agents, in Smith NT, Corbascio AN (eds): *Drug Interactions in Anesthesia.* Philadelphia, Lea & Febiger, 1986, chap 19. Used by permission.

Table 4–3. Biosynthesis and Metabolism of Catecholamines

Catecholamine		Enzyme	Enzyme Inhibitors
Phenylalanine			
↓	←	Hydroxylase	
Tyrosine			
↓	←	Hydroxylase	←α-methyl-p-tyrosine
DOPA	Rate limiting		
↓	←	Decarboxylase	←α-methyldopa (Aldomet)
Dopamine			
↓	←	β-hydroxylase	←Disulfiram (Antabuse)
Norepinephrine	Rate limiting		
↓	←	*N*-methyltransferase	
Epinephrine			
↓	←	COMT[†]	←Pyrogallol, Tropolone
Metanephrine			
↓	←	MAO	←MAO inhibitor (Pargyline)
Vanillylmandelic acid			

From Wona KC, Everett JD: Sympathomimetic drugs, in Smith NT, Corbascio AN (eds): *Drug Interactions in Anesthesia.* Philadelphia, Lea & Febiger, 1986, chap 7. Used by permission.

[†]COMT = catechol-O-methyltransferase.

reduction in demand of analgesic requirements and a significant reduction in pain scores.[31a]

Muscle Relaxants. Prolonged apnea following succinylcholine administration has been described in patients receiving MAOI agents.[32] A decrease in plasma cholinesterase content may be responsible for this interaction; since pregnancy also reduces the plasma cholinesterase activity, this drug effect may be heightened in obstetric population.

Lithium Carbonate

Lithium has become a very popular medication for the treatment of recurrent depression. *Interactions of lithium with a few agents used during general anesthesia are important. Lithium can prolong the activity of succinylcholine, pancuronium,*[33] *and barbiturates.* Lithium rapidly crosses the placenta and can also affect neonates .[34]

Serotonin reuptake inhibitors (SSRIs) have been used increasingly in recent times. Serotonin is an important neurotransmitter as well modulator in both peripheral and central nervous systems. Both selective serotonin receptor agonists and antagonists have been used. Some of these agents have been used for migraine headaches, vascular disorders, neuropathic pain, nausea, and vomiting. However, SSRIs are popular mainly in the area of psychological illness, especially major depression. Because of their popularity, interactions with other medications as well as anesthetic agents are extremely important. Important pharmacologic interactions have been observed while treating the women with serotonergic drugs if they are taking serotonin inhibitors (e.g., fluoxetine).

The Serotonin Syndrome

The serotonin syndrome, a potentially life-threatening symptom complex, has been described with chronic use of SSRIs and interaction with other serotonergic drugs. Clinical features include disorientation, confusion, agitation, restlessness, fever, shivering, diaphoresis, diarrhea, hypertension, tachycardia, ataxia, hyperreflexia, and myoclonus movements. All are related to exaggerated serotonin effects both peripherally and centrally.

Anesthetic Implications

SSRIs are eliminated by hepatic biotransformation involving the cytochrome P450 and its isoenzymes (2DG, 1A2, 2C, 3A4). These medications, as well as some of their metabolites, can inhibit the cytochrome P450 isoenzymes. Thus, plasma concentrations of any drugs that rely on hepatic metabolism and clearance will increase. One should carefully follow any parturient who are on chronic SSRI therapy: (1) preoperative coagulation data should be evaluated; (2) sedative effects of benzodiazepines may be prolonged; and (3) serotonergic drugs such as meperidine, pentazocine, and dextromethorphan may predispose women to serotinin syndrome. SSRIs such as fluoxetine (Prozac) can antagonize the effects of the mu-opiate morphine, resulting in a decreased duration of analgesia; on the other hand, fluoxetine does not interfere with kappa-opiate drugs such as pentazocine. The popular sympathomimetic medication in obstetrics is ephedrine, and excitatory interaction has been reported after its use in cases taking fluoxetine. Because the SSRIs inhibit the cytochrome P450, amide local anesthetic metabolism may be inhibited; hence, proper precautions are necessary while using higher concentrations and volumes of local anesthetic in women taking SSRIs. Some of the SSRIs possess α_1 adrenergic antagonism. Exaggerated hypotension following spinal anesthesia has been reported following the use of Risperidone.

Tocolytic Drugs

These drugs are commonly used for the treatment of preterm labor. They work by relaxing the uterus. Different groups of agents that have been used are (l) magnesium sulfate; (2) β-mimetic agents; (3) calcium channel blockers, e.g., nifedipine; (4) prostaglandin synthetase inhibitors, e.g., indomethacin; and oxytocin antagonists, e.g., atosiban.

Magnesium Sulfate

In many institutions in the United States, magnesium sulfate has become the tocolytic drug of choice. It might be the ideal agent for diabetic patients as well as for those with cardiac problems.

Magnesium sulfate can interact with both depolarizing and nondepolarizing muscle relaxants.[35] *It can also reduce the minimum alveolar concentration of general anesthetics. Magnesium will cross the placenta freely and can cause neonatal hypotonia, hyporeflexia, and respiratory depression. Calcium can be used as a specific antagonist.* Obstetric cases receiving magnesium sulfate may need less general anesthetic, and they should be carefully monitored with a blockade monitor if muscle relaxants are used.

β-*Mimetic Drugs*

These are the most popular of all tocolytic agents; ritodrine and terbutaline are the most commonly used of these drugs. Terbutaline is favored because it is less expensive, with similar incidences of side effects. Because of their various side effects, drug interactions related to β-mimetic agents are extremely important.

Central Nervous System. β-Mimetic drugs will stimulate the CNS and can cause agitation, restlessness, and tremors.

Cardiovascular System. *Tachycardia, hypotension, and tachyarrhythmias are due to a direct effect of the drugs as well as an indirect effect from hypokalemia,which may be associated with the use of these drugs.*

Respiratory System. *Pulmonary edema is one of the most complex problems associated with β-mimetic therapy.* Its incidence has been noted to be as high as 5%.[36] The mechanism is not known, but three factors may be important: (l) left ventricular dysfunction, (2) low colloidal oncotic pressure,[37] and (3) increased pulmonary capillary permeability due to infection.[38] Volume expansion with *large amounts of fluid can increase the incidence of pulmonary edema.*

Metabolic Changes. *Hyperglycemia, hyperinsulinemia, and consequent hypokalemia* are possible side effects. Ketoacidosis can occur mainly in diabetic parturients.

Tachycardia can be worsened in the presence of other β-agonist drugs such as epinephrine, ephedrine, and parasympatholytic drugs such as atropine and can increase the chance of tachyarrhythmias. *Phenylephrine (Neo-Synephrine) may be indicated to treat hypotension in such cases. Halothane must be avoided if general anesthesia is used. Hypokalemia can also prolong the effect of nondepolarizing muscle relaxants.*[39]

Calcium Channel Blockers

Nifedipine has been used successfully as a tocolytic drug. *Calcium channel blockers will potentiate the myocardial depressant effect of inhalational anesthetics.*[40] They also will potentiate the various actions of dantrolene. Uterine hemorrhage can be a potential problem. An important drug interaction between the Ca-channel blocker (nifedipine) and magnesium has been reported. Severe hypotension with cardiovascular collapse may occur.

Prostaglandin Inhibitors

Prostaglandin inhibitors like indomethacin can affect platelet function and can interfere with coagulation. Regional anesthesia may be contraindicated in such situations.

Oxytocin antagonist, Atosiban has recently been tried as a tocolytic agent. It has been found to be somewhat effective without causing significant maternal or neonatal side effects.

Hypotensive Drugs

Hydralazine

Hydralazine will cause reflex tachycardia and can potentiate the effects of other drugs that are associated with maternal tachycardia.

Nitroglycerin

Nitroglycerin can be used for the treatment of hypertension or occasionally for uterine relaxation. It can affect the neuromuscular blockade produced by pancuronium.[41]

Nitroprusside

Consideration of cyanide toxicity should be addressed when nitroprusside is used for a long time in large doses.

Trimethaphan

Trimethaphan, a ganglion blocker, has been used to treat hypertension in pre-eclamptic cases. *The drug interaction of trimethaphan and non-depolarizing muscle relaxants has been described.*[42]

Uterotonic Agents

Different groups of agents are used to increase uterine contraction after delivery.

Oxytocin

Oxytocin is a commonly used agent for placental expulsion and the treatment of uterine atony.[43] *Naturally occurring oxytocin is Pitocin combined with vasopressin and other polypeptide hormones and is secreted by the posterior pituitary gland Synthetic oxytocin has a different effect on the cardiovascular system from naturally occurring oxytocin.* Synthetic oxytocin (Pitocin) is associated with hypotension, whereas pitressin (naturally occurring oxytocin) will be associated with hypertension. Hypotension is well tolerated in healthy women because this effect is transient. However, severe problems have been noted in women with severe hypovolemia.[44] A large bolus dose (more than 2 units) of Pitocin should be avoided, and for therapeutic reasons it should be used intravenously in dilute concentration.

Synthetic oxytocin (Pitocin) can cause antidiuretic responses in large doses (100 mU or more).[45] Water intoxication, along with an abundant volume of hypotonic solution, has been described following the infusion of massive doses of oxytocin. Use of isotonic saline solution in place of 5% glucose in water should diminish the risk of water intoxication.

Ergot Alkaloids

Ergonovine maleate (Ergotrate) and methylergonovine maleate (Methergine) are used for tetanic uterine contraction and are the drugs of choice when oxytocin fails to produce adequate uterine contraction. *However, in contrast to synthetic oxytocin, these agents will cause maternal hypertension by causing direct peripheral vasoconstriction. Severe hypertension with cerebral hemorrhage has been described when intravenous Methergine is administered in combination with other vasoactive drugs* such as *ephedrine and phenylephrine.*[46]

Prostaglandin

$PGF_{2\alpha}$ is the drug of choice if uterine contraction is not effective following the use of Pitocin and Methergine. *Transient hypertension, severe bronchoconstriction, and pulmonary vasoconstriction have been described following the use of* $PCF_{2\alpha}$.[47] Careful attention is needed while using $PCF_{2\alpha}$ in patients receiving vasopressors or agents that cause bronchoconstriction (Propranolol HCl [Inderal]).

Local Anesthetics

Of the two groups of local anesthetics (ester vs. amide) *ester local anesthetics are mainly associated with allergic reactions because of the metabolic product para-aminobenzoic acid.*

Chloroprocaine is the ideal local anesthetic to use in the presence of fetal distress and acidosis. *Mean in vitro half-lives of 11 ± 2.8 and 15.4 ± 5.2 seconds have been described for maternal and fetal plasma, respectively, whereas the in vivo half-life was found to be 3.1 ± 1.6 minutes* in maternal plasma.[48] Only one case of maternal grand mal seizures has been reported, this was associated with abnormal cholinesterase activity. In this case the dibucaine number was zero.[49]

Interesting drug interactions have been described in association with chloroprocaine. Bupivacaine's effectiveness has been observed to be shortened when it is used after chloroprocaine.[50] The mechanism is not known. The effects of μ-receptor agonist drugs such as fentanyl and morphine have also been observed to be shortened following the use of chloroprocaine.[51] Chloroprocaine or its metabolites may act as a μ-receptor antagonist.

The use of bicarbonate in combination with a local anesthetic has become popular because of faster onset. Several mechanisms have been suggested. Increased pH, with a more basic form of the local anesthetic and the effect of CO_2 have been proposed.[51a] Using 8:4 mEq of bicarbonate, the solution should be 1 in 10ml for lidocaine, 1 in 20ml for 2-chloroprocaine, and 0.1ml in 20ml for bupivacaine. The possibility of precipitation, especially with bupivacaine, should be kept in mind.

Narcotics

The *use of agonist-antagonist medication either parenterally or epidurally in women addicted to narcotics can trigger an acute abstinence syndrome* characterized by tachycardia, tachypnea, diaphoresis, hypotension, abdominal cramps, and agitation and apprehension.[52]

Anti-Fungal Drugs

Azole, an anti-fungal drug, works by inhibition of a fungal cytochrome P450. Azole is a potent inhibitor of midazolam hydroxylation and thus can increase the concentration of midazolam.

Drugs Used for Fetal Indications

At the present time, different agents have been used maternally to treat fetal arrhythmias. These abnormal rhythms in the fetus are usually due to defects in the conduction system that are either anatomic or related to viral infection. Digoxin, verapamil, quinidine, procainamide, and propranolol have been used in mothers in the hope that these drugs will ultimately reach the fetus via the placenta. Important drug interactions may involve cardiogenic drugs and agents that may be used for maternal indications. *Maternal plasma levels should be monitored for therapeutic digoxin levels. The plasma potassium concentration is also important because low plasma potassium levels exacerbate digoxin toxicity. Mothers receiving β-blockers may need higher doses of ephedrine to treat hypotension following regional anesthesia. On the other hand, ephedrine might be detrimental in the presence of fetal tachyarrythmias; smaller doses of phenylephrine (Neo-Synephrine) may be indicated* in such a situation. However, if there is associated congenital fetal bradycardia, Neo-Synephrine use should be contraindicated.

Drug interactions are complex, and a thorough knowledge is necessary because various agents may be used for both maternal and fetal indications.

References

1. Pillinger CB, Adamson R: Antibiotic blockade of neuromuscular function. *Annu Rev Pharmacol* 1972; 12:169.
2. Miller RD, Smith NT: Neuromuscular blocking agents, in Smith NT, Corbascio AN (eds): *Drug Interactions in Anesthesia.* Philadelphia, Lea & Febiger, 1986.
3. Bruckner J, Thomas KC, Bikhazi GB: Neuromuscular drug interactions of clinical importance. *Anesth Analg* 1980; 59:678.
4. Julien RM: Lidocaine in experimental epilepsy: Correlation of anticonvulsants effect with blood concentrations. *Electroencephalogr Clin Neurophysiol* 1973; 34:639.
5. Fariello RG: Epileptogenic properties of enflurane and their clinical interpretation. *Electroencephalogr Clin Neurophysiol* 1980; 48:595.
6. Bovill JG: Adverse drug interactions in anesthesia, *J Clin Anesth* 1997; 9:35.

6a. Gaffney TE, Chidsey CA, Braunwald E: Study of the relationship between the neurotransmitter store and adrenergic nerve block induced by reserpine and guanethidine. *Circ Res* 1963; 12:264.

7. Poulton TJ, James FM III, Lookridge O: Prolonged apnoea following trimethaphan and succinylcholine. *Anesthesiology* 1979; 50:54.
8. Michel R, Adams AP: Acute amphetamine abuse: Problems during general anesthesia for neurosurgery. *Anaesthesia* 1979; 34:1016.
9. Wilkerson RD: Cardiovascular effects of cocaine: Enhancement by yohimbine and atropine. *J Pharmacol Exp Ther* 1989; 248:57.
10. Derlet RW, Albertson TE: Potentiation of cocaine toxicity with calcium channel blockers. *Am J Emerg Med* 1989; 7:464.
11. Jackson JE, Powell JR, Wandell M, et al: Cimetidine decreases theophylline clearance. *Am Rev Respir Dis* 1981; 123:615.

12. Hirshman CA, Krieger W, Littlejohn G, et al: Ketamine-aminophylline-induced decrease in seizure threshold. *Anesthesiology* 1982; 56:464.
13. Takaori M, Loehning RW: Ventricular arrhythmias during halothane anaesthesia: Effect of isoproterenol, aminophylline and ephedrine. *Can Anaesth Soc J* 1965; 12:275.
14. Doll DC, Rosenberg H: Antagonism of neuromuscular blockade by theophylline. *Anesth Analg* 1979; 58:139.
15. Belani KG, Anderson WW, Buckley JJ: Adverse drug interaction involving pancuronium and aminophylline. *Anesth Analg* 1982; 61:473.
16. Buchanan N, Hurwitz S, Butler P: Asthma—a possible interaction between hydrocortisone and theophylline. *S Afr Med J* 1979; 56:1147.
17. Lofgren RP, Gilbertson RA: Cimetidine and theophylline. *Ann Intern Med* 1982; 96:378.
18. Klotz U, Reimann 1: Delayed clearance of diazepam due to cimetidine. *N Engl J Med* 1980; 302:1012.
19. Feely J, Wilkinson GR, McAllister CV, et al: Increased toxicity and reduced clearance of lignocaine by cimetidine. *Ann Intern Med* 1982; 96:592.
20. Feely J, Wilkinson GR, Wood AJJ: Reduction of liver blood flow and propranolol metabolism by cimetidine. *N Engl J Med* 1981; 304:692.
21. Snyder SH: The dopamine hypothesis of schizophrenia. *Am J Psychiatry* 1976; 133:197.
22. Jackson CL, Smith D: Analgesic properties of mixtures of chlorpromazine with morphine and meperidine. *Ann Intern Med* 1956; 45:640.
23. Wallis R: Potentiation of hypnotics and analgesics. Clinical experience with chlorpromazine. *NY State J Med* 1955; 55:243.
24. Gilman AG, Goodman LS, Gilman A (eds): *The Pharmacological Basis of Therapeutics,* ed 6. New York, Macmillan Publishing Co Inc, 1980.
25. Eggers GN, Corssen G, Allen C: Comparison of vasopressor responses in the presence of phenothiazine derivatives. *Anesthesiology* 1959; 20:261.
26. Janowsky DS, Janowsky EC: Methscopolamine as a preanesthetic medication (letter). *Can Anaesth Soc J* 1976; 23:334.
27. Moore DC, Bridenbaugh LD: Chlorpromazine: A report of one death and eight near fatalities following its use in conjunction with spinal, epidural and celiac plexus block. *Surgery* 1956; 40:543.

28. Boakes AJ: Vasoconstrictors in local anesthetics and tricyclic antidepressants, in Graham-Smith DG (ed): *Drug Interactions.* Baltimore, University Park Press, 1977.
29. Jenkins LC, Graves HB: Potential hazards of psychoactive drugs in association with anesthesia. *Can Anaesth Soc J* 1976; 22:334.
30. Rogers KJ: Role of brain monoamines in the interaction between pethidine and tranylcypromine. *Eur J Pharmacol* 1971; 14:86.
31. Eade NR, Renton KW: Effect of monamine oxidase inhibitors on the n-demethylation and hydrolysis of meperidine. *Biochem Pharmacol* 1970; 19:2243.
31a. Rosenblatt WH, Cioffi AM, Sinaka R, et al: An analgesic adjunct to patient-controlled analgesia. *Anesth Analg* 1991; 73:553.
32. Bodley PO, Halwax K, Potts L: Low pseudocholinesterase levels complicating treatment with phenelzine. *Br Med J* 1969; 3:410.
33. Vizi ES, Illes P, Ronai A, et al: The effect of lithium on acetylcholine release and synthesis. *Neuropharmacology* 1972; 11:521.
34. Wilbanks GD, Bressler B, Peete CH Jr, et al: Toxic effects of lithium carbonate in a mother and newborn infant. *JAMA* 1970; 213:865.
35. Ghoneim MM, Long JP: Interaction between magnesium and other neuromuscular blocking agents. *Anesthesiology* 1970; 32:23.
36. Benedetti TJ: Life threatening complications of beta-mimetic therapy for preterm labor inhibition. *Clin Perinatol* 1986; 13:843.
37. Grospietsch G, Fenske M, Birndt J, et al: The renin-angiotensin-aldosterone system, antidiuretic hormone levels and water balance under tocolytic therapy with fenoterol and verapamil. *Int J Gynaecol Obstet* 1980; 17:590.
38. Hatjis CG, Swain M: Systemic tocolysis for premature labor is associated with an increased incidence of pulmonary edema in the presence of maternal infection. *Am J Obstet Gynecol* 1988; 159:723.
39. Miller RD, Roderick L: Diuretic-induced hypokalemia and apancuronium neuromuscular blockade and its antagonism by neostigmine. *Br J Anaesth* 1978; 50:541.
40. Kates RA, Kaplan JA, Gylon RA, et al: Hemodynamic interactions of verapamil and isoflurane. *Anesthesiology* 1983; 59:132.
41. Glisson SN, El Etr AA, Lum R: Prolongation of pancuronium-induced neuromuscular blockade byintravenous infusion of nitroglycerin. *Anesthesiology* 1979; 51:47.
42. Wilson SL, Miller RM, Wright C: Prolonged neuromuscular blockade associated with trimethaphan: A case report. *Anesth Analg* 1976; 55:353.

43. Rall TW, Schliefer LS: Oxytocin, prostaglandins and ergot alkaloids, in Gilman AC, Goodman LS, Rall TW,et al (eds): *Pharmacologic Basis of Therapeutics,* ed 7. New York, Macmillan Publishing Co Inc, 1985, pp 867-880.
44. Weis FR, Peak J: Effects of oxytocin on blood pressure during anesthesia. *Anesthesiology* 1974; 40:189.
45. Munsick RA: The pharmacology and clinical application of various oxytocic drugs. *Am J Obstet Gynecol* 1965; 93:442.
46. Abouleish E: Postpartum hypertension and convulsion after oxytocic drugs. *Anesth Analg* 1976; 55:813.
47. Greely WJ, Leslie JB, Reves JG: Prostaglandin and the cardiovascular system. A review and update. *J Cardiothorac Anesth* 1987; 1:331.
48. Kuhnert BR, Kuhnert PM, Philipson EH, et al: The half-life of 2-chloroprocaine. *Anesth Analg* 1986; 65:273.
49. Smith AR, Dongzin H, Resano F: Grand mal seizures after 2-chloroprocaine epidural anesthesia in a patient with plasma cholinesterase deficiency. *Anesth Analg* 1987; 66:677.
50. Corke BC, Carlson CG, Dettbarn WD: The influence of 2-chloroprocaine on the subsequent analgesic potency of bupivacaine. *Anesthesiology* 1984; 60:25.
51. Malinow AM, Mokriski BLK, Wakefield ML: Does pH adjustment reverse nesacaine antagonism of post cesarean epidural fentanyl analgesia? *Anesth Analg* 1988; 67(suppl):137.
51a. Bokesch PM, Raymond SA, Strichartz GR: Dependence of lidocaine potency on pH and PCO_2. *Anesth Analg* 1987; 66:9.
52. Weintraub SJ, Naulty JS: Acute abstinence syndrome after epidural injection of butorphanol. *Anesth Analg* 1985; 64:452.

5
Uteroplacental Blood Flow

Maintenance of uteroplacental blood flow is the hallmark for fetal well-being; hence an in-depth knowledge of this subject is essential for individuals taking care of pregnant women.

Uterine blood flow is determined by the equation

$$\frac{\text{Uterine arterial pressure} - \text{uterine venous pressure}}{\text{Uterine vascular resistance}}$$

Hence any condition that will *significantly decrease mean maternal arterial pressure or significantly increase uterine vascular resistance* will decrease uteroplacental blood flow and, ultimately, umbilical blood flow.

At term, 10% of the cardiac output (700 mL/min) supplies the uterus. The placental vasculature remains maximally dilated; thus placental blood flow will mainly depend upon perfusion pressure.

Measurement of Uteroplacental Blood Flow

Because of the absence of practical noninvasive techniques, most of the data regarding uteroplacental blood flow came from animal experiments. A group from Finland originally studied human intervillous and myometrial blood flow by using radioactive xenon (^{133}Xe)[1]. This technique recently has been banned by the World Health Authority. More recently, Doppler ultrasound measurement of uterine and umbilical arterial velocity waveforms have been used with some success.[2] The ratio of the peak systolic waveform and diastolic trough of blood flow velocity (S/D) has been observed in different studies, and a *high S/D ratio is associated with reduced placental perfusion* (Fig. 5-1).

Fetal oxygen transfer also depends on oxygen affinity and the oxygen-carrying capacity of maternal and fetal blood. The oxygen carrying capacity will ultimately depend on hemoglobin concentration and the oxyhemoglobin dissociation curve (oxygen affinity). *The oxygen dissociation curve is shifted to the left in the fetus as compared with the mother.* The hemoglobin concentration of fetal blood is high (15 g/100 mL) when compared with the mother (12 g/100 mL). Hence, the higher oxygen affinity as well as the higher oxygen-carrying capacity of fetal blood benefits the fetus by increasing oxygen uptake across the placenta.

Clinical Implications of the Uteroplacental Circulation

The uteroplacental circulation is directly involved with respiratory gas exchange in neonates. Fetal oxygenation will depend on the uterine vein oxygen content and umbilical vessel blood flow. Because of fetal reserve and the different compensatory mechanisms, animal studies support the contention that healthy fetuses can tolerate a decrease of 40% to 50% oxygen delivery without any untoward effect.[3] Animal

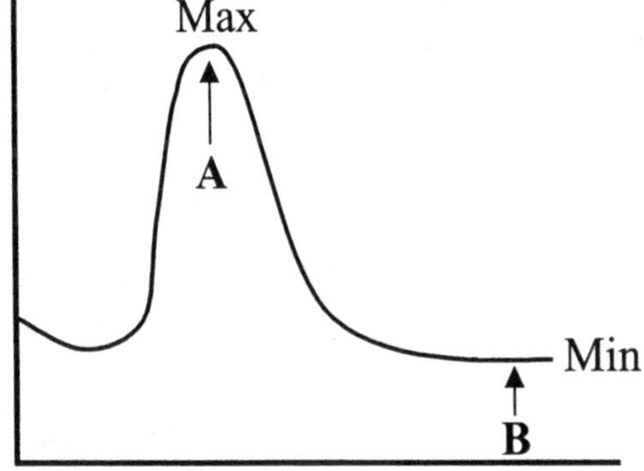

Pulsatility Index = A – B / Mean

Pourcelot Ratio = A – B / A

Systolic/Diastolic = A/B

Figure 5-1. Umbilical blood flow velocity.

studies have shown that fetal oxygen delivery averages 24 mL O_2/min/kg and that oxygen consumption is 3 mL O_2/min/kg. Compensation takes place either by increased oxygen extraction or by redistribution of the fetal circulation. Stark et al. showed an increased production of fetal vasopressin[4] in hypoxic situations. Vasopressin might play a role in redistribution of the fetal circulation.

Carbon dioxide (CO_2) exchange will depend upon umbilical as well as uterine blood flow. Acute respiratory acidosis can be caused by an accumulation of CO_2 because of a decrease in either uterine or umbilical blood flow. *Maternal hypocapnia, on the other hand, will be associated with fetal hypoxia and acidosis. Three mechanisms have been suggested for this: (1) maternal hypocapnia ($<$25 mm Hg) will cause uterine and umbilical vessel vasoconstriction*[5]*; (2) mechanical hyperventilation will increase intrathoracic pressure and reduce venous return as well as cardiac output and thus*

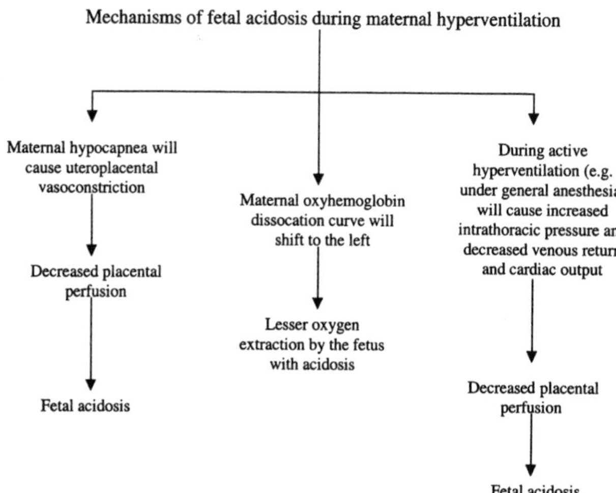
Mechanisms of fetal acidosis during maternal hyperventilation
Maternal hypocapnea will cause uteroplacental vasoconstriction
Decreased placental perfusion
Fetal acidosis
Maternal oxyhemoglobin dissocation curve will shift to the left
Lesser oxygen extraction by the fetus with acidosis
During active hyperventilation (e.g. under general anesthesia) will cause increased intrathoracic pressure and decreased venous return and cardiac output
Decreased placental perfusion
Fetal acidosis

Figure 5-2. Mechanisms of fetal acidosis during maternal hyperventilation.

reduce uteroplacental blood flow[6] (Fig. 5-2); and *(3) maternal alkalosis will shift the oxygen-hemoglobin dissociation curve to the left, and thus the fetus will have difficulty extracting oxygen.*[7]

Factors That Can Alter Uteroplacental Blood Flow

As mentioned previously, uteroplacental blood flow depends mainly on perfusion pressure. Important factors that decrease uterine blood flow are as follows:

Uterine Contraction

Uterine contraction reduces uteroplacental blood flow. Contractions can be measured by observing intrauterine pressure. An intrauterine pressure of 20 mm Hg will not affect uteroplacental blood flow, whereas a pressure of

30 mm Hg will reduce the perfusion by 50% and contractions associated with an intrauterine pressure of 40 mm Hg will completely stop intervillous perfusion.[8] This stoppage of circulation usually does not affect the fetus because the contraction is short-lived; however, if the reserve is already compromised or if there is tetanic contraction, fetal asphyxia can occur.

Decreased Uterine Blood Flow

Decreased mean maternal artery pressure will reduce uterine artery blood flow and ultimately uteroplacental blood flow. *Aortocaval compression by the large gravid uterus (supine position) is one of the main causes of decreased uterine blood flow.* Besides this important factor. other factors that can significantly decrease uterine blood flow are (1) sympathectomy from regional anesthesia and (2) hypovolemia from severe hemorrhage.

Pathological Conditions

The three most important maternal pathological states that reduce the placental perfusion considerably are (1) *pregnancy induced hypertension* (pre-eclampsia), (2) diabetes, and (3) overdue dates or postmature pregnancy.

Pharmacological Agents

Intravenous Induction Agents

Thiopental, Methohexital. In animal studies, *thiopental*[9] and *methohexital*[9] reduced uteroplacental blood flow by reducing maternal systolic and diastolic pressures. However, in clinical situations, induction of general anesthesia for cesarean section has been associated with a reduction in placental blood flow of 35% and no drop in mean maternal artery blood pressure. *Release of catecholamines due to light anesthesia has been suggested to be the main reason for this change in uteroplacental blood flow.*[10]

Diazepam. In doses of 0.5 mg/kg, diazepam did not affect the mean maternal arterial pressure or uteroplacental blood flow.[11] Larger doses, however, reduced uteroplacental blood flow by reducing maternal arterial pressure. Midazolam has the same effect.

Ketamine. Animal studies showed a decrease in uteroplacental blood flow due to an increase in mean maternal artery blood pressure following the use of ketamine at doses between 0.7 and 0.5 mg/kg.[12,13] However, in humans, clinical doses of 1 mg/kg did not affect the clinical or the acid-base status of neonates following either vaginal delivery or cesarean section.[14,15]

Etomidate, Propofol. McCollum and Dundee compared four induction agents, thiopental, etomidate, methohexital, and propofol in equipotent doses.[16] Propofol was associated with the greatest drop in mean arterial pressure, whereas etomidate was observed to be the most cardiostable agent. Hence, one should expect a larger drop in uteroplacental blood flow with propofol than with etomidate.[16,17]

Inhalation Agents

Halothane. Animal experiments support the view that light and moderately deep anesthesia (1 and 1.5 minimum alveolar concentration (IMAC)) will maintain uteroplacental blood flow by uterine vasodilation even though there is a slight decrease in maternal artery blood pressure.[18] However, a deep level of anesthesia (2 MAC) will significantly reduce uteroplacental blood flow by decreasing the mean maternal artery blood pressure.[18]

Isoflurane. Animal studies with isoflurane have shown similar results as those with halothane.[18]

Methoxyflurane. Because of its property of less uterine relaxation, methoxyflurane did not increase uteroplacental blood flow even when administered in low concentrations. In high concentrations it decreased uteroplacental blood flow via decreased maternal arterial pressure.[19]

Enflurane. Like halothane and isoflurane, light and moderate degrees of enflurane anesthesia did not alter maternal cardiovascular function and performance, uteroplacental blood flow, fetal cardiovascular function, or fetal acid-base status.[20] Enflurane in concentrations of more than 1 vol/100 mL produced dose-related maternal and fetal bradycardia, decreased uteroplacental blood flow, and fetal acidosis.[21]

Desflurane and Sevoflurane

The newer inhalational anesthetics, such as desflurane and sevoflurane, are associated with more precise control over maintenance of anesthesia; hence a more rapid recovery is possible. Interestingly, their pharmacokinetics is similar to that of nitrous oxide, and they may be used instead of nitrous oxide. In obstetric anesthesia these agents would be used only for a short time and in low concentrations; hence, the cardiovascular, respiratory, or hepatorenal problems should be insignificant.[22]

Desflurane is resistant to biodegradation, whereas sevoflurane has the potential for biodegradation. The degradation of sevoflurane by soda lime can produce a toxic product. The MAC–awake is 2.4% for desflurane and 0.61% for sevoflurane. In equipotent MAC there are no differences in the degree of uterine relaxation. A recent study compared isoflurane and sevoflurane for general anesthesia for cesarean section. Sevoflurane and isoflurane at equianesthetic concentrations (0.46 MAC hr) were observed to produce similar drops in blood pressure and heart rate changes during the operation. Blood loss and uterine tone were similar. No differences were observed in neonatal neurobehavioral outcome.[23]

Local Anesthetics

In vitro studies on human uterine arteries obtained from pregnant and nonpregnant uteri showed that high doses of the local anesthetics lidocaine and mepivacaine (400 to 1,000 μg/mL) caused uterine artery vasoconstriction only in specimens obtained from pregnant uteri.[22a] This vasoconstriction could not be prevented by prior treatment with phenoxybenzamine. In in vivo studies in pregnant sheep, a dose-related, transient decrease in uterine blood flow was observed when injecting 20-, 40-, and 80-mg bolus doses of lidocaine or mepivacaine into the dorsal aorta.[23a] One of the limitations of these studies was that a high dose of local anesthetics could only be achieved in a clinical situation by injecting local anesthetics directly in a vein while performing epidural anesthesia. *Higher blood levels can also be achieved with a paracervical block, and this may be associated with severe fetal bradycardia.*[24] *The mechanisms of fetal bradycardia are* (1) *uterine vasoconstriction due to large amounts of local anesthetics as well as* (2) *direct depression of the fetal heart by local anesthetics.* When less lidocaine (blood level, 2 to 4 µg/mL) is used, close to the clinical blood concentration during epidural anesthesia, no significant decrease in uterine blood flow was observed even after prolonged infusion (2 hours).[25] Ropivacaine and bupivacaine do not cause vasoconstriction or reduce uteroplacental blood flow in therapeutic doses.[25a] On the other hand, cocaine is associated with a significantly higher degree of uterine vasoconstriction and reduced uteroplacental blood flow. Intravenous injections of 0.5 to 1 mg/kg of cocaine in sheep reduced uterine blood flow by 48% to 65% with an associated increase in maternal blood pressure.[26]

Pharmacological Agent Added to the Local Anesthetic

Epinephrine is frequently added to local anesthetics to intensify the sensory and motor blockade as well as prolong the duration of anesthesia. Epinephrine possesses both α- and β-mimetic effects on adrenergic receptors. *Fifteen micrograms of epinephrine has been suggested as an intravascular test dose.*[27] *The addition of epinephrine (5 µg/mL) has also been shown to decrease vascular uptake of local anesthetics.*[28] *Low blood levels of epinephrine, as can occur from systemic absorption from the epidural space, may decrease the mean arterial pressure because of its β-mimetic effect and can reduce uteroplacental blood flow*[29] unless the blood pressure is corrected. On the other hand, the injection of epinephrine intravascularly will cause uterine vasoconstriction in a dose-dependent manner.[30]

Vasopressors

In parturients, ephedrine, which has mainly a β-mimetic effect, has been the drug of choice for the treatment of hypotension following regional anesthesia or from other pharmacological agents or hypovolemia following blood loss. *Ephedrine will increase the blood pressure by both ionotropic and chronotropic effect on the heart without decreasing the uterine blood flow. On the other hand, vasopressors,* which have mainly α-mimetic effects *(mephentermine, metaraminol, methoxamine), will increase the blood pressure with a significant reduction in uterine blood flow.*[31] However, recent studies in normal parturients have shown that phenylephrine, when used in small incremental doses, corrects the decrease in maternal blood pressure without affecting the acid-base values of neonates.[32a]

Antihypertensive Agents

Hydralazine. In animal studies, hydralazine decreased maternal blood pressure with an associated increase in uteroplacental blood flow.[33] In parturients with pre-eclampsia, hydralazine decreased maternal blood pressure; however, there was no increase in intervillous blood flow even in the presence of increased umbilical vein blood flow.[34]

Nitroglycerin. In pregnant sheep, nitroglycerin administered after phenylephrine-induced hypertension decreased maternal artery blood pressure and caused an increase in uteroplacental blood flow.[35]

Nitroprusside. In animal studies, nitroprusside decreased maternal artery blood pressure with an associated decrease in uteroplacental blood flow.[36]

Trimethaphan (Arfonad). A ganglionic blocking agent, trimethaphan can decrease maternal blood pressure with a decrease in uteroplacental blood flow.

Verapamil. In animals, calcium channel blockers like verapamil will decrease maternal arterial pressure and cause a reduction in uteroplacental blood flow.[37]

β-*Adrenergic Blocking Drugs*

Propranolol (Inderal). This drug has been used in the treatment of pregnancy-induced hypertension, thyrotoxicosis, idiopathic hypertrophic obstructive cardiomyopathy, and supra-ventricular tachycardia. Use of propranolol can cause fetal (1) bradycardia, (2) hypoglycemia, (3) intrauterine growth retardation, (4) respiratory depression, and (5) hyperbilirubinemia.

Esmolol. Maternally administered esmolol produces β-adrenergic blockade and hypoxemia in fetal sheep. Also, possibly because of rapid placental transfer, esmolol can cause direct fetal bradycardia.[38]

Tocolytic Drugs

Magnesium Sulfate, β-Mimetics, Calcium Channel Blockers, Prostaglandin Inhibitors. Uteroplacental blood flow will depend ultimately on the mean maternal artery blood pressure. By relaxing the uterus, these agents can increase uteroplacental blood flow provided that maternal artery blood pressure is maintained at a normal level.

Epidural and Subarachnoid Opiates

Epidural and subarachnoid opiates, except meperidine. should not affect the uteroplacental blood flow.[39,40]

Different anesthetic techniques and agents will affect uteroplacental blood flow and ultimately fetal well-being. Hence, appropriate knowledge of uteroplacental physiology and pathology is important for the obstetric anesthesiologist.

References

1. Jouppila R, Jouppila P, Hollman A, et al: Effect of segmental extradural analgesia on placental blood flow during normal labour. *Br J Anaesth* 1978; 50:563.
2. Marx GF, Patel S, Berman J, et al: Umbilical blood flow velocity waveforms in different maternal positions and with epidural analgesia. *Obstet Gynecol* 1986; 68:61.
3. Wilkening RB, Meschia G: Fetal oxygen uptake, oxygenation, and acid-base balance as a function of uterine blood flow. *Am J Physiol* 1983; 24:749.
4. Stark RI, Wardlaw SL, Daniel SS, et al: Vasopressin secretion induced by hypoxia in sheep: Developmental changes and relationships to β-endorphin. *Am J Obstet Gynecol* 1982; 143: 204.

5. Motoyama EK, Rivard G, Acheson F, et al: Adverse effect of maternal hyperventilation on the foetus. *Lancet* 1966; 1:286.
6. Levinson G, Shnider SM, deLorimier AA: Effects of maternal hyperventilation on uterine blood flow and fetal oxygenation and acid-base status. *Anesthesiology* 1974; 40:340.
7. Parer JT, Eng M, Aoba H, et al: Uterine blood flow and oxygen uptake during maternal hyperventilation in monkeys at cesarean section. *Anesthesiology* 1970; 32:130.
8. Abouleish E: Transfer of drugs across the placenta, in Abouleish E (ed): *Pain Control in Obstetrics.* Philadelphia, JB Lippincott, 1977, p 37.
9. Cosmi EV, Condorelli S, Scarpelli EM: Fetal asphyxia induced by sodium thiopental, thiamylal and methohexital (abstract IV, 3/12). Presented at the Fourth European Congress of Perinatal Medicine. Prague, 1974.
10. Jouppila P, Kuikka J, Jouppila R: Effect of induction of general anesthesia for cesarean section on intervillous blood flow. *Acta Obstet Gynecol Scand* 1979; 58:249.
11. Mofld M, Brinkman CR III, Assali NS: Effects of diazepam on uteroplacental and fetal hemodynamics and metabolism. *Obstet Gynecol* 1973; 41:364.
12. Levinson G, Shnider SM, Gildea JE, et al: Maternal and foetal cardiovascular and acid-base changes during ketamine anaesthesia in pregnant ewes. *Br J Anaesth* 1973; 45:1111.
13. Craft JB, Coaldrake LA, Yonekura JL: Ketamine, catecholamines, and uterine tone in pregnant ewes. *Am J Obstet Gynecol* 1983; 146:429.
14. Meer FM, Downing JW. Coleman AJ: An intravenous method of anaesthesia for caesarean section. Part II. Ketamine. *Br JAnaesth* 1973; 45:191.
15. Hodgkinson R, Marx GF, Kim SS, et al: Neonatal neurobehavioral tests following vaginal delivery under ketamine, thiopental and extradural anesthesia. *Anest Analg* 1977; 56:548.
16. McCollum JSC, Dundee J: Comparison of induction characteristics of four intravenous anesthetic agents. *Anaesthesia* 1986; 4:995.
17. Fahy LT, Van Mourik GA, Utting JE: A comparison of the induction characteristics of thiopentone and propofol. *Anaesthesia* 1985; 40:934.
18. Palahniuk RJ, Shnider SM: Maternal and fetal cardiovascular and acid-base changes during halothane and isoflurane anesthesia in the pregnant ewe. *Anesthesiology* 1974; 41:462.

19. Smith JB, Manning FA, Palahniuk RJ: Maternal and foetal effects of methoxyflurane anaesthesia in the pregnant ewe. *Can Anaesth Soc J* 1975; 22:449.
20. Shnider SM, Wright RG, Levinson G, et al: Plasma norepinephrine and uterine blood flow changes during endotracheal intubation and general anesthesia in the pregnant ewe (abstract). Presented at the Annual Meeting of the American Society of Anesthesiologists, Chicago, 1978, p 115.
21. Cosmi EV: Drugs, anesthetics and the fetus, in Scarpelli EM, Cosmi EV (ed): *Reviews in Perinatal Medicine,* vol 1. Baltimore, University Park Press, 1976, p 191.
22. Eger EI: New inhaled anesthetics. *Anesthesiology* 1994; 80:906
22a. Gibbs CP, Noel SC: Human uterine artery responses to lidocaine. *Am J Obstet Gynecol* 1976; 126:313.
23. Gambling DR, Sharma SK, White PF et al: Use of sevoflurane during elective cesarean birth. A comparison with isoflurane and spinal anesthesia. *Anesth Analg* 1995; 81:90.
23a. Greiss FC Jr, Still JG, Anderson SG: Effects on the local anesthetic agents on the uterine vasculatures and myometrium. *Am J Obstet Gynecol* 1976; 124:889.
24. Asling JH, Shnider SM, Margolis AJ, et al: Paracervical block anesthesia in obstetrics. II. Etiology of fetal bradycardia following paracervical block anesthesia. *Am J Obstet Gynecol* 1970; 107:626.
25. Biehl D, Shnider SM, Levinson G: The direct effect of circulatory lidocaine on uterine blood flow and foetal well-being in the pregnant ewe. *Can Anaesth Soc J* 1977; 24:445.
25a. Santos AC, Arthur GR, Wlody D, et al: Comparative systemic toxicity of ropivacaine and bupivacaine in nonpregnant and pregnant ewes. *Anesthesiology* 1995; 82:734.
26. Moore TR, Sorg J, Key TC, et al: Effects of intravenous cocaine on uterine blood flow and cardiovascular parameters in the pregnant ewe (abstract). Presented at the Annual Meeting of the Society for Gynecologic Investigation, Phoenix, Ariz, 1985, p 175.
27. Moore DC, Batra MS: The components of an effective test dose prior to epidural block. *Anesthesiology* 1981; 55:693.
28. Scott DB, Jebson PJR, Braid DP, et al: Factors affecting plasma levels of lignocaine and prilocaine. *Br J Anaesth* 1972; 44:1040.
29. Bonica JJ: Circulatory effects of peridural block. II. Effects of epinephrine. *Anesthesiology* 1974; 34:514.
30. Hood DD, Dewan DM, Rose JC, et al: Maternal and fetal effects of intravenous epinephrine-containing solutions in gravid ewes. *Anesthesiology* 1986; 4:610.

31. Ralston DH, Shnider SM, deLorimier AA: Effects of equipotent ephedrine, metaraminol, mephentermine and methoxamine on uterine blood flow in the pregnant ewe. *Anesthesiology* 1974; 40:354.
32. Ramanathan S, Grant GJ: Phenylephrine for the treatment of maternal hypotension due to epidural anesthesia. *Acta Anaesthesiol Scand* 1988; 32:559.
33. Brickman CR III, Assah NS: Uteroplacental hemodynamic response to antihypertensive drugs in hypertensive pregnant sheep, in Lindheimer MD, Katz AI, Zuspan FP (eds): *Hypertension in Pregnancy.* New York, John Wiley & Sons Inc, 1976, pp 363–375.
34. Jouppila P, Kirkinen P, Koivula A, et al: Effects of dihydralazine infusion on the fetoplacental blood flow and maternal prostanoids. *Obstet Gynecol* 1985; 65:115.
35. Craft JB, Co EG, Yonekura ML: Nitroglycerin therapy for phenylephrine-induced hypertension in pregnant ewes. *Anesth Analg* 1980; 59:494.
36. Ring G, Krames E, Shnider SM, et al: Comparison of nitroprusside and hydralazine in hypertensive pregnant ewes. *Obstet Gynecol* 1977; 50:598.
37. Murad SHN, Tabsh KMA, Shilyanski G, et al: Effects of verapamil on uterine blood flow and maternal cardiovascular function in the awake pregnant ewe. *Anesth Analg* 1985; 64:7.
38. Ducey JP, Knapp KG: Maternal esmolol administration resulting in fetal distress and cesarean section in term pregnancy. *Anesthesiology* 1992; 77:829.
39. Rosen MA, Hughes SC, Curtis JD, et al: Effects of epidural morphine on uterine blood flow and acid-base status in the pregnant ewe (abstract). *Anesthesiology* 1982; 57:383.
40. Craft JB Jr, Coaldrake LA, Bolan JC, et al: Placental passage and uterine effects of fentanyl. *Anesth Analg* 1983; 62:894.

6
Physiology of Labor and Delivery

▼

Labor and delivery are complex processes involving different organ systems orchestrated in expelling the fetus and placenta from the mother. This process has been divided into three specific stages:

1. *The first stage starts from the latent phase of labor (progressive cervical dilatation associated with regular uterine contraction) and terminates at the time of full dilatation of the cervix.*
2. *The second stage starts from full dilatation of the cervix and terminates at the time of the delivery of the infant.*
3. *The third stage starts from delivery of the infant and terminates at the time of expulsion of the placenta.*

Pain of Parturition

Pain during the first stage of labor is mediated through the afferent nerve supply of the uterus via the sympathetic nerve, which ultimately reaches the T10-L1 segments of the spinal cord. The first stage of labor pain has been described as referred pain. This can be explained by the common neuronal pool supplying both the uterus and the anterior abdominal wall (Fig. 6-1). *In summary, pain during the first stage of labor is mediated by the T10-L1 spinal segments, whereas second-stage pain is carried by the S2, S3, and S4 spinal segments.*

The nerves from the uterus together with other autonomic nerve fibers from the cervix form the interior hypogastric plexus; fibers from this plexus traverse along the iliac vessels as the right and left hypogastric nerves. These nerves ultimately communicate with the superior hypogastric nerve and reach the sympathetic chain either directly or via the aortic plexus. These finally reach the spinal cord via the posterior nerve root ganglion. Some of the nerve fibers from the ovary, uterine ligaments, and fallopian tubes travel via ovarian nerves and ultimately reach the spinal cord via the aortic plexus and sympathetic chain. The nerves in the spinal cord relay to

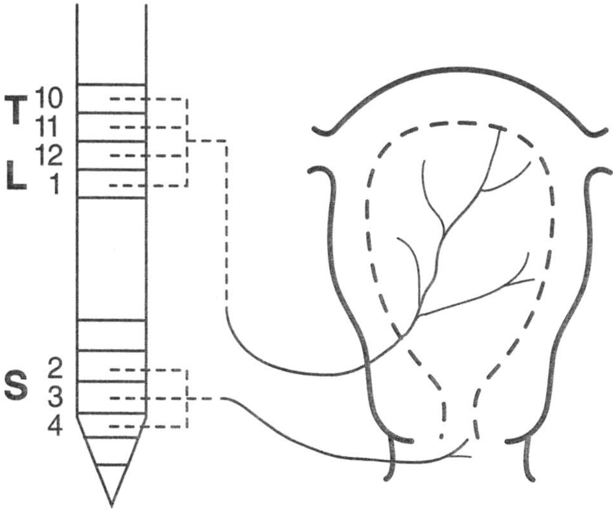

Figure 6-1. Pain pathways for the first and second stages of labor.

neurons of the posterior horn cells and ultimately reach the central nervous system via the lateral spinothalamic tract.

Pain during the second stage of labor follows a different pathway from the first stage of labor. Pain for the second stage of labor is carried by the pudendal nerve (S2, S3, S4). This nerve originates from the sacral plexus and accompanies the pudendal vessels across the ischial spine where the nerve can be blocked.

Relief of Labor Pain (Not Related to Medication)

The McGill pain questionnaire ranks labor pain in the upper part of the pain scale between that of cancer pain and amputation of a digit[1] (Fig. 6-2). Although systemic medications and

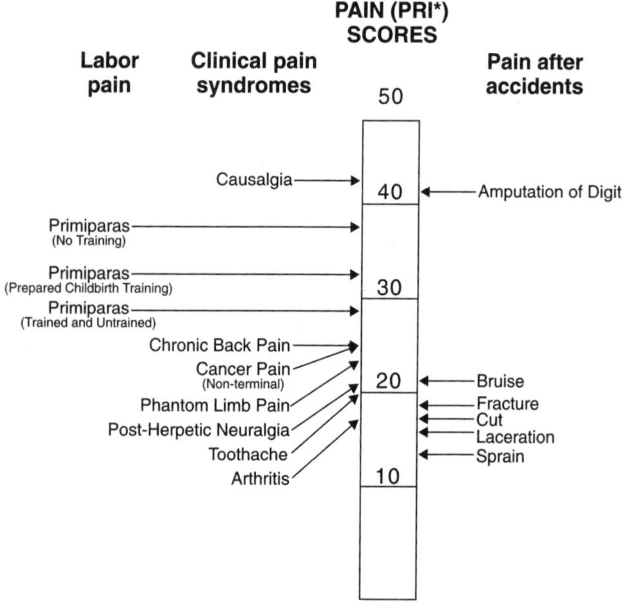

Figure 6-2. Comparison of pain scores by using the McGill pain questionnaire. (Adapted from Melzack R: *Pain* 1984; 19:321.)

regional anesthetics have become popular in recent years, other techniques that do not involve medication have also been tried in different centers with varied success. These techniques include hypnosis, psychoanalgesia (natural childbirth and psychoprophylaxis), the Leboyer technique, acupuncture, and transcutaneous electrical nerve stimulation (TENS).

Hypnosis

Hypnosis has been used for relief of labor pain for a long time. The advantages of this technique include minimal maternal and fetal physiological interference; however, the major disadvantage is related to its relatively small success rate.

Psychoanalgesia

Natural Childbirth

Dick-Read in 1940 originated this concept and tried to make it popular.[2] He explained the mechanism of labor pain in relation to anxiety and fear and preached a fearless approach to labor to minimize the pain.

Psychoprophylaxis

Lamaze is the originator of this psychoanalgesic technique, and it became very popular among women who tried to avoid medications during labor and delivery. This technique involves a proper education of parturients regarding "positive" conditioned reflexes. The advantages of this procedure include the avoidance of any medications, which disturb the maternal physiology, as well as avoidance of fetal depression from narcotics. However, the success rate of this technique varies considerably, and parturients may request systemic medications or regional analgesia when using this technique. Interestingly, a study shows that parturients prepared for delivery under psychoprophylaxis need less analgesia than do unprepared parturients.[3]

Leboyer Technique

In 1975 the French obstetrician Leboyer described "birth without violence."[4] According to the author the psychological birth trauma of the neonate can be reduced by avoiding noise, bright lights, and other stimulation of the delivery room. Hence Dr. Leboyer believes in delivering the baby in a silent semidark room and also avoiding stimulation of the newborn immediately after the delivery. In Boston Hospital for Women, Leboyer delivery was popular among a few obstetricians. Parturients received either systemic medication, local anesthetic via the epidural route, or no medication. Anesthesiologists and neonatologists faced a few problems: (1) problems with neonatal temperature and (2) improper lighting for adequate evaluation of the babies. This technique is seldom used in Brigham and Women's Hospital at the present time.

Acupuncture

Acupuncture techniques have been used in China both for surgery as well as for pain relief; however, there is no evidence of this technique being used for pain relief of labor and delivery. Wallis and colleagues used this technique in parturients without adequate success.[5]

Transcutaneous Electrical Nerve Stimulation

TENS has been used for chronic pain therapy as well as relief of acute postoperative pain. Although the mechanism is not exactly known, the different hypotheses that have been put forward are (1) modulation of the pain impulse reaching the substantia gelatinosa and (2) liberation of endogenous opioids.[6,7]

TENS has been used for the relief of labor pain with variable success. Skin electrodes of conductive adhesive are placed over the T10-L1 spinal region bilaterally; TENS can also be applied in the sacral area during the second stage of labor (Fig. 6-3). Because of its inconsistent success, this technique has never become popular in this country.

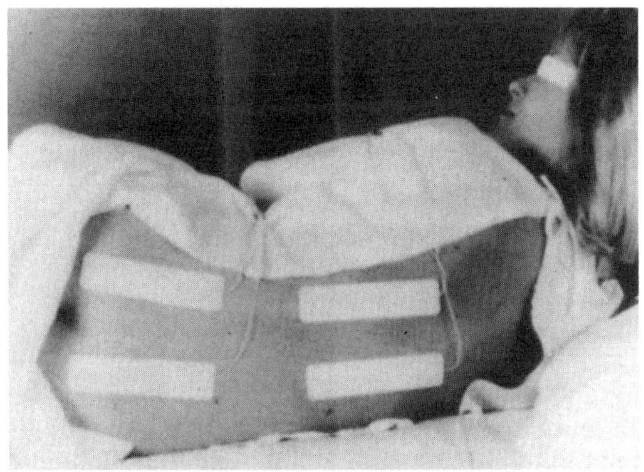

Figure 6-3. Placement of TENS electrodes on a patient's back. (From DeVore JS, Hughes SC: Psychologic and alternative techniques for obstetric anesthesia, in Shnider SM, Levinson G (eds): *Anesthesia for Obstetrics.* Baltimore, Williams & Wilkins, 1987. Used by permission.)

Water Birth

Another natural childbirth option that has become popular is water birth. Water birth provides a calm, relaxing atmosphere for both the expectant mother and her newborn.

Ultimate success from the techniques described above vastly depends upon the parturients' own motivation; hence the success of these methods varies widely, and thus these modes have never been universally accepted.

References

1. Melzack R: The myth of painless childbirth. *Pain* 1984; 19:32.
2. Dick-Read G: *Childbirth Without Fear,* ed. 2. New York, Harper & Row Publishers Inc, 1959.
3. Scott JR, Rose NB: Effect of psychoprophylaxis (Lamaze preparation) on labor and delivery in primiparas. *N Engl J Med* 1976; 294:1205.

4. Leboyer F: *Birth Without Violence.* London, Wildwood House, 1975.
5. Wallis, Shnider SM, Palahniuk RJ, et al: An evaluation of acupuncture analgesia in obstetrics. *Anesthesiology* 1984; 41:596.
6. Bundsen P, Peterson LE, Selstam U: Pain relief in labor by transcutaneous electrical nerve stimulation: A prospective matched study. *Acta Obstet Gynecol Scand* 1981; 60:459.
7. Scanlon RA, Viernstein MC, Long DM: Reduction of postoperative pain and narcotic use by transcutaneous electrical nerve stimulation. *Surgery* 1980; 87:142.

7
Relief of Labor Pain by Systemic Medication

▼

Narcotics
 Morphine
 Meperidine
 Alphaprodine (Nisentil)
 Fentanyl
 Remifentanil
Sedatives and/or Tranquilizers
 Barbiturates
 Tranquilizers
  Phenothiazines
  Benzodiazepines
Dissociative Medications
Amnestic Agents
Neuroleptanalgesia
Agonist and Antagonist Agents
Remifentanil
Inhalation Analgesia

Systemic medications have been used exclusively or in association with psychoanalgesia for relief of labor pain during both the first and second stages of labor. These drugs can be classified in the following manner:

1. Narcotics
2. Sedatives and/or tranquilizers
3. Dissociative medications
4. Amnestic drugs
5. Neuroleptanalgesia
6. Agonist-antagonist medications

Narcotics

Narcotics are popular agents for the relief of labor pain either in an early stage before the administration of epidural analgesia or throughout the first and second stages of labor. Because of their faster action and more reliable plasma concentrations, most of these agents are used intravenously. The various narcotics that can be used are as follows:

Morphine

One of the most effective pain relievers, morphine used to be a popular agent; however, because of the *possibility of a higher incidence of neonatal respiratory depression* this agent is not popular for obstetric patients at the present time. It is used either intramuscularly (5 to 10 mg) or intravenously (2 to 3 mg), and its peak effect occurs at 1 to 2 hours and 20 minutes, respectively.[1]

Meperidine

This is the most commonly used drug at the present time because of its fast onset. It is used both intramuscularly (50 to 100 mg) and intravenously (25 to 50 mg), and its time of onset is 40 to 50 minutes and 5 to 10 minutes, respectively. Meperidine rapidly crosses the placenta and attains fetal and maternal equilibrium within 6 minutes.[2] An interesting observation associated with maternally administered meperidine *was the higher incidence of neonatal respiratory depression when the delivery took place during the second and third hour of drug administration. No significant respiratory depression of neonates was observed when delivery took place within 1 hour or 4 hours after drug administration.*[3] Kunhert et al. did an extensive study to explain this interesting observation; these authors measured umbilical cord and neonatal urine concentrations of meperidine and normeperidine *and found that neonatal urine meperidine concentrations showed the highest amount of drug transfer to fetal tissues after 2 to 3 hours of maternal administration* (Fig. 7-1).[4] Normeperidine, a metabolite of meperidine, reached its highest fetal concentration after 4 hours of maternal administration (Fig. 7-2). They also

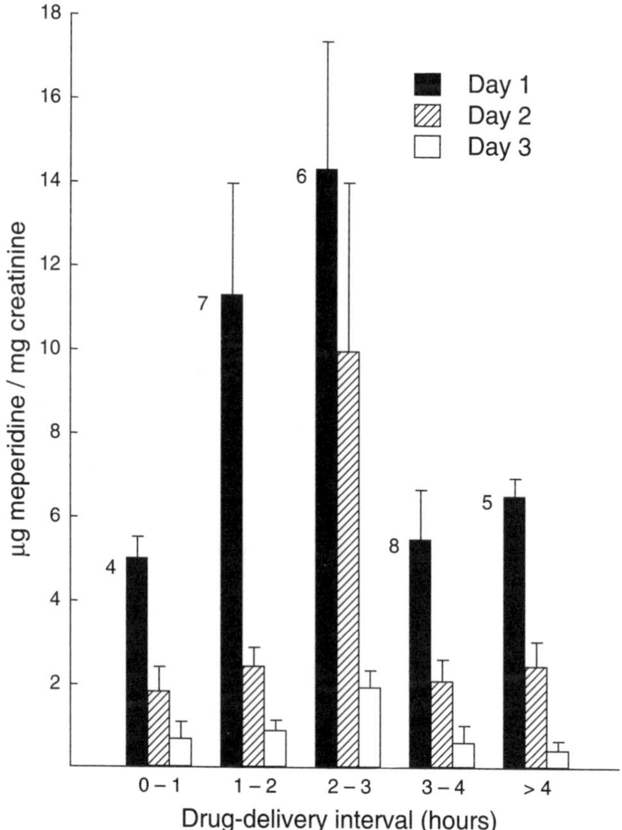

Figure 7-1. Relationship between the meperidine delivery interval and urinary excretion of meperidine by the neonate. (Adapted from Kuhnert BR, Kuhnert PM, Tu AL, et al: *Am J Obstet Gynecol* 1979; 133:909.)

observed poor Brazelton neonatal neurobehavioral scores at both 12 hours and 3 days of age; according to these authors this is related to normeperidine. *Thus, the immediate fetal effect that is observed after the maternal administration of meperidine as shown by low Apgar scores most probably is*

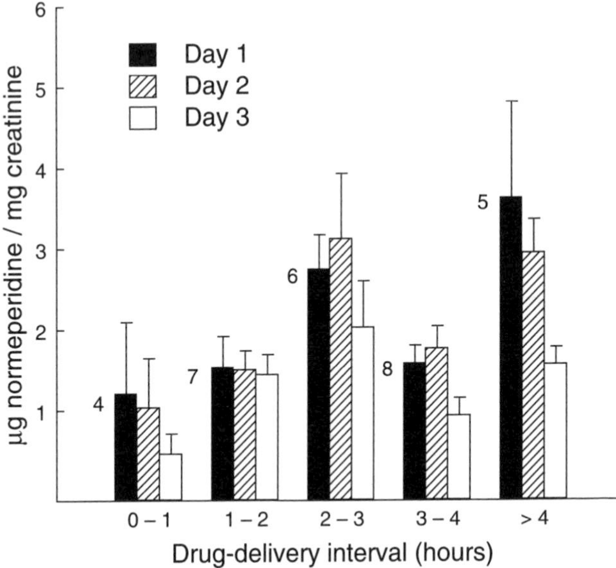

Figure 7-2. Relationship between the meperidine delivery interval and urinary excretion of normeperidine by the neonate. (Adapted from Kuhnert BR, Kuhnert PM, Tu AL, et al: *Am J Obstet Gynecol* 1979; 133:909.)

related to the direct effect of meperidine; on the other hand, delayed neonatal neurobehavioral changes are probably related to the metabolic product normeperidine. Recently neonatal neurobehavior change has been observed from normeperidine excreted from breast milk.[5]

Alphaprodine (Nisentil)

Because of its faster onset and short duration of action, alphaprodine used to be a popular drug among obstetricians, but *this agent was associated with a sinusoidal fetal heart rate pattern.* This drug is not available at the present time.

Fentanyl

Fentanyl is a rapid-acting and short-lasting narcotic, and 100 μg of fentanyl is equipotent to 10 mg of morphine and 100 mg of meperidine. This agent can be used intramuscularly (50 to 100 μg) or intravenously (25 to 50 μg) and will have its peak effect in 7 to 8 minutes and 3 to 5 minutes, respectively. *Interestingly, Eisele and colleagues used 1 μg/kg of fentanyl intravenously before cesarean section and found no differences in Apgar scores, in umbilical cord acid-base values, or in neurobehavioral scores between medicated and control groups.*[6] The main disadvantage of this agent is its short duration: it only lasts for 1 to 2 hours even if used intramuscularly.

Remifentanil

Remifentanil, a new ultra short-acting opioid receptor agonist produces analgesia, however it is quickly metabolized by nonspecific esterases. It crosses the placenta, but it is rapidly metabolized by the neonate. It has been used as a continuous intravenous infusion or patient controlled infusion with some success.[6a] This may be a proper alternative when neuraxial technique is contraindicated. In one report authors used 0.1 mcg/kg/min to 0.2 mcg/kg/min with success.

Sedatives and/or Tranquilizers

These agents can be used either to allay apprehension and anxiety or in conjunction with narcotics to decrease the incidence of nausea and/or vomiting.

Barbiturates

Barbiturates are seldom used at the present time because of their adverse effects in neonates when used in high doses.

Tranquilizers

Phenothiazines

Hydroxyzine (Vistaril) and promethazine (Phenergan) have been used extensively in obstetric cases. These agents possess effective anxiolytic as well as antiemetic properties *and can decrease the beat-to-beat variability of the fetal heart rate.*

Benzodiazepines

These agents are effective anxiolytic, hypnotic, anticonvulsant, as well as amnestic drugs.

Diazepam. A popular anxiolytic drug, diazepam has been used extensively in obstetric practice. In small doses (2.5 to 10 mg) diazepam did not affect Apgar scores or neonatal acid-base values; however, lower Scanlon neurobehavior scores were observed at 4 hours.[7] *In larger doses diazepam can produce neonatal hypotonia, lethargy and hypothermia. Sodium benzoate, which is used as a buffer in the injectable solution, can displace the bilirubin from albumin and can cause hyperbilirubinemia.* Diazepam still remains the drug of choice to treat convulsions following local anesthetic toxicity or in eclamptic patients.

Midazolam. Because of its fast onset and short half-life this agent has become very popular in nonobstetric cases. Because of its potent anterograde amnestic effect, one has to be careful when using it for parturients.[8]

Dissociative Medications

Ketamine has been used as an induction agent during general anesthesia for cesarean section. In small intravenous doses (10 to 15 mg) it may be a useful analgesic drug. The possibility of delirium and hallucinations during emergence from cesarean section following large doses of ketamine may be a problem. The use of diazepam during induction can decrease the incidence of this drawback. Other untoward side effects include hypertension, increased salivation, as well as increased involuntary movements. An *increased intensity of uterine contractions has also been observed following the use of ketamine*

(*>1 mg/kg intravenously*)[9]; neonatal depression can also occur in this dose range.

Amnestic Agents

Scopolamine (hyoscine) is a potent amnestic agent and also possesses mild sedative properties. It was used in combination with morphine for "twilight sleep." Scopolamine crosses the placenta and can cause fetal tachycardia and a loss in beat-to-beat variability.

Neuroleptanalgesia

Innovar (droperidol, 2.5 mg/mL, plus fentanyl, 0.05 mg/mL), although extensively used in general surgical cases, has never become popular in the obstetric population.

Agonist and Antagonist Agents

Butorphanol (Stadol) and nalbuphine are extremely popular at the present time for the relief of labor pain. One to 2 mg of butorphanol has been found to be as effective as 40 to 80 mg of meperidine for relieving labor pain. Butorphanol was associated with less drowsiness as well as less nausea and/or vomiting. *However, the use of butorphanol was associated with a 75% incidence of a transient sinusoidal fetal heart rate pattern.*[10] Because of the problem with the sinusoidal pattern, although benign, as well as maternal somnolence, butorphanol is rarely used at Brigham and Women's Hospital at the present time. Nalbuphine (Nubain), 10 mg intravenously, has become the drug of choice. In a double-blind randomized study using intravenous increments of nalbuphine, 3 mg, vs. meperidine, 15 mg, by patient-controlled analgesia during the first stage of labor, better maternal analgesia was observed with nalbuphine; there were no differences between the two in the maternal or neonatal side effects.[11]

Sedatives, tranquilizers, and narcotics have been used in parturients for a long time; newer agents might be more effective and less detrimental to both mother and baby.

Remifentanil

Remifentanil is the newest opiate marketed for intravenous use. A case report that included three patients was published from England. The authors used patient-controlled intravenous remifentanil for pain during labor for three thrombocytopenic parturients. A bolus of 0.5 mcg/kg with a lockout period of 2–3 min allowed successful demand anesthesia with each contraction. The authors mentioned that there was an initial period during which the expectant mothers learned to anticipate the next contraction and to deliver a bolus close to thirty seconds before the initiation of the contraction. In such cases remifentanil was associated with excellent analgesia, and the doses ranged from 426–1050 mcg/hour. They reported one episode of maternal sedation and fetal heart rate decelerations, which may have been due to excessive demand dosing; however, as the authors mentioned, mothers and neonates tolerated remifentanil without problems. Remifentanil has a unique advantage because of its rapid metabolism by tissue esterase; hence it does not accumulate in the fetus.[11a]

Inhalation Analgesia

Inhalation analgesia is still being used in different parts of the United States. At Brigham and Women's Hospital inhalation analgesia by mask is not used, for fear of maternal aspiration.

In the United Kingdom inhalation analgesia has been used with great success during both the first stage as well as the second stage of labor. *Entonox is a mixture of 50% oxygen and 50% nitrous oxide delivered in a cylinder.* This is connected with a mask for use by the parturient. *One of the main problems with this agent (entonox) is the possibility of separation of the gas mixture when the temperature reaches −7°C*; in such a situation parturients will inhale 100% oxygen first, followed by nitrous oxide, and this can cause severe complications. Parturients can self-administer this agent; however, constant communication between the woman and the administrator is absolutely vital. One should start to inhale 30 seconds before the onset of the contraction so that an adequate brain concentration can be achieved at the peak of the uterine contraction. Besides N_2O, the other inhalation agents that have been used are methoxyflurane and trichloroethylene (Trilene). Enflurane 1% with oxygen or isoflurane 0.75% in oxygen have been compared with N_2O/O_2 (50%) for relief of labor pain and found to be more effective than N_2O/O_2 mixture. However, these agents never became popular in the United States. Two recent inhalational agents, desflurane and seroflurane, are undergoing trials. Desflurane, because of its extreme stability from biodegradation, may be a better choice in obstetric anesthesia.[12]

The effect of the inhalation agents on uterine activity and neonates will depend upon the concentrations of the agents used. In smaller concentrations, no detrimental effect on uterine contraction or neonates has been observed. If general anesthesia is ever indicated for vaginal delivery, then one must take all precautions (nonparticulate antacid, preoxygenation, cricoid pressure, endotracheal tube with an inflated cuff) to avoid any complication. *Occasionally a high concentration of inhalation anesthetics may be necessary to relax the uterus for manipulation by the obstetrician.*[13] Sevoflurane or desflurane also may be used. *Major indications for these manipulations are (1) extraction of the head during a breech delivery, (2) internal version and extraction of the second baby during the delivery of twins, (3) extraction of a retained placenta, and (4) reduction of uterine inversion.* To minimize postpartum bleeding, one should immediately shut off the inhalation anesthetics following uterine relaxation.

References

1. Way WL, Costley EC, Way EL: Respiratory sensitivity of the newborn infant to meperidine and morphine. *Clin Pharmacol Ther* 1965; 6:454.
2. Shnider SM, Way EL, Lord MJ: Rate of appearance and disappearance of meperidine in fetal blood after administration of narcotic to the mother. *Anesthesiology* 1966; 17:227.
3. Shnider SM, Moya F: Effects of meperidine on the newborn infant. *Am J Obstet Gynecol* 1964; 89:1000.
4. Kuhnert BR, Kuhnert PM, Tu AL, et al: Meperidine and normeperidine levels following meperidine administration during labor II. Fetus and neonate. *Am J Obstet Gynecol* 1979; 133:909.

5. Whittels B, Scott DT, Sinatra RS: Exogenous opioids in human breast milk and acute neonatal neurobehavior: A preliminary study. *Anesthesiology* 1990; 73:864.
6. Eisele JH, Wright R, Rogge P: Newborn and maternal fentanyl levels at cesarean section. *Anesth Analg* 1982; 61:179.
7. Rolbin SH, Wright RG. Shnider SM, et al: Diazepam during cesarean section—effects on neonatal Apgar scores, acid-base status, neurobehavioral assessment and maternal and fetal plasma norepinephrine levels (abstract). Presented at the Annual Meeting of the American Society of Anesthesiologists, New Orleans, 1977, p 449.
8. Kanto J, Aaltonen L, Erkkola R: Pharmacokinetics and sedative effect of midazolam in connection with cesarean section performed under epidural analgesia. *Acta Anaesthesiol Scand* 1984; 28:116.
9. Marx GF: Postpartum uterine pressure with different doses of ketamine. *Anesthesiology* 1979; 50:163.
10. Hatjis CG, Meis PJ: Sinusoidal fetal heart rate pattern associated with butorphanol administration. *Obstet Gynecol* 1986; 67: 377.
11. Frank M, McAteer EJ, Cattermole R, et al: Nalbuphine for obstetric analgesia: A comparison of nalbuphine with pethidine for pain relief in labour when administered by patient controlled analgesia. *Anaesthesia* 1987; 42:697.
11a. Jones R, Pegrum A, Stacey RGW: Patient-controlled analgesia using remifentanil in the parturient with thrombocytopenia. *Anaesthesia* 1999; 54:459.
12. Jones RM: Desflurane and seroflurane: Inhalation anesthetics for this decade. *Br J Anaesth* 1990; 65:527.
13. Munson ES, Majer WR, Caton D: Effects of halothane cyclopropane and nitrous oxide on isolated human uterine muscle. *J Obstet Gynecol Br Commonw* 1969; 76:27.

8
Spinal Opiates in Obstetrics

Subarachnoid and epidural opiates have become extremely popular for pain relief for both labor and delivery as well as cesarean section. *Interestingly, spinal opioids have physicochemical properties very similar to local anesthetics,*[1] as shown in Table 8-1. *Low pKa and high lipid solubility will be associated with a rapid onset of pain relief, whereas low lipid solubility, because of higher concentrations of drug in the cerebrospinal fluid (CSF), will increase the chance of delayed respiratory depression (morphine).* The site and mechanism of action are different. Presynaptic and postsynaptic receptors in the substantia gelatinosa of the dorsal horn of the spinal cord have been cited as the major site of action for spinal opiates,[1] whereas blockade of the axonal membrane of the spinal nerve roots and of the anterior and posterior horn cells is the mechanism of action for local anesthetics. Consequently, *spinal opiates can produce "selective" blockade of pain without blocking the sympathetic nervous system and thus can maintain a stable cardiovascular system.*

Table 8-1. Physicochemical Properties of Opioids vs. Local Anesthetics

Drug	Molecular Weight (Bases)	pKa (25°C)	Partition Coefficient[†]
Local anesthetics[‡]			
Procaine hydrochloride	236	8.9	0.02[§]
Lidocaine hydrochloride	234	7.9	2.9[§]
Bupivacaine hydrochloride	288	8.1	27.5[§]
Etidocaine hydrochloride	276	7.7	141[§]
Opioids[‡]			
Morphine sulfate	285	7.9[¶]	1.42[‖]
Meperidine hydrochloride	247	8.5	38.8[‖]
Methadone hydrochloride	309	9.3	116[‖]
Fentanyl citrate	336	8.4	813[‖]
Sufentanil citrate	386	8.0	1,778[‖]
(−)Lofentanil *cis*-oxalate	408	7.8	1,450[‖]
β-Endorphin	3,300	—	—
Remifentanil HCl	413	7.07	17.9

Adapted from Cousins MJ, Mather LE: *Anesthesiology* 1984; 61:277.
[†]*n*-Heptane and octanol partition coefficients are strongly correlated for similar compounds in a log-log relationship.
[‡]Commonly used forms.
[§]*n*-Heptane/pH 7.4 buffer, partition coefficient.
[¶]Tertiary amino group.
[‖]Octanoll/pH 7.4 buffer, partition coefficient.

There are different varieties of opiate receptors, e.g., μ, δ, κ, and σ, and these are bound to different opioid agonists. *μ-Receptors bind to β-endorphin, and this is associated with analgesia, respiratory depression, and euphoria.* The δ-receptors are associated with the epileptic, behavioral, and sedative effects of opioids. These receptors bind to enkephalins more specifically than β-endorphin. The κ- and σ-receptors are specifically bound to ketocyclozocine and *N*-allylnormetaz-ocine, respectively. *The κ-receptor is associated with analgesia, miosis, and sedation,* whereas σ-receptors mediate dysphoria, hallucinations, and respiratory and vasomotor stimulation. Opiate receptors present in areas of the nervous system that are important for nociception and affect.[2]

Use of Spinal Opiates

Labor and Delivery

Epidural Opiates

When used alone, epidural opioids may provide satisfactory pain relief if used in higher doses. Morphine, 7.5 mg, provided satisfactory pain relief only during the first stage of labor[3] (Fig. 8-1). The use of up to 100 mg of meperidine was associated with adequate but a brief duration of pain relief,[4] and this was also observed in the case of fentanyl. One hundred to 200 μg of fentanyl provided quick but a short duration of pain relief.[5] Alfentanil provided inadequate pain relief for the first

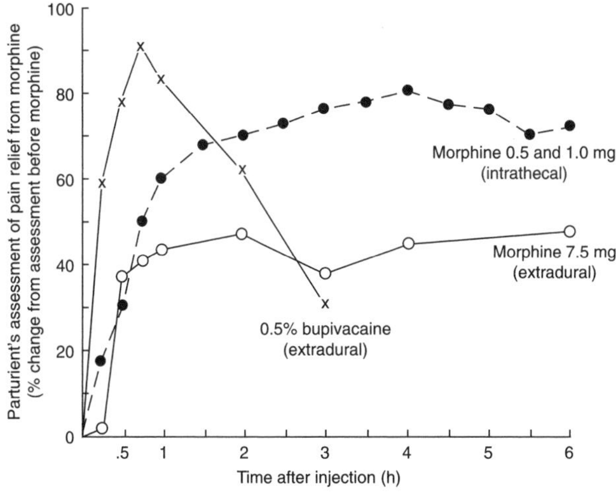

Figure 8-1. Maternal pain relief during the first stage of labor after extradural administration of 0.5% bupivacaine, 7.5 mg epidural morphine, or 0.5 and 1 mg intrathecal morphine. (Adapted from Abboud TK, Shnider SM, Dailey PA, et al: *Br J Anaesth* 1984; 56:1358.)

stage of labor when used in a bolus dose of 30μg/kg followed by a 30-μg/kg/hr infusion.[6] Epidural sufentanil was associated with adequate pain relief of optimal duration when used in a dose of 40 to 50μg.[7] Mixtures of epidural opiates and local anesthetics have become very popular in recent years because of several advantages: (1) they were found to be effective for both the first and second stages of labor, (2) one can reduce the doses of both the local anesthetics and the narcotics and consequently minimize the side effects, and (3) there is a possible synergistic effect. At the present time, continuous infusion is used more often than the intermittent technique. The most popular mixture is the combination of bupivacaine, 0.125%, with fentanyl, 1 to 2μg/mL, at an infusion rate of 8 to 10mL/hr. With this dose regimen, no loss of beat-to-beat fetal heart rate variability was observed,[8] and neonatal neurobehavioral scores were also found to be within normal limits. A few investigators used bupivacaine in a lower concentration of 0.0625% with 2μg/mL of fentanyl and achieved adequate pain relief with minimal motor blockade.[9] Sufentanil has also been used in a 1-μg/mL dose with 0.125% bupivacaine at a rate of 10 mL/hr and provided excellent analgesia for both the first and second stages of labor.[10] At Brigham and Women's Hospital we compared a 0.125% bupivacaine infusion mixed with either 2μg/mL of fentanyl or 5μg/mL of alfentanil delivered at a rate of 10mL/hr.[11] Compared to fentanyl and sufentanil, alfentanil crosses the placenta in larger amounts in fetal side because of its low pKa and low lipid solubility.

The mixture of bupivacaine and alfentanil was associated with better perineal analgesia without increasing the rate of using forceps, and neurobehavioral scores were within normal limits. However, alfentanil because of higher placental transfer can affect the neonates if it is used for a long time. Butorphanol has also been used with 0.0625% bupivacaine to achieve adequate pain relief.[12] Butorphanol, however, may be associated with sinusoidal fetal heart rate. At the present time patient controlled epidural analgesia (PCEA) has become popular as it showed less physicians' intervention compared to continuous epidural infusion. PCEA with background infusion has shown to be more effective than PCEA alone.[12a]

Subarachnoid Opiates

Subarachnoid morphine, 0.5 to 1 mg, was associated with adequate pain relief mainly for the first stage of labor and to a certain extent for the second stage.[13] However, there were several disadvantages: a slower onset (45 to 60 minutes) of pain relief as well as side effects. The combination of 0.25 mg of morphine and 25 μg of fentanyl provided a faster onset[14]; however, the side effects of subarachnoid morphine still remain a major problem. Ten milligrams of subarachnoid meperidine was tried via a 32-gauge catheter for pain relief during labor.[15] The mean duration of pain relief was 136 ± 58 minutes, and there were only a few maternal side effects; however, no neonatal problems were observed. Intrathecal opiates might be beneficial in situations where an absolutely stable cardiovascular system is essential, e.g., pregnant women with severe Eisenmenger's syndrome or the tetralogy of Fallot.[16]

Combined Spinal/Epidural (CSE)

A combined spinal/epidural has become popular in recent years. A 4½-inch, 17-gauge epidural needle is introduced into the epidural space. A 4$\frac{11}{16}$-inch, 25-gauge Whitacre spinal needle is passed via the epidural needle into the subarachnoid space and then wait for the CSF. Intrathecal opioid mixed with local anesthetic is injected at this time. The spinal needle is withdrawn and the epidural catheter is inserted. Sufentanil in doses of 10 μg has been very effective. The addition of epinephrine did not extend the analgesic duration. The addition of 10 μg of sufentanil and 2.5 mg of bupivacaine prolonged the duration of analgesia. Use of 25 mcg of fentanyl mixed with 2.5 mg of bupivacaine has become popular at the present time.

Cesarean Section

Epidural Opiates

Different epidural opioids have been used for both intrapartum and postpartum pain relief. Fentanyl, 50 to 100 μg, has been used with different local anesthetics for better intraoperative pain relief as well as postoperative pain relief.[18] The addition of fentanyl was associated with more intense sensory anesthesia as well as a lower incidence of nausea and vomiting during manipulation of the uterus.[19] Neonatal neurobehavior examinations were within normal limits. Twenty micrograms of sufentanil was used in combination with 0.5% bupivacaine and epinephrine, 1:200,000.[20] The addition of sufentanil was associated with better intraoperative as well as postoperative pain relief as compared with 0.5% bupivacaine alone.

Epidural morphine (3 to 5 mg) has become the most popular agent for postoperative pain relief.[21] The duration of pain relief varies between 12 and 24 hours. Side effects commonly noted are pruritus, nausea, and vomiting. *A rare but important complication of intraspinal morphine is delayed respiratory depression. The incidence of this problem has been suggested to be 1 in 1,000.[22] Close postoperative monitoring of these women is important.* An unusual complication that has been described following the use of epidural morphine is the recurrence of herpes simplex virus infection.[23] The etiology is unknown but may be related to central stimulation of the trigeminal nerve ganglion by the epidural morphine. *Epidural opioids (μ-agonists, e.g., morphine, fentanyl) may not be effective if these agents are used following 2-chloroprocaine.[24,25] The mechanism is not known; however, an anti-μ–specific antagonist effect by chloroprocaine and its metabolites has been suggested.[26]*

Subarachnoid Opiates

Intrathecal opioids have also been used during the introduction of local anesthetics for both intraoperative and postoperative pain relief. Fentanyl, 10 μg, mixed with local anesthetic will provide excellent intraoperative and a short duration of postoperative pain relief.[27] Morphine at a dose between 0.1 and 0.3 mg has been shown to provide a prolonged period of postoperative pain relief (18 to 27 hours).[28,29] A combination of 5 μg fentanyl, 0.1 mg morphine, and 12 mg of 0.75% hyperbaric bupivacaine provided excellent intraoperative and postoperative pain relief.[30] Pruritus, nausea, and vomiting are not uncommon following the use of intrathecal morphine, and *one should also be aware of delayed respiratory depression.* Recently Thi and colleagues used 1 mg/kg meperidine for cesarean section successfully. Side effects included hypotension, nausea, and pruritus. Addition of small doses of clonidine with morphine was found to increase the duration of postoperative analgesia as well as reduced the use of additional narcotics.[30a]

Treatment of Side Effects

Various specific antagonists like naloxone, naltrexone, and nalmefene have been used to treat side effects, especially those following the administration of intraspinal morphine.[31–33] Naloxone infusion at a rate of 0.5 mg/hr has been observed to be effective; naltrexone, 6 mg orally, and nalmefene, 0.4 mg/70 kg intravenously, have also been used with success. Besides these specific antagonists, other medications that have been used are diphenhydramine (Benadryl) for the treatment of itching and metoclopramide, transdermal scopolamine, and droperidol for nausea and vomiting. The administration of κ-agonist/μ-antagonist agents like nalbuphine may also be suitable because this will reverse the unpleasant side effects without interfering with pain relief.[34]

Monitoring

Proper monitoring of patients following intraspinal opiate administration is essential. *Immediate and delayed respiratory depression should be treated promptly.* The use of oxygen saturation, end-tidal P_{CO_2}, and apnea monitors has been advised by a number of authors. However, these devices may not be reliable in every situation; hence close nursing supervision is ideal for these patients.

Newer Drugs

Stimulation of brainstem neurons is accompanied by the spinal release of norepinephrine with associated analgesia.[35] The intraspinal administration of an α-adrenergic agonist will produce analgesia by inhibiting the release of substance P and thus preventing nociceptive neuron firing produced by noxious stimuli.[36] One of the main advantages of α-adrenergic agonist drugs is the absence of respiratory depression, pruritus, and nausea and vomiting. Clonidine, an α-adrenergic agonist, is currently going through trials and shows promise. Four hundred to 800μg of clonidine provided adequate pain relief without any adverse side effects.[37] These drugs can also be used in combination with local anesthetics as well as opiates.

Recently, because of the popularity as well as practicality of the CSE technique, different agents have been tried as an adjuvant to local anesthetic. Two medications that warrant mentioning are (1) clonidine and (2) neostigmine.

Clonidine, a spinal alpha-2 adrenoreceptor agonist, has been tried by the intrathecal route. In one study 0.125% bupivacaine mixed with 75mcg of clonidine was used epidurally. This study found no neonatal problem according to the Apgar scores. However, the authors cautioned regarding the effect of clonidine in neonates, especially related to hypotomia and drowsiness. Since the elimination of clonidine is prolonged, these symptoms may appear within 24 hours of drug administration.[38] Recently clonidine in 50mcg dose was used intrathecally mixed with 2.5mg bupivacaine and 10mcg sufentanil, with or without neostigmine. The authors did not use neurobehavioral testing for neonatal outcome.[39] Such testing may be important before the use of intrathecal clonidine becomes more popular.

Neostigmine may be an interesting agent for spinal analgesia. The doses of neostigmine, however, must be optimal, as higher doses may be associated with nausea and lower extremity weakness. The doses as well as the optimal mixture of neostigmine, clonidine, opioids and bupivacaine are under study.[40]

Intraspinal opiates have made a significant change in the practice of obstetric anesthesia. For labor and delivery, one can use a very low concentration of local anesthetic combined with intrathecal opiates to achieve minimal motor blockade. For cesarean section, intraspinal opiates are associated with intense pain relief both during and after surgery. Even with all these advantages, the side effects, especially delayed respiratory depression, remain the major problem. However, use of smaller doses of intrathecal morphine have significantly reduced the incidences of this problem.

References

1. Cousins MJ, Mather LE: Intrathecal and epidural administration of opioids. *Anesthesiology* 1984; 61:276.
2. Ramanathan S: *Obstetriec Anesthesia.* Philadelphia, Lea & Febiger, 1988, p 81.
3. Hughes SC, Rosen MA, Shnider SM, et al: Maternal and neonatal effects of epidural morphine for labor and delivery. *Anesth Analg* 1984; 63:319.
4. Baraka A, Maktabi M, Nouehid R: Epidural meperidine-bupivacaine for obstetric analgesia. *Anesth Analg* 1982; 61:652.
5. Carrie LES, O'Sullivan GM, Seegobin R: Epidural fentanyl in labour. *Anaesthesia* 1981; 36:965.
6. Heytens L, Cammu H, Cammu F: Extradural analgesia during labor using alfentanil. *Br J Anaesth* 1987; 59:331.
7. Steinberg RB, Powell GM, Hu X, et al: Epidural sufentanil for analgesia for labor and delivery. *Reg Anaesth* 1989; 14:225
8. Mokriski BLK, Malinow AM, St. Amant MC, et al: Epidural narcotic analgesia for labor and fetal heart variability (abstract). *Anesthesiology* 1989; 71:856.
9. Chestnut DH, Owen CL, Bates NJ, et al: Continuous infusion epidural analgesia during labor: A randomized, double-blind comparison. *Anesthesiology* 1988; 68:754–759.
10. Phillips G: Continuous infusion epidural analgesia in labor: The effect of adding sufentanil to 0.125% bupivacaine. *Anesth Analg* 1986; 67:462.
11. Ray N, Datta S, Johnson MD, et al: Low dose alfentanil versus fentanyl with bupivacaine for continuous epidural infusion for labor (abstract). *Anesthesiology* 1990; 73:933.
12. Rodriguez J, Abboud TK, Reyes A, et al: Continuous infusion epidural analgesia during labor: A randomized, double-blind comparison of 0.0625% bupivacaine/0.0002% butorphanol versus 0.125% bupivacaine (abstract). *Anesthesiology* 1989; 71:84.

13. Abboud TK, Shnider SM, Dailey PA, et al: Intrathecal administration of hyperbaric morphine for the relief of pain in labor. *Br J Anaesth* 1984; 56:1351.
14. Leighton BL, DeSimone CA, Norris MC: Intrathecal narcotics for labor revisited: The combination of fentanyl and morphine intrathecally provides rapid onset of profound, prolonged analgesia. *Anesth Analg* 1989; 69:122.
15. Boreen S, Norris MC, Mingy D, et al: Intrathecal meperidine for labor analgesia. *Reg Anaesth* 1990; 15(suppl):8.
16. Abboud TK, Raya J, Noueihed R, et al: Intrathecal morphine for relief of labor pain in a parturient with pulmonary hypertension. *Anesthesiology* 1983; 59:477.
17. Reference deleted in proof.
18. Johnson C, Oriol N, Feinstein D: Onset of action between bupivacaine 0.5% vs bupivacaine 0.5% plus fentanyl 75 μg (abstract). *Anesthesiology* 1989; 71:843.
19. Ackerman WE, Juneja MM, Colclough GW, et al: Epidural fentanyl significantly decreases nausea and vomiting during uterine manipulation in awake patients undergoing cesarean section (abstract). *Anesthesiology* 1988; 69:679.
20. Vertommen J, Vandermeulen E, Shnider SM, et al: The effect of the addition of epidural sufentanil to bupivacaine 0.5% for elective cesarean section (abstract). *Anesthesiology* 1989; 71:868.
21. Rosen MA, Hughes SC, Shnider SM, et al: Epidural morphine for the relief of postoperative pain after cesarean section. *Anesth Analg* 1983; 62:666.
22. Leicht CH, Hughes SC, Dailey PA, et al: Epidural morphine sulfate for analgesia after cesarean section: A postoperative report of 1000 patients (abstract). *Anesthesiology* 1986; 65:366.
23. Crone L, Conly JM, Clark KM, et al: Recurrent herpes simplex virus labialis and the use of epidural morphine in obstetrics. *Anesth Analg* 1988; 67:318.
24. Kotelko DM, Thigpen JW, Shnider SM, et al: Postoperative epidural morphine analgesia after various local anesthetics (abstract). *Anesthesiology* 1983; 59:413.
25. Malinow AM, Mokurski BLK, Wakefield ML: Does pH adjustment reverse nesacaine antagonism of postcesarean epidural fentanyl analgesia? *Anesth Analg* 1988; 67(suppl):1376.
26. Camann WR, Hartigan PM, Gilbertson LI, et al: Chloroprocaine antagonism of epidural opioid analgesia: A receptor-specific phenomenon? *Anesthesiology* 1990; 73:860–863.
27. Hunt CO, Naulty JS, Bader AM, et al: Perioperative analgesia with subarachnoid fentanyl-bupivacaine for cesarean delivery. *Anesthesiology* 1989; 71:535.

28. Abouleish E, Rawal N, Fallon K, et al: Combined intrathecal morphine and bupivacaine for cesarean section. *Anesth Analg* 1988; 67:370.
29. Chadwick HS, Ready LB: Intrathecal and epidural morphine sulphate for post cesarean section analgesia. *Anesthesiology* 1988; 68:925.
30. Naulty JS: Cesarean delivery analgesia with subarachnoid bupivacaine, fentanyl and morphine (abstract). *Anesthesiology* 1989; 71:864.
30a. Nguyen TV, Orhiague G, Ngu TH, Bonnett F: Spinal anesthesia with neperidine as the sole agent for cesarean delivery. *Reg Anesth* 1994; 19(6):386–389.
31. Rawal N, Scholt U, Cahlstrom B, et al: Influence of naloxonc infusion on analgesia and respiratory depression following epidural morphine. *Anesthesiology* 1986; 64:194.
32. Abboud TK, Afrasiabi A, Davidson J, et al: Prophylactic oral naltrexone with epidural morphine: Effect on adverse reactions and ventilatory responses to carbon dioxide. *Anesthesiology* 1990; 72:233.
33. Kohieczko KM, Jones JG, Barrowcliffe MP, et al: Antagonism of morphine-induced respiratory depression with nalmefene. *Br J Anaesth* 1988; 61:318.
34. Latasch L, Probst S, Dudziak R: Reversal by nalbuphine of respiratory depression caused by fentanyl. *Anesth Analg* 1984; 63:814.
35. Yaksh TL, Hammond DL, Tyce GM: Functional aspects of bulbospinal monoaminergic projections in modulating processing of somatosensory information. *Fed Proc* 1981; 40:2786.
36. Kuraishi Y, Hirota N, Sato Y: Noradrenergic inhibition of the release of substance P from the primary afferents in the rabbit spinal dorsal horn. *Brain Res* 1985; 359:177.
37. Mendez R, Eisenach JC, Kashtan K: Epidural clonidine analgesia after cesarean section. *Anesthesiology* 1990; 73:848.
38. Cigarini MD, Kaba A, Bonnet F, et al: Epidural clonidine combined with bupivacaine for analgesia in labor effects on mother and neonate. *Reg Anesth* 1995; 20:113.
39. D'Angelo R, Dean L, Meister G, et al: Labor analgesia from spinal neostigmine combined with spinal sufentanil, bupivacaine, and clonidine. *Anesthesiology* 1999 Suppl A17.
40. Hood DD, Eisenach JC, Tong C, et al: Cardiorespiratory and spinal cord blood flow effects of intrathecal neostigmine methysulfate, clonidine, and their combination in sheep. *Anesthesiology* 1995; 82:428.

9
Effect of Maternally Administered Anesthetics and Analgesics on Neonates and Neurobehavioral Testing

Regional Anesthesia
Spinal and General Anesthesia
Paracervical Block
Pudendal Block
Intrathecal Narcotics
Systemic Medication
Narcotic Antagonists
General Anesthesia
Intravenous Agents
Inhalational Agents

Apgar scores and neonatal acid-base values at the time of delivery used to be the main criteria to evaluate the effects of maternally administered drugs on neonates. Neurobehavior tests have become popular in recent years to observe subtle changes as well as the delayed effect of maternally administered medications. Various neurobehavioral examinations used include: the Graham-Rosenblith scale,[1] the Prechtl-Beintema neurological examination,[2] the Bayley scales,[3] the Brazelton neonatal behavioral examination,[4] the Scanlon early neonatal neurobehavioral scale (ENNS),[5] and the Amiel-Tison/Barrier/Shnider (ABS)[6] neurological and adaptive capacity scoring system. Although based on the Prechtl-Beintema[2] neurological examination, the Brazelton neurobehavioral examination is one of the most thorough tests existing at the present time. The state of consciousness is recognized before evaluation of each item, and habituation to different stimuli is an important part of this examination. However, one of the disadvantages of Brazelton's examination[4] is that it takes 45 minutes to complete the evaluation when performed by an experienced person. Scanlon et al.[5] devised a simple, less time-consuming test by adapting different elements from the Prechtl-Beintema[2] neurological examination as well as Brazelton's neonatal[4] behavioral assessment scale. Scanlon's examination (ENNS) (Table 9-1) also recognizes the state of consciousness before each individual observation. Habituation to pin prick, light, and sound are included in this study. Tone is also observed in this study by a pull to sitting, arm recoil, Moro response, etc. Statistical analysis for ENNS is performed by the chi-square and the Fisher exact tests, as well as by an analysis of covariant comparisons between high and low scores. The last test that has been added to the list of neurobehavioral examinations is the ABS scoring system.[6] The ABS test is quicker than other examinations. *It mainly stresses neonatal tone* and at the present time is only used for early screening of newborn activity.

Regional Anesthesia

Neonatal effects from regional anesthesia can occur mainly from two sources: (1) *indirectly from reduced uteroplacental perfusion due to hypotension, which can happen from sympathetic blockade,* and (2) *local anesthetics or narcotics that are used in regional anesthetic techniques.*

Maternal hypotension is associated with fetal acidosis; however, we observed that if maternal hypotension is corrected within 2 minutes, the drop in maternal blood pressure does not affect the Apgar scores or neonatal neurobehavioral scores as determined by the ENNS scoring system.[7] Hollmen and associates observed the effect of maternal hypotension on neonatal acid-base values and ENNS scores following epidural anesthesia for cesarean section.[8] They noted a significant correlation between maternal hypotension (lasting more than 3 minutes) and fetal acidosis as well as weak rooting and sucking reflexes in the babies. *Obviously, the duration and degree of*

Table 9–1. Scanlon's Neurobehavioral Test Scoring System

State

The infant's state is scored as follows:

Awake States

A-1 The eyes may be opened or closed, the eyelids fluttering, the infant drowsy or semidozing. The activity level is variable, with interspersed mild startles from time to time. The infant reacts to sensory stimuli, but delay in response is often seen. State change after stimulation is frequently noted.

A-2 The eyes are open. There is considerable motor activity with thrusting movements of the extremities and even a few spontaneous startles. The infant reacts to external stimulation with an increase in startles or motor activity, but discrete reactions are difficult to distinguish because of general high activity level. Intermittent fussing does not result in a change of state.

A-3 There is an alert, bright look. The infant seems to focus attention on the source of stimulation, such as an object to be sucked, or visual or auditory stimuli. Impinging stimuli may break through, but with some delay.

A-4 This state is characterized by intense crying, which is difficult or impossible to break through with stimulation.

Sleep States

S-1 There is light sleep with the eyes closed, a low activity level with random movements, and startles or startle equivalents. The baby responds to internal and external stimuli with startle equivalents, often with a resulting change of state.

S-2 Deep sleep with no spontaneous activity except for startles or startle equivalents, usually at regular intervals. External stimuli produce startles with some delay. Suppression of startles is rapid, and state changes

Table 9–1 (cont.).

State (cont.)

are less likely. During an examination, state is recorded eight times, immediately prior to each specific test.

Specific Tests

1. *Response to Pin Prick*

With the infant supine, the examiner pricks the sole of the subject's foot lightly with a pin. The response has two components:

a) Local flexion of the in-volved limb (withdrawal) plus a generalized re-sponse characterized by trunk and limb motion, color changes, crying, etc. Only the magnitude of the local withdrawal is scored in the response category as follows:

0 No response
1 Weak or delayed response
2 Fairly brisk response, perhaps delayed, but more vigorous than 1
3 Vigorous, brisk response, easily elicited

b) The response decrement score is recorded as the number of stimuli required before alteration of either the local withdrawal response or the general response, whichever comes first.

2. *Tone Evaluation*

a) *Pull to Sitting*

The infant is gently pulled by his hands to the sitting position, and the movement of his head is observed. Scoring is based on the observed. Scoring is based on the following criteria for head control against gravity:

0 No evidence of head control
1 Weak head control; unable to maintain head erect
2 More control; had held in erect position for short period
3 Marked control; head consistently held erect

b) *Arm Recoil*

The infant's forearms are gently extended and suddenly released by the examiner. The recoil is scored as follows:

0 Absent
1 Weak recoil, to as much as 45 degrees
2 More marked recoil
3 Very strong, rapid recoil, usually with overshoot

c) *Truncal Tone*

The infant is suspended horizontally by the examiner's hand under its abdomen. The test is scored as follows:

0 Complete floppiness
1 Weak attempt to extend either hips or

Continued.

Table 9-1 (cont.).

Specific Tests (cont.)

neck; weak trunk straightening
- 2 Stronger neck or hip extension; vigorous trunk straightening
- 3 Rigidity of neck, trunk, and hips

d) *General Body Tone*

A composite score is assigned for the subjec-tive evaluation of the infant's muscle tone as follows:
- 0 Minimal or absent tone
- 1 Weak tone
- 2 Average tone
- 3 Strong tone

3. *Rooting*

The skin of the cheek or the corner of the mouth is gently stroked by the examiner's finger. The infant is observed for head turning and lip movement while supine with his head in the midline. Scoring is as follows:
- 0 No response
- 1 Lip movements only or weak, incomplete head turning
- 2 Full head turn toward stimulus with much lip movement (even if somewhat delayed)
- 3 Vigorous turning and sucking lip movements

4. *Sucking*

With the infant in a supine position, the examiner inserts the proximal joint of his index finger into the infant's mouth. Sucking is scored as follows:
- 0 No response
- 1 1 to 3 sucks
- 2 Strong sucks, 3 to 10 per group
- 3 Long periods of vigorous sucking

5. *Moro Response*

This response is elicited by a rapid, short head drop with the infant in the supine position. The scoring of the infant's optimal Moro response, a response which is usually observed after the first or second stimulus application, is as follows:
- 0 No response
- 1 Slow response with weak arm movements, encirclement incomplete
- 2 Moderately rapid response, complete encirclement
- 3 Full, rapid response with encirclement

Stimulus applications are repeated at 5-second intervals and the number counted. The examiner notes the number of stimuli required until the

Table 9-1 (cont.).

Specific Tests (cont.)

first maximal response, and then the number until this stereotyped "best" response is observably altered.

Response decrement is recorded as the number of maneuvers performed from the infant's optimal Moro response until this response becomes different.

6. *Response Decrement to Light in Eyes*

   The light from a flashlight is shined briefly into the infant's eyes at approximately 5-second intervals. The examiner records the number of stimuli applied before the infant's initial response, usually a blink, is observably modified.

7. *Response to Sound*

   Either a ball or a rattle is sounded a few inches from the infant's ear, out of visual range. The response is observable movement or activity, and the infant's maximal response to the stimulus is scored as follows:

   0 No response
   1 Slight change in activity level in response to sound
   2 Some head turning towards sound; searching, alert behavior
   3 Definite searching; almost immediate response to sound

   The sound stimulus is repeated at approximately 5-second intervals, with the examiner counting the number of applications. Note is made of the number of stimuli required until the optimal response first occurs. The stimulus applications are repeated and counted until the optimal response is observably changed. Response decrement to sound is recorded as the number of stimuli needed from the first optimal response to visible alteration of this "best" response.

8. *Placing*

   With the infant in the upright position, the leg is raised until the dorsum of the foot touches a protruding bassinet edge. Scoring is based on flexion of the stimulated leg and placing of the stimulated foot on the edge as follows:

   0 No response
   1 Minimal flexion and extension of leg; foot not placed
   2 Full response, difficult to elicit, foot placed

Continued.

Table 9-1 (cont.).

Specific Tests (cont.)

3 Full response, easily and rapidly elicited

9. *Alertness*
This is a composite, more subjective score that includes the most alert periods during the entire exam. It takes into account head turning toward a variety of environmental stimuli, widening of eyes, "bright-looking" face, shutting out of interfering activity, etc.
   0 Dull or absent response to most stimuli
   1 Several short or one moderately long attentive period including at least one A-2 state score during the exam
   2 Many fairly long attentive periods including at least one A-3 state score during the exam
   3 Alerting responses to almost all stimuli, either environmental or applied

10. *General Assessment*
This is the examiner's appraisal of the infant's performance on the entire examination. Assessment is scored either *A*bnormal, *B*orderline, *N*ormal or *S*uperior. The reasons for putting an infant into this category, such as which scores or tests made up the assessment, are noted.
The dominant state score is entered, and the number of state changes is recorded as the lability. The comment space is used to describe any unusual aspect of the examination, any untoward events or interruptions, and such difficult to-quantitate variables as body color changes and abnormal movements.

*From Browns WU, Scanlon JW, Weiss JB: *Anesthesiology* 1974; 40:121. Used by permission.

maternal hypotension will be important determinant factors for fetal hypoxia and consequently neonatal neurobehavioral changes. Early treatment of maternal hypotension is important and becomes absolutely essential in a situation in which there is already decreased placental perfusion (diabetes, preeclampsia, postdate pregnancy, etc.).

Scanlon et al, by using the ENNS scoring system, first observed a lower muscle strength and tone in babies follow-

ing the use of maternal epidural lidocaine and mepivacaine for vaginal delivery as compared with babies whose mothers received low spinal, local, or no anesthesia.[9] The same authors did not observe this problem in a subsequent study following the use of bupivacaine. *The low muscle tone phenomenon was explained by (1) impaired transmission of conducted impulses at the neuromuscular junction and (2) depression of spinal reflex activity. However, subsequent studies using the ENNS as well as the ABS scoring systems did not note any changes in neonates following the use of lidocaine or mepivacaine for epidural anesthesia.*[10,11] The new amide local anesthetics were not associated with neonatal neurobehavioral changes. There are several studies that observed the effect of other local anesthetics like bupivacaine, 2-chloroprocaine, and etidocaine and detected no adverse neurobehavioral scores following either vaginal delivery or cesarean section[12] (Table 9-2).

Spinal and General Anesthesia

Hodgkinson and colleagues compared neonates whose mothers received either spinal anesthesia with tetracaine or general anesthesia with induction agents such as thiopental and ketamine. They observed better overall ENNS scores in babies whose mothers received spinal anesthesia as compared with neonates of mothers who received general anesthesia on both the first and second days.[13]

Paracervical Block

There are several sources reporting ENNS scores following paracervical blockade. Parturients receiving local infiltration or spinal anesthesia acted as a control group. In one study no differences were found between the groups,[14] whereas in the second study the neonates whose mothers received paracervical blocks had a slower response decrement to repeated pin pricks, Moro maneuvers, and light flashes.[15] The exact mechanism of the observed differences is not clear.

Table 9–2. Summary of Selected Neurobehavioral Studies

Year	Reference	Local Anesthetic	Neurobehavioral Test and Findings
1974	Scanlon et al.	Lidocaine, mepivacaine	Scanlon ENNS: decreased muscle tone up to 8 hr, "floppy but alert"
1976	Scanlon et al.	Bupivacaine	Scanlon ENNS: no change from nonepidural group
1976	Tronick et al.	Mepivacaine, lidocaine	Scanlon ENNS and serial Brazelton NBAS: CLE[†] resulted in poorer motor organization
1977	Corke	Bupivacaine	Scanlon ENNS: no difference from control group
1977	Hodgkinson et al.	Chloroprocaine	Scanlon ENNS: compared chloroprocaine epidural with ketamine or thiopental for vaginal delivery and chloroprocaine performed best
1978	McGuinness et al.	Bupivacaine	Scanlon ENNS: compared epidural bupivacaine with spinal tetracaine for cesarean delivery; no difference
1980	Datta et al.	Bupivacaine, chloroprocaine, etidocaine	Scanlon ENNS: no difference in elective cesarean delivery; CLE
1981	Rosenblatt et al.	Bupivacaine	Brazelton NBAS: decreased organization and alertness for 6 wk
1982	Abboud et al.	Bupivacaine, Lidocaine, chloroprocaine	Scanlon ENNS: no difference with any vs. non-CLE controls
1983	Abboud et al.	Lidocaine	Scanlon ENNS: no difference compared with non-CLE controls

Table 9–2 (cont.).

Year	Reference	Local Anesthetic	Neurobehavioral Test and Findings
1983	Abboud et al.	Bupivacaine, chloroprocaine, lidocaine	Scanlon ENNS: No differences; CLE for elective cesarean delivery
1984	Kuhnert et al.	Lidocaine, chloroprocaine	Brazelton NBAS: at 5 hr chloroprocaine better than lidocaine for motor cluster
1984	Kileff et al.	Bupivacaine, lidocaine	Scanlon ENNS: no difference at 4 and 24 hr for elective cesarean delivery
1985	Kuhnert and Linn	Chloroprocaine	Brazelton NBAS: at 3 days less improvement in regulation of state vs. nondrug controls
1988	Kuhnert et al.	Bupivacaine, chloroprocaine	Brazelton NBAS: bupivacaine better than chloroprocaine in orientation and regulation of state

*From Arcario TJ, Thomas RL: Fetal Distress, in Datta S (ed): *Anesthetic and Obstetric Management of High Risk Pregnancy.* Chicago, Mosby Year Book, 1991. Used with permission from Elsevier.

†CLE = continuous lumbar epidural analgesia; NBAS = neurobehavior assessment score.

Pudendal Block

The neonatal local anesthetic concentration will vary following a pudendal block, depending upon the dose of local anesthetic as well as the time interval between the start of infiltration and delivery of the baby. Merkow and colleagues observed neonatal neurobehavioral effects following bupivacaine-, mepivacaine-, and chloroprocaine-induced pudendal blocks.[16] ENNS testing was performed at 4 and 24 hours of age. At 4 hours, infants whose mothers received mepivacaine for a pudendal block had a better decremental response; however, this difference did not exist by 24 hours. The implication of this difference is unknown at the present time.

Intrathecal Narcotics

Epidural and subarachnoid narcotics combined with local anesthetics have become a popular technique for both labor and delivery including cesarean section. The combination of narcotic and local anesthetic has been associated with a faster onset of pain relief, intense sensory anesthesia, as well as postpartum pain relief. Morphine, fentanyl, sufentanil, and alfentanil have all been used successfully. Neurobehavioral tests (ENNS and NACS [neonatal adaptive capacity score]) have been performed in a few studies in which the authors did not find any neonatal effects, provided that the doses were within the therapeutic range.[17–19]

Systemic Medication

Systemic medication has been observed to affect neonatal neurobehavioral tests. Brazelton compared neonatal breastfeeding ability as well as weight gain in infants whose mothers received either less than 60 mg or more than 150 mg of barbiturates.[4] The higher doses of barbiturates affected the neonatal ability to breastfeed and delayed the onset of weight gain. Kron and colleagues also observed a decrease in both sucking ability as measured by sucking pressure and volume consumed by infants whose mothers received 100 mg of secobarbital when compared with the control group.[20]

Diazepam in doses of 2.5 to 10 mg prior to cesarean section decreased the muscle tone variables of the ENNS at 4 hours after birth; however, this change disappeared by 24 hours of life.[21]

Meperidine used to be the most commonly used narcotic for the relief of labor pain. Various studies have observed its neonatal effects following maternal administration. Hodgkinson et al. observed depression of most items of the ENNS at both 24 hours and 48 hours of life in the neonates whose mothers received between 50 and 150 mg of meperidine; there was also a correlation between the degree of depression and the total amount of meperidine used.[22] Brower and colleagues compared neonatal electroencephalograph (EEG) patterns in two groups[23]: (1) a control group where the parturients did not receive meperidine and (2) a study group where the mothers received meperidine alone or in combination with prome-thazine and/or diazepam. EEG patterns were observed during olfactory, visual, tactile, and auditory stimulation. The authors noticed an alteration in the EEG tracing only during auditory stimulation in the neonates whose mothers received meperidine. Kron and colleagues observed less effective sucking in the neonates whose mothers received meperidine as compared with mothers who inhaled nitrous oxide for the relief of labor pain.[20] The complete study regarding the effect of maternally administered meperidine on neonates was performed by Lieberman and colleagues.[24] The authors divided the neonates into three groups: (1) those whose mothers did not receive any medication, (2) those whose mothers received 100 to 150 mg of meperidine on request, and (3) those whose mothers received epidural bupivacaine, 0.375%, for pain relief during labor. When the NBAS (neurobehavior assessment score) scoring system was used, no differences were observed among the groups until the third day postdelivery, when the authors found an impaired habituation to ringing in the neonates whose mothers received meperidine during labor. Unfortunately, the importance of this isolated difference is not known.

Borgstedt and Rosen examined both the EEG patterns and the Prechtl-Beintema scoring system in two groups of neonates[25]: (1) those whose mothers did not receive any systemic medication and (2) those whose mothers received morphine or meperidine with phenobarbital or promethazine. The majority of the babies had drug-related EEG changes when compared with the unmedicated group. Using butorphanol or meperidine in parturients for pain relief in labor, Hodgkinson and colleagues did not observe any differences in ENNS values between the two groups of neonates.[26]

Narcotic Antagonists

Naloxone, a specific narcotic antagonist, will cross the placenta and reach the neonate; hence different investigators, just before the delivery of the infants, administered intramuscular naloxone to mothers who received narcotics during labor to improve neonatal neurobehavioral scores.[27] Although prior maternal naloxone administration improved the neonatal ventilatory response to carbon dioxide, it did not improve the neurobehavioral scores of the neonates. Others have tried the administration of intramuscular naloxone to infants immediately after delivery, and this technique improved ENNS scores.[28] However, most authorities, including the Academy of Pediatrics, do not recommend naloxone treatment for newborns unless there is respiratory depression related to maternal narcotic administration.[29] Naloxone can alter the amount of neonatal circulatory enkephalins and endorphins, which might be important for neonatal adaptation to sensory stimuli and stress as well as for maintenance of circulatory homeostasis.

General Anesthesia

Intravenous Agents

The effect of general anesthesia on neonatal neurobehavioral scores depends upon several factors, e.g., the agents themselves, the total amount used for induction and maintenance, and the duration of the operative procedure to deliver the infant. Hodgkinson and colleagues compared neurobehavioral scores in three groups of neonates following vaginal delivery or cesarean section: (1) those whose mothers received thiopental, (2) those whose mothers received ketamine, and (3) those whose mothers received epidural or spinal anesthesia.[13,30] On day 1, infants of mothers who received ketamine for induction had higher ENNS scores in overall assessment, habituation to pin prick, and alertness as compared with mothers who received thiopental for induction. By the second day, these differences were found to have disappeared. Etomidate, an intravenous induction agent, is cardiovascularly more stable and in therapeutic doses is not associated with neonatal neurobehavioral changes. Propofol, a new intravenous induction agent, has been compared with thiopental. No differences in neonatal neurobehavioral examinations were observed between the drugs. However, the neonates whose mothers received regional anesthesia scored better than the groups receiving ketamine and thiopental up to 48 hours of life.

Inhalational Agents

The addition of small amounts of inhalational anesthetics during cesarean section until delivery of the baby did not affect the ENNS scores.[31]

Although it is obvious from the above discussion that some maternally administered medications can affect neonatal neurobehavior scores, all differences have been found to disappear within a few days. Hence the long-term effect of changes in the neonatal neurobehavioral examination is not known at present. Interestingly, a few long-term studies fail to show any adverse effects. On the other hand, it is always important to recognize the subtle effects of any medication, especially when medications are new and before they are widely used in pregnant women.

References

1. Rosenblith JF: The modified Graham behavior test for neonates: Test-retest reliability, normative data, and hypotheses for future work. *Biol Neonate* 1961; 3:174.
2. Prechtl JFR, Beintema D: The neurological examination of the full term infant. *Clin Dev Med* (*London*) 1964, no 12.
3. Bayley N: *Manual for the Bayley Scale of Infants Development.* New York, Psychological Corp, 1969.
4. Brazelton TB: Psychological reaction of the neonate: II. Effect of maternal medication on the neonate and his behavior. *J Pediatr* 1961; 58:513.
5. Scanlon JW, Browns WU, Weiss JB: Neurobehavioral responses of newborn infants after maternal epidural anesthesia. *Anesthesiology* 1974; 40:121.

6. Amiel-Tison C, Barrier G, Shnider SM: A new neurological scoring system (abstract). Presented at the 11th World Congress of Obstetrics and Gynecology, Tokyo, October 1979.

6a. Blair JM, Hill DA, Fee JPH. Patient-controlled analgesia for labour using remifentanil: A feasibility study. *Br J Anaesth* 2001; 87:A15

7. Corke BC, Datta S, Ostheimer GW: Spinal anesthesia for cesarean section: The influence of hypotension on neonatal outcome. *Anaesthesia* 1982; 37:658.

8. Hollmen AI, Jouppila R, Kaivista M, et al: Neurological activity of infants following anesthesia for cesarean section. *Anesthesiology* 1978; 48:350.

9. Scanlon JW, Ostheimer GW, Brown WU, et al: Neurobehavioral responses and drug concentrations in newborns after maternal epidural anesthesia with bupivacaine. *Anesthesiology* 1976; 45:400.

10. Kileff ME, James FM III, Dewan MD, et al: Neonatal neurobehavioral responses after epidural anesthesia for cesarean section using lidocaine and bupivacaine. *Anesth Analg* 1984; 63:413.

11. Abboud TK, Moore MJ, Jacobs J, et al: Epidural mepivacaine for cesarean section, maternal and neonatal effects. *Reg Anaesth* 1987; 12:76.

12. Datta S, Corke BC, Alper MH, et al: Epidural anesthesia for cesarean section: A comparison of bupivacaine, chloroprocaine and etidocaine. *Anesthesiology* 1980; 52:48.

12a. Ferrante FM, Rosinia FA, Gordon DG, et al. The role of continuous background infusions in patient-controlled epidural analgesia for labor and delivery. *Anesth Analg* 1994; 79:80

13. Hodgkinson R, Bhatt M, Kim SS, et al: Neonatal neurobehavioral tests following cesarean section under general and spinal anesthesia. *Am J Obstet Gynecol* 1978; 132:670.

14. Britt I, Lindbach F, Ingebjorg S: Neurobehavioral responses of infants after paracervical block during labor. *Acta Obstet Gynecol Scand* 1979; 58:41.

15. Nesheim BI, Lindback E, Storm-Mathisen I, et al: Neurobehavioral response of infants after paracervical block during labour. *Acta Obstet Gynecol Scand* 1979; 58:41.

16. Merkow AJ, McGuinness GA, Erenberg A, et al: The neonatal neurobehavioral effects of bupivacaine, mepivacaine and 2-chloroprocaine used for pudendal block. *Anesthesiology* 1980; 52:309.

17. Baraka A, Noueihid R, Hajj S: Intrathecal injection of morphine for obstetric analgesia. *Anesthesiology* 1981; 54:136.

18. Hughes SC, Rosen MA, Stefani SJ, et al: Maternal and neonatal effects of epidural morphine for labor (abstract). Presented at the Annual Meeting of the Society for Obstetric Anesthesia and Perinatology, San Diego, 1981, p 31.
19. Hunt CO, Naulty S, Malinow AM, et al: Epidural butorphanol-bupivacaine for analgesia during labor and delivery. *Anesth Analg* 1989; 68:323.
20. Kron RE, Ipsen J, Goddard KE: Consistent individual differences in the nutritive sucking behavior of the human newborn. *Psychosom Med* 1968; 30:151.
21. Rolbin SH, Wright BG, Shnider SM: Diazepam during cesarean section—Effects on neonatal assessment and maternal and fetal plasma norepinephrine levels (abstract). Presented at the Annual Meeting of the American Society of Anesthesiology, New Orleans, 1977, p 449.
22. Hodgkinson R, Bhatt M, Want CH: Double blind comparison of the neurobehavior of neonates following administration of different doses of meperidine to the mother. *Can Anaesth Soc J* 1978; 25:405.
23. Brower KR, Crowell DH, Leung P, et al: Neonatal electroencephalographic patterns as effects by maternal drugs administered during labor and delivery. *Anesth Analg* 1978; 57:303.
24. Liebermann BA, Rosenblatt DB, Belsey E, et al: The effects of maternally administered pethidine or epidural bupivacaine on the fetus and newborn. *Br J Obstet Gynaecol* 1979; 86:598.
25. Borgstedt AD, Rosen MG: Medication during labor correlated with behavior and EEG of the newborn. *Am J Dis Child* 1968; 115:21.
26. Hodgkinson R, Huff RW, Hayashi RH, et al: Double blind comparison of maternal analgesia and neonatal neurobehavior following intravenous butorphanol and meperidine. *J Int Med Res* 1979; 7:224.
27. Hodgkinson R, Bhatt M, Grewal G, et al: Neonatal neurobehavior in the first 48 hours of life. Effect of the administration of meperidine with and without naloxone in the mother. *Pediatrics* 1978; 62:294.
28. Bonta BW, Gagliardi JO, Williams V, et al: Naloxone reversal of mild neurobehavioral depression in normal newborn infants after routine obstetric analgesia. *J Pediatr* 1979; 94:102.
29. American Acadamy of Pediatrics Committee on Drugs: Naloxone use in newborns. *Pediatrics* 1980; 65:667.
30. Hodgkinson R, Marx GF, Kim SS, et al: Neonatal neurobehavioral tests following vaginal delivery under ketamine, thiopental and extradural anesthesia. *Anesth Analg* 1977; 56:548.

30b. Paech KJ, Pavy TJG, Orlikowski CEP: Postcesarean analgesia with spinal morphine, clonidine or their combination. *Anesth Analg* 2004; 98:1460
31. Warren TH, Datta S, Ostheimer GW, et al: Comparison of the maternal and neonatal effects of halothane, enflurane and isoflurane for cesarean delivery. *Anesth Analg* 1983; 62:516.

10
Fetal Monitoring

▼

Fetal Heart Rate Monitoring
- Baseline Heart Rate
- Baseline Variability
- Fetal Heart Rate Pattern (Periodic Changes)
  - *Early Decelerations*
  - *Variable Decelerations*
  - *Late Decelerations*

Biophysical Profile
- Nonstress Test
- Contraction Stress Test or Oxytocin Challenge Test

Assessment of Fetal Maturity

One of the most important goals for the anesthesiologist caring for a pregnant women should be to maintain the uteroplacental unit and fetus in optimal condition. Hence, an adequate knowledge of uterine activity and fetal monitoring is important. Different devices are used for the intrapartum assessment of uterine activity as well as fetal well-being.

Assessment of uterine activity is important in predicting the normal progress of labor and also fetal well-being.[1] Parameters related to uterine activity are (1) baseline uterine tone and amplitude, (2) duration of contractions, and (3) the interval between contractions. Normal baseline tone varies between 8 and 20mmHg and increases to between 25 and 75mmHg during contractions. However, the peak pressure can rise to 130mmHg with bearing-down efforts in the second stage of labor. A contraction can last from 30 to 90 seconds, and the interval between contractions normally varies from 2 to 3 minutes. A tocodynamometer can measure the parameters of uterine activity when placed on the abdominal wall.[2]

However, one of the major limitations of external tocodynamometry is the possible reception of inaccurate data from improper positioning of the instrument on the abdominal wall. Internal monitoring is more accurate and reliable, and it measures both amniotic fluid and intrauterine pressure.[3] The prerequisites of internal monitoring include (1) engagement of the presenting part, (2) adequate cervical dilatation, and (3) ruptured membranes. Internal measurement of uterine activity is commonly used in high-risk cases (e.g., diabetes, postmaturity) as well as in parturients receiving epidural analgesia for the relief of labor pain.

Fetal Heart Rate Monitoring

The baseline heart rate, beat-to-beat variability (short and long term), and the fetal heart rate pattern (periodic changes) are the most important variables that should be followed in recording the fetal heart rate.

Baseline Heart Rate

The normal baseline fetal heart rate varies between 120 and 160 beats per minute (BPM), and it is modulated by parasympathetic and sympathetic nerve activity (Fig. 10-1).

Fetal tachycardia is diagnosed when the baseline escalates above 160 BPM. The major causes of fetal tachycardia are:

1. *Fetal hypoxia due to any cause*
2. *Maternal fever, most often associated with infection*
3. *Maternal administration of sympathomimetic drugs, e.g., ephedrine, β-mimetic drugs for tocolysis (terbutaline), epinephrine*
4. *Maternal administration of parasympatholytic drugs, e.g., atropine, phenothiazines*
5. *Maternal hyperthyroidism*
6. *Fetal anemia*
7. *Fetal tachyarrythmias*

Fetal bradycardia is defined as a fetal heart rate less than 100 BPM. The following are major causes:

1. *Fetal head compression or umbilical cord compression*

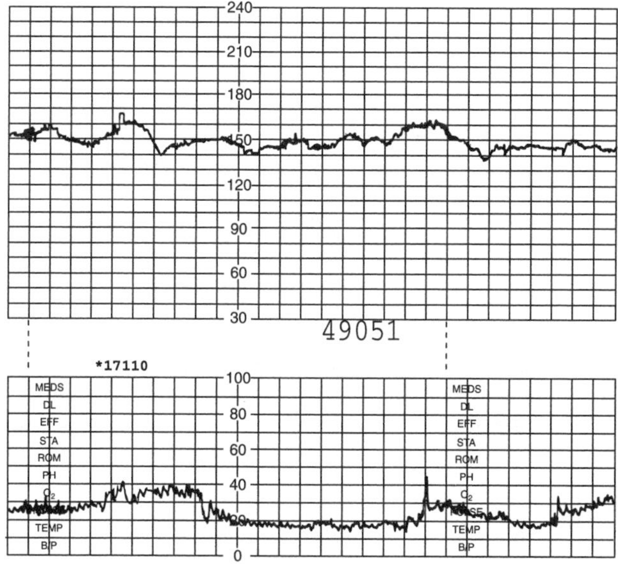

Figure 10–1. Normal fetal heart rate pattern.

2. *Maternal administration of parasympathomimetic drugs, e.g., neostigmine*
3. *Maternal administration of β-blockers, e.g., propranolol*
4. *Prolonged fetal hypoxia for any reason*
5. *Fetal congenital heart block*
6. *Combined spinal epidural technique, especially in parturients with decreased ureteroplacental blood flow.*

Baseline Variability

Baseline variability is generally recognized as the single most important parameter for the recognition of intrauterine fetal well-being. Baseline variability is due to a constant battle between the fetal sympathetic (increasing the heart rate) and parasympathetic systems (decreasing the heart rate). The presence of good baseline variability is an indicator of intact central nervous system as well as normal cardiac functions.

Baseline variability has been classified into (1) short-term variability, representing a beat-to-beat difference of 5 to 15 beats, and (2) long-term variability, which generally shows a frequency of 3 to 5 cycles per minute. *Fetal heart rate variability can be a very accurate indicator if it is used by direct fetal electrocardiogram monitoring.* Short-term variability is more important in predicting fetal well-being. Various factors that can affect this are as follows (Fig. 10-2):

1. *Maternal administration of narcotic drugs, e.g., meperidine (Demerol), morphine, alphaprodine (Nisentil), or butorphanol, which work by depressing the fetal central nervous system*
2. Maternally administered sedatives and hypnotics, e.g., barbiturates, diazepam, phenothiazines, or promethazine (Phenergan), which also affect the fetal central nervous system

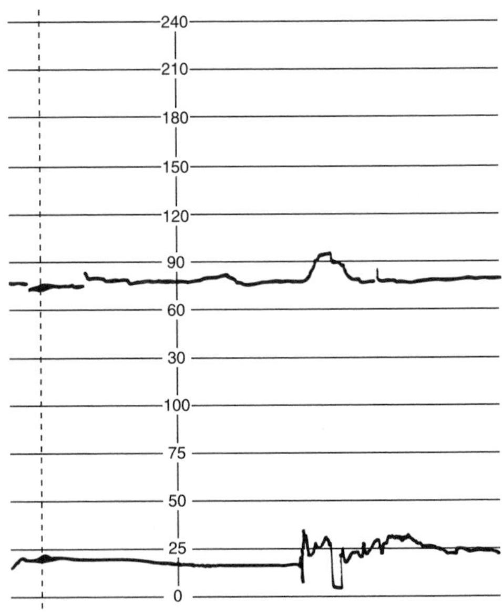

Figure 10-2. Decreased variability of the fetal heart rate.

3. Maternally administered parasympatholytic drugs, e.g., atropine or phenothiazines
4. *The use of inhalational anesthetics*
5. *Fetal sleep cycle*
6. Extreme prematurity
7. Fetal tachycardia

Fetal Heart Rate Pattern (Periodic Changes)

Periodic changes are defined as transient accelerations or decelerations of short duration of the fetal heart rate followed by a return to baseline levels. There are three categories of decelerations: early, variable, and late.

Early Decelerations

Characteristics of early decelerations (Fig.10-3) are as follows:

1. *Uniform. U-shaped deceleration*
2. Slow onset and slow return to baseline
3. *Exact mirror image of uterine contractions in duration*
4. Acceleration of the fetal heart not preceding the onset of a contraction or following the end of a contraction
5. Fetal heart rate usually not falling below 20 to 30 BPM
6. *Good beat-to-beat variability*

Two mechanisms for early deceleration that have been suggested are (1) *fetal head compression with increased intracranial pressure* (Fig. 10-4) and (2) *increased volume of blood entering the fetal circulation during contractions, thus triggering the baroceptor reflex activity. Both of these mechanisms are vagally mediated and can be prevented by atropine.*[4]

Variable Decelerations

This is the most common of all fetal heart rate patterns (Fig. 10-5), and the characteristics of this pattern are a follows:

1. Variability in duration
2. Variability in shape and size
3. Variability in time

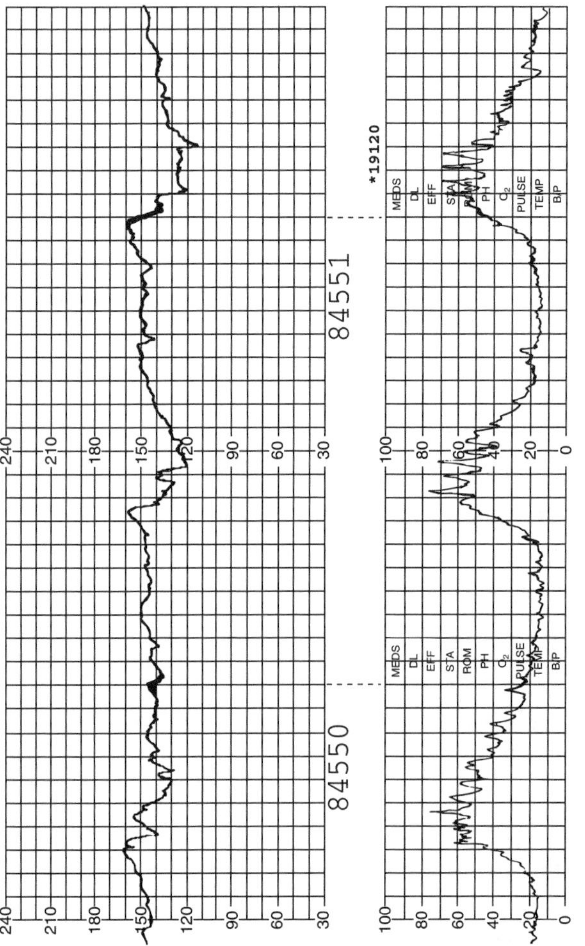

Figure 10–3. Early decelerations.

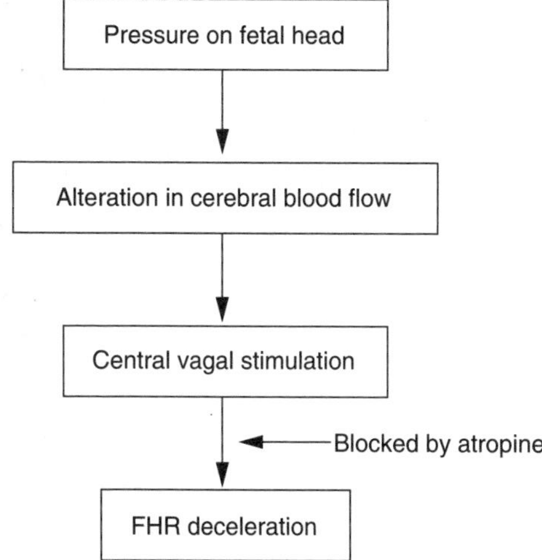

Figure 10–4. Mechanism of early decelerations (FHR = fetal heart rate). (Adapted from Freeman RK, Garite TS: *Fetal Heart Rate Monitoring.* Baltimore, Williams & Wilkins, 1981.)

This is probably caused by compression of the umbilical cord against the fetal body parts, e.g., head, neck, or shoulder. Because the maximum pressure on the cord is generated at the time of uterine contractions, the pattern coincides with uterine contraction. These decelerations are usually very abrupt in relation to both the onset and the return to baseline levels. Depending upon the magnitude of the decrease in the fetal heart rate, the variable decelerations have been further subdivided into (1) mild (duration less than 30 seconds and deceleration not below 80 BPM), (2) moderate (regardless of the duration, the fetal heart rate is less than 80 BPM), and (3) severe (duration greater than 60 seconds and a fetal heart rate less than 70 BPM). Occasionally, variable decelerations can change to late decelerations or severe fetal bradycardia.

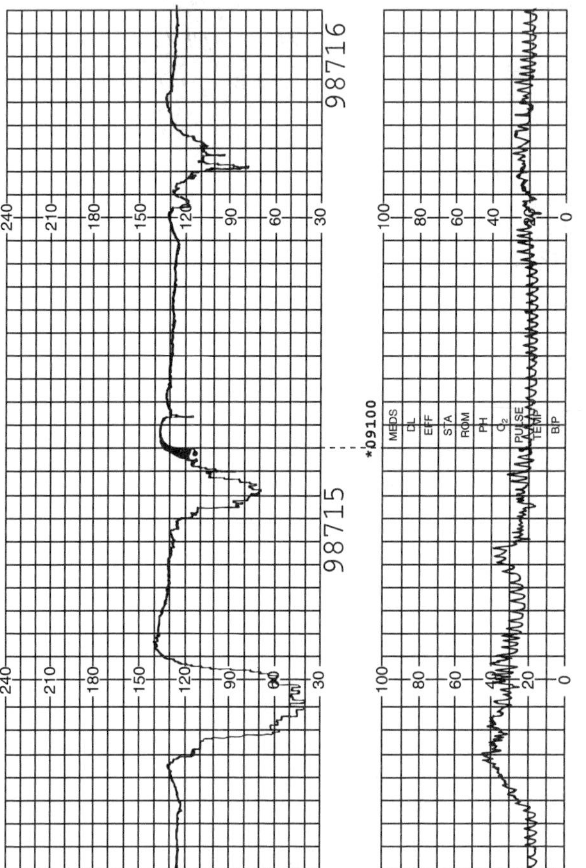

Figure 10–5. Variable decelerations.

Late Decelerations

Definitely a sign of uteroplacental insufficiency, late decelerations (Fig. 10-6) are characterized by the following:

1. The onset of deceleration usually starts 30 seconds or more after the onset of uterine contraction.
2. The peak of the deceleration arrives long after uterine contraction.
3. The onset and return are gradual and smooth.
4. The drop in fetal heart rate usually varies between 10 and 20 BPM and rarely falls lower than 30 to 40 BPM.
5. Although not always, there is a correlation between the magnitude of decelerations and the degree of fetal hypoxia. *The major cause of late decelerations is reduced placental perfusion, as can be seen during supine hypotensive syndrome because of aortocaval compression, severe hypotension following regional anesthesia, abruptio placentae, postmaturity, diabetes mellitus; pre-eclampsia/eclampsia, etc.*

Besides these three main patterns, the other patterns that have been described are prolonged decelerations and a sinusoidal pattern.

Prolonged decelerations may be associated with a loss of variability and a baseline fetal heart rate below 70 BPM; once the duration exceeds 2 to 3 minutes, urgent intervention is usually necessary.

A *sinusoidal pattern* is associated with a sine wave pattern above and below the baseline with a cyclicity of about 4 to 8 minutes. Actually, there is an increased long-term variability. *One of the major causes of this pattern is the severe fetal anemia usually associated with Rh incompatibly. A benign sinusoidal pattern has been associated with narcotics like alphaprodine (Nisentil) or butorphanol (Stadol).*

Besides fetal heart rate monitoring, fetal scalp pH sampling is also very important in making an ultimate judgement of fetal well-being.[5,6] *Normal fetal scalp pH varies between 7.25 and 7.32; mild acidosis is documented when the pH varies between 7.20 and 7.24; and severe acidosis is noted when the pH becomes lower than 7.20.* A good correlation has been observed between severity of the fetal heart rate pattern and fetal

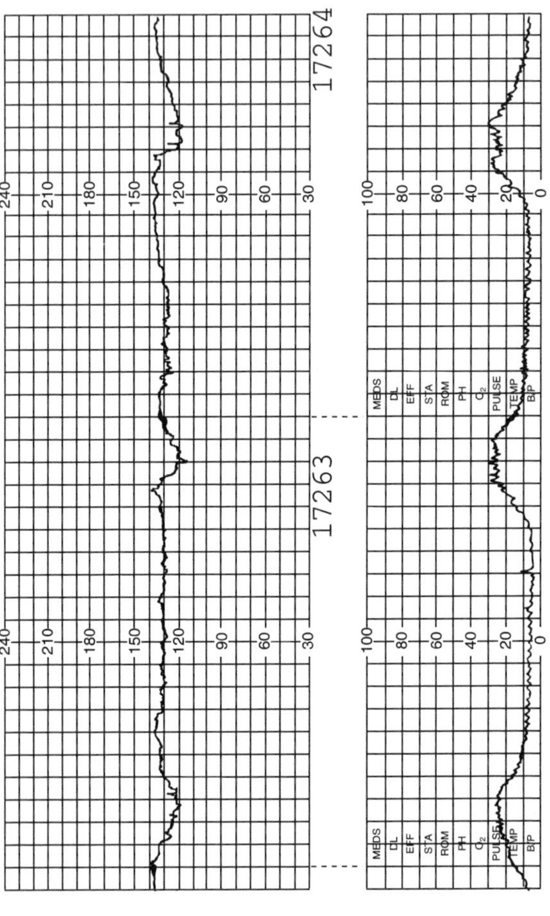

Figure 10–6. Late decelerations. (Adapted from Martin R: Prepartum and intrapartum fetal monitoring, in Datta S (ed): *Anesthetic and Obstetric Management of High Risk Pregnancy*. Chicago, Mosby–Year Book, 1991.)

acidosis as observed by fetal scalp pH. At the present, most obstetricians are in favor of confirming fetal compromise as shown in fetal heart rate monitoring by routine sampling of fetal scalp pH.

Biophysical Profile

Peripartum evaluation of the high-risk fetus is done by evaluation of immediate biophysical activities: (1) fetal movement, (2) fetal tone, (3) fetal breathing movements, (4) heart rate activity, and (5) volume of amniotic fluid.[7] The first four parameters reflect the presence of normal fetal central nervous system activity, whereas amniotic fluid volume is an indicator of long-term or chronic fetal compromise. These parameters are all measured by ultrasound except for the fetal heart rate. The variables are scored 2 if normal and 0 if abnormal. Fetal heart rate activity is measured by nonstress testing and the oxytocin challenge test.

Nonstress Test

This involves the detection of changes in the fetal heart rate and fetal movement in association with uterine contraction.

Usually this test is described as reactive if there are two fetal movements in 20 minutes with accelerations of the fetal heart rate of at least 15 BPM. The test is described as nonreactive in the absence of fetal movement and accelerations of the fetal heart rate.

Contraction Stress Test or Oxytocin Challenge Test

In the presence of a nonreactive nonstress test, the oxytocin challenge test becomes an important issue. Intravenous oxytocin is used, beginning at a rate of 0.5–1.0 units/min, to induce three adequate uterine contractions within a 10-minute period. The oxytocin challenge test is considered to be positive if persistent late decelerations exist, whereas the test is interpreted as negative in the presence of normal fetal heart rate tracings. *The oxytocin challenge test is contraindicated if there is history of classical cesarean section or placenta previa and if the parturient is at risk of premature labor.*

A poor biophysical score (5 or less out of 10) indicates that close supervision of the fetus is necessary.

Assessment of Fetal Maturity

Phospholipids, the major components of lung surfactant, are produced by fetal alveolar cells in a sufficient amount by 36 weeks' gestation. The *lecithin/sphingomyelin ratio (L/S) is commonly used to predict fetal lung maturity and is said to be normal when the ratio is 2 in normal pregnancies. For diabetic parturients, the ratio should be at least 3.5 or higher.* Measurements of saturated phosphotidylcholine are occasionally used in normal parturients; the normal value is 500 mg/dL, whereas in diabetics it is 1,000 mg/dL.

Recently, the TD_x fetal lung maturity (FLM) test has become popular.[8] It is expressed in milligrams of surfactant per gram of albumin (the cutoff value is 50 mg/g).

A FLM value of <50 mg/g indicates immature lung, between 50 and 70 mg/g is borderline, and >70 mg/g predicts adequate lung maturity. In the author's institution, FLM is not used in diabetic parturients.

In summary, an adequate knowledge of the detection of normal uterine activity and fetal well-being is necessary so that anesthetic techniques do not interfere with uterine activity, the fetoplacental unit, or above all, the fetus.

References

1. Caldeyro-Barcia R, Posserio JJ: Physiology of uterine contractions. *Clin Obstet Gynecol* 1960; 3:386.
2. Reynold SRM, et al: Recording uterine contraction patterns in pregnant women: Applications of strain gauge in multi-channel tocodynamometer. *Science* 1947; 106:427.
3. Williams EA, Stallworthy JA: A simple method of internal tocography. *Lancet* 1952; 1:330.
4. Freeman RK, Gartie TJ (eds): *Fetal Heart Rate Monitoring.* Baltimore, Williams & Wilkins, 1981, pp 63–83.

5. James LS: Acid-base status of human infants in relation to birth asphyxia and the onset of respiration. *J Pediatr* 1958; 52:379.
6. Saline E, Schneider D: Biochemical supervision of the foetus during labour. *J Obstet Gynaecol Br Commonw* 1967; 74:799.
7. Manning FA, et al: Fetal biophysical profile scoring: A prospective study in 1184 high-risk patients. *Am J Obstet Gynecol* 1981; 140:289.
8. Russell JC, et al: Multicenter evaluation of TD_x test for assessing fetal lung maturity. *Clin Chem* 1989; 35:1005.

11 Relief of Labor Pain by Regional Analgesia/Anesthesia

Epidural Analgesia
- Anatomy of the Epidural Space
- Contents of the Epidural Space
- Site of Action
- Test Dose
- Techniques
  - *Segmental block*
  - *Complete block*

Possible Problems
- Asymmetrical Sensory Block
- Diminishing Analgesia
- Dense Motor Block
- Patchy Block
- Miscellaneous

Local Anesthetic Alone vs. Local Anesthetic and Narcotic Infusion

Contraindications

Monitoring Following the Administration of Epidural Analgesia

Effects of Epidural Analgesia
- Progress of Labor
  - *Effect of the addition of epinephrine to the local anesthetic*
- Uteroplacental Perfusion
- Fetal Effects

Complications of Epidural Analgesia and Anesthesia

Parasthesia

Accidental Dural Puncture

Subdural Injection

Massive Epidural Analgesia

Accidental Intravascular Injection

Cardiovascular Toxicity of Local Anesthetic

Backache

Methemoglobinemia

Broken Epidural Catheter

Neurological Complications

Obstetric causes

Anesthesia-related causes

Treatment of Headache Following Accidental Dural Puncture

Contraindications to Blood Patches

Spinal Anesthesia

Combined Spinal/Epidural (CSE)

Caudal Anesthesia

Paracervical Block

Lumbar Sympathetic Block

Pudendal Block

It is well accepted, at the present time, that regional analgesia and anesthesia (i.e., epidural, caudal, or spinal), if properly administered and maintained and if there is no maternal hypotension, will not affect the uterine blood flow. Joupilla, Hollman, and colleagues have extensively studied, with xenon 112, the effect of regional anesthesia for labor or cesarean section on uteroplacental perfusion.[1,2] Healthy parturients in labor showed a 35% increase in intervillous blood flow following the administration of either 10 mL of 0.25% bupivacaine or 2% chloroprocaine (Fig. 11-1).[1] In parturients with pre-eclampsia,the epidural injection of 10 mL of 0.25% bupivacaine resulted in a much more significant improvement in intervillous blood flow.[2] The increase amounted to 77%.

These findings most probably related to an increased amount of circulating endogenous catecholamines due to the stress of labor pain, which will decrease placental blood flow.[3] Epidural analgesia will decrease catecholamine concentrations and thus indirectly can increase placental blood flow. Preliminary investigations in animals with epidural opiates

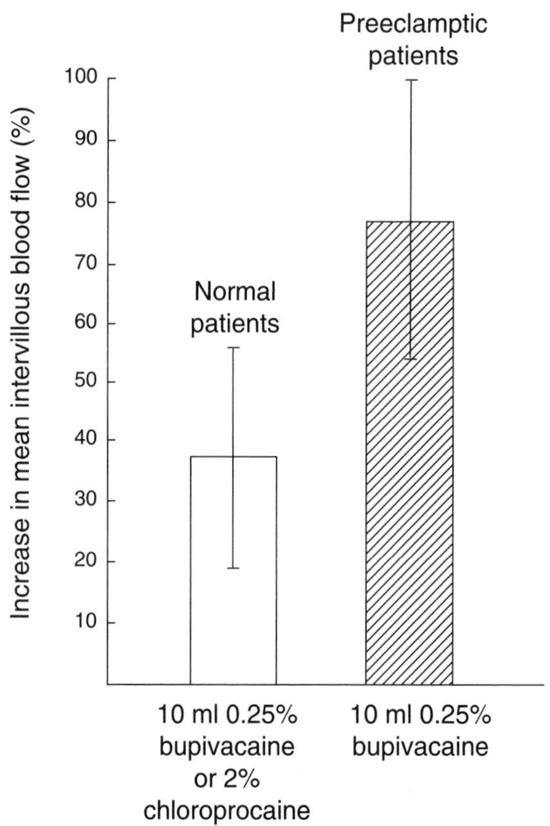

Figure 11-1. Percent increase in mean intervillous blood flow values (±SE) after epidural anesthesia for labor in normal parturients. (Adapted from Hollmen A, Jouppila R, Jouppila P, et al: *Br J Anaesth* 1982; 54:837.)

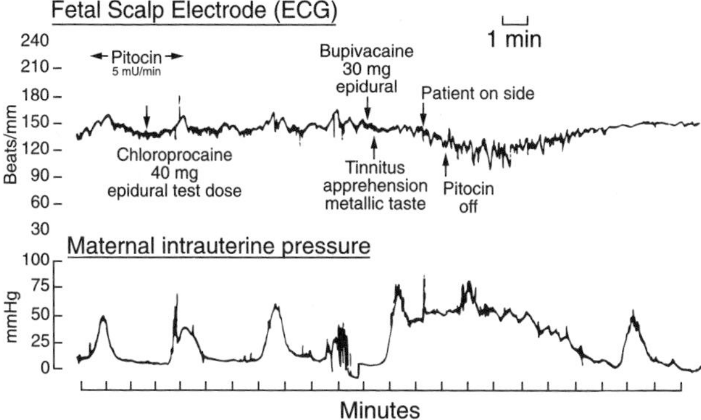

Figure 11-2. Tetanic uterine contraction occurring after inadvertent intravenous injection of bupivacaine. (Adapted from Greiss FC, Still JG, Anderson SG: *Am J Obstet Gynecol* 1976; 124:889.)

showed no significant changes in uterine blood flow, and no changes in any maternal or fetal cardiovascular or acid-base variable. Regional analgesia may affect uterine activity and the course of labor either directly or indirectly. *In the concentrations generally achieved in the clinical situation, there seems to be no direct effect of local anesthetics on uterine contractility. However, the high concentrations that might be achieved with an accidental intravascular injection or paracervical injection or paracervical block may increase uterine tone as well as decrease uterine blood flow* (Fig. 11-2).[4]

Table 11-4 summarizes the techniques used for the relief of labor pain.

Epidural Analgesia

This is a very useful procedure for both the first and second stages of labor. It offers greater versatility of effect when compared with any other anesthetic methods for labor and delivery. Before discussing the various techniques, it is necessary to address the different steps that are involved in initiating epidural anesthesia.

Table 11-4. Techniques Used for Relief of Labor Pain

First Stage	Second Stage
(1) Epidural analgesia	(1) Epidural analgesia
(2) Continuous spinal analgesia and anesthesia	(2) Spinal anesthesia
(3) Combined spinal epidural technique (CSE)	(3) Combined spinal epidural technique (CSE)
(4) Caudal analgesia	(4) Caudal analgesia
(5) Paracervical block	(5) Pudendal nerve block
(6) Bilateral sympathetic block	

Anatomy of the Epidural Space

Recent cryomicrotome studies have advanced the knowledge of epidural spaces for the anesthesiologist. The epidural space is a potential space. Contents of the epidural space as described by Hogan are contained in a series of metamerically and circumferentially discontinuous compartments separated by zones where the dura contacts the canal wall. *As dura for the most part does not adhere to the canal,* the catheters and solution pass through the empty areas without restriction. Dura tapers off inferior to the L4–L5 disc in the sacral canal, and the space is usually filled by the epidural fat.[4a] One of the interesting findings of cryomicrotome study is the presence of fat pad in the triangular space between the ligamenta flava and dura. Hogan observed no midline fibrous septum. However, the presence of midline fatty tissue can cause patchy or unilateral block. When unilateral block occurs, it is usually on the right side.[4b] The distance from the skin to the epidural space has been observed using ultrasound and magnetic resonance examination. The depth varies considerably from 3–9 cm; the average depth is 4.5–5.5 cm.

The epidural space is a potential space, triangular in shape, with the apex facing posteriorly (Fig. 11-3) that lies between the dura mater and the ligamentum flavum. The epidural space extends from the base of the skull to the sacral hiatus *and is bounded* in the following manner:

1. Superiorly by the dura adherent to the skull at the foramen magnum. *The clinical implication of this is related to the absence of total spinal anesthesia via the epidural route.*
2. Inferiorly by the sacrococcygeal ligament at the level the S2–3 interspace.
3. Anteriorly by the posterior longitudinal ligament.
4. Posteriorly by the ligamentum flavum.
5. Laterally by the dural cuffs, pedicles, and lamina.

Contents of the Epidural Space

I. Anterior and posterior nerve roots with their coverings.
II. Blood vessels that supply the spinal cord.
   A. The posterior spinal artery, which originates from the inferior cerebellar artery and supplies the posterior columns and posterior horns.
   B. The anterior spinal artery, which originates from the two vertebral arteries at the foramen magnum and supplies the anterior portion of the spinal cord.
   C. The *artery of Adamkiewicz, which is the major feeder of the anterior spinal artery and arises from one intercostal or lumbar artery in the T8–L3 region. It supplies the lower two thirds of the spinal cord.*
   D. The vertebral veins, which drain blood from the vertebral column and the nervous tissue and ultimately form the vertebral venous plexus. They run via the anterolateral part of the epidural space and ultimately

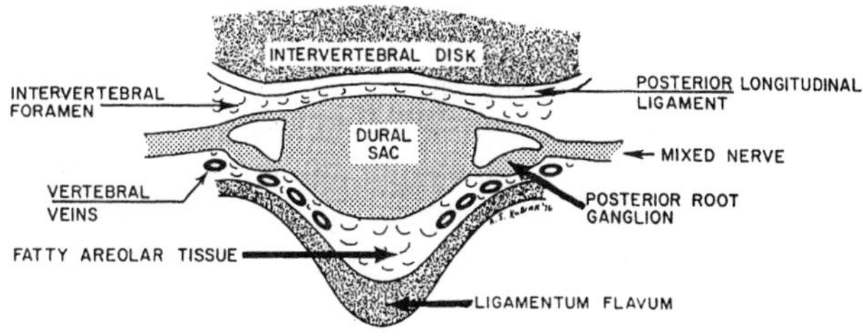

Figure 11–3. Contents of the epidural space. (From Abouleish E: *Pain Control in Obstetrics.* Philadelphia, JB Lippincott, 1977, p 261. Used by permission.)

drain into the azygos vein. This venous connection is associated with important clinical implications: *during pregnancy due to obstruction of the inferior vena cava, epidural and azygos vein blood flow is markedly increased. A small dose of local anesthetic injected accidentally into the epidural vein, especially during labor, can reach the heart in a higher concentration*[5] *and thus increase the chances of myocardial depression.*

III. *Fatty areolar tissue.*

Fatty tissue is deposited between the nervous and vascular structures.

At the Brigham and Women's Hospital, every effort is made to consult the parturient before induction of epidural anesthesia and informed consent is signed by the patient. The majority of anesthesiologists prefer to perform the technique by placing the woman on her side, except for obese women, for whom a sitting position is preferred.

Site of Action

The *site of action* of the local anesthetic during epidural analgesia is not exactly known; however, several sites have been suggested: (1) *spinal roots, the most important site;* (2) mixed spinal nerve; (3) dorsal root ganglion; and (4) the *spinal cord, which might be the ultimate site of action and plays an important role in regression of the block. Observation of the fetal heart rate is of paramount importance before the introduction of epidural anesthesia.* Five hundred to 1000ml of Ringer's lactate solution is used for acute volume replacement unless contraindicated, and 30 mL of Bicitra is given routinely before the induction of epidural analgesia. At Brigham and Women's Hospital, the Weiss modification of the Tuohy needle is routinely used. The majority of anesthesiologists in the author's institution use the technique of loss of resistance by air; however, a few prefer the "hanging-drop" technique. The technique of loss of resistance with saline and the Tuohy needle is used routinely in many institutions in this country. The L2–3 or L3–4 interspace is usually used *(a line drawn from the top of the iliac crest coincides with either the L4–5 inter-*

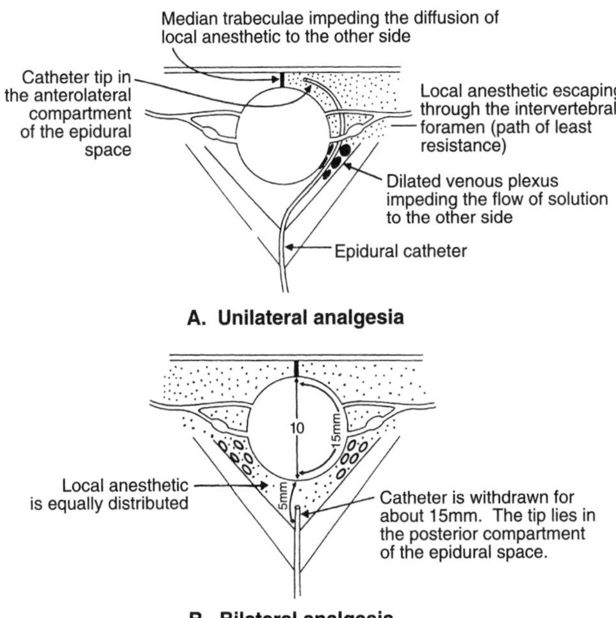

Figure 11–4. Placement of the epidural catheter and explanation of a unilateral block. (Adapted from Abouleish E: *Pain Control in Obstetrics.* Philadelphia, JB Lippincott, 1977, p 282.)

space or the L4 spinous process) for introduction of the epidural needle. Once the space is identified by using either the loss-of-resistance or the hanging-drop technique, 3 to 5 cm of the epidural catheter is inserted into the space. *Personally, I do not insert more than 3 cm of the catheter unless the patient is obese. This technique will reduce the incidence of a unilateral block* (Fig. 11-4).

Test Dose

An ideal test dose should be able to detect both accidental intravascular and subarachnoid injections of local anes-

thetics. Moore and Batra originally suggested that the use of 15 µg of epinephrine (1 : 200,000) with local anesthetic will detect accidental intravascular injections in nonpregnant patients by showing tachycardia.[6] The heart rates of the 175 patients increased from a mean of 79 ± 14 to 111 ± 15 beats per minute. The heart rate increased within 23 ± 6 seconds following the injection and returned to baseline within 32 ± 33 seconds. However, Moore and Batra used this test dose only in nonpregnant cases who were undergoing elective surgery and were under the influence of heavy premedication. When *using 3 mL of 0.5% plain bupivacaine via the epidural route in 100 parturients in active labor, Cartwright and colleagues[7] observed heart rate increases of more than 20 beats per minute in 24 women and more than 30 beats per minute in 12 women in the following 60 seconds even though the catheters were not intravascular.* Leighton and colleagues, using 15 µg of epinephrine intravenously in term parturients, observed heart rate increases of greater than 25 beats per minute that lasted longer than 15 seconds in only 50% of cases.[8] From these studies it became obvious that, in pregnant women, 15 µg of epinephrine might not be sensitive or specific enough to rule out accidental intravascular injection. On the other hand, Abraham and colleagues, in search of an ideal test dose for both accidental intravascular and subarachnoid injections, used 3 mL of 1.5% hyperbaric lidocaine mixed with epinephrine (1 : 200,000) via an epidural catheter[9] (Fig. 11-5). The maternal heart rate increased from 76 ± 2 to 109 ± 6 if the solution was injected intravenously, and the sensory anesthesia reached the S2 level in 1.45 ± 0.12 minutes if the solution was accidentally injected in the subarachnoid space. Hence, the use of epinephrine, 15 µg, for the diagnosis of accidental intravascular injections remains controversial. If epinephrine is used in the laboring women as a test dose, one must observe first the maternal heart rate at base-to-peak uterine contraction. Then one can interpret the effect of intravenous epinephrine. Recently Leighton and colleagues examined air as a useful clinical indicator of intravenous placement of the epidural catheter. Using 1 mL of air through the epidural catheter and monitoring heart tones with a Doppler ultrasound probe, these authors observed only a 2%

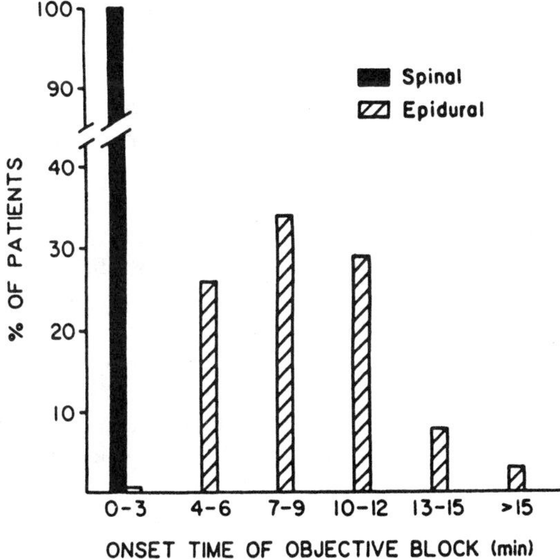

Figure 11-5. Time to onset of objective sensory loss (to pin prick) following epidural and spinal administration of a hyperbaric 1.5% lidocaine solution. (From Abraham RA, Harris AP, Maxwell LG: *Anesthesiology* 1986; 64:116. Used by permission.)

false-positive rate.[10] None of the 303 parturients in their study developed any complications due to the injection of 1 mL of air; the authors concluded that air, with precordial Doppler detection, is a safe and effective test for identifying intravenously located epidural catheters. We have to wait for the reaction of the anesthesiology community on the use of air as an indicator of intravascular injections. In the meantime, while looking for an ideal test dose, one has to be extra careful in preventing and diagnosing an incorrect placement of the epidural catheter:

1. For elective cases, unless contraindicated, one can use an epinephrine (15 μg)-containing solution as a test dose. *A continuous electrocardiograph (ECG) monitor is essential to detect tachycardia. In this respect, one must remember that*

parturients who are being treated with β-blocking drugs may not show tachycardia even when the epinephrine is intravascular.[11]

2. *Negative aspiration findings may not exclude intravascular catheter placement because the catheter may be against vein wall and because aspiration can collapse the vein lumen.* Aspiration immediately following the injection of local anesthetic may be more effective in recognizing intravascular catheter placement because the local anesthetic will push the vein wall away and may also dilate the blood vessels; placing the catheter 45 to 50 degrees below the patient's body level at this stage can help the blood to flow through the catheter if it is intravascular. Local anesthetics should be injected only 3 to 5 mL at a time, and the signs and symptoms of intravascular injection should be closely monitored.

Techniques

Pain relief with the epidural technique can be obtained in two ways: the *segmental block technique* with intermittent injections and the *complete block technique* with intermittent injections or continuous infusion.

Segmental Block

A *segmental block* may be used in the first stage to limit the extent of sensory analgesia to the T10–L1 segments. As labor progresses to the second stage, analgesia can be extended to block the sacral innervation. A full top-up dose is given for this purpose while the woman is in the sitting position for about 5 minutes. A higher concentration of local anesthetic may be used at this stage to achieve motor block and perineal relaxation if a forceps delivery is planned or if cesarean section becomes necessary. However, one of the main disadvantages of this technique is that *perineal pain relief* (S2–S5) *cannot always* be *guaranteed.* For delivery, local infiltration, a pudendal block, or a low subarachnoid block may be needed.

Complete Block

A *complete block* (T10–S5) can provide sensory analgesia from T10 to S5 from the very first dose, but the incidence of hypotension is higher than when a segmental block is used. Good nursing care is mandatory to help the parturient coordinate her "pushing" with every contraction at the second stage. The incidence of forceps delivery may be higher. Routine monitoring of maternal vital signs, the fetal heart rate, and uterine contractions are essential during epidural analgesia. Drugs commonly used are bupivacaine, 0.0625%, 0.125% to 0.25%. The complete-block technique can be achieved by using either the *intermittent technique* or continuous infusion. The intermittent technique needs reinforcement every 1½ to 2 hours or if the patient is uncomfortable. A sensory level of analgesia is maintained from T10 to S5.

Continuous infusion for epidural analgesia in obstetrics was first described in 1963.[12] However, the technique did not become popular, mainly because of the lack of availability of proper instruments as well as local anesthetics. With the advent of better mechanical infusion pumps as well as better local anesthetics, continuous infusion has indeed become the technique of choice for vaginal delivery. Different authors have compared the intermittent injection technique with continuous epidural infusion (CEI), and the recognized advantages of CEI are as follows[13]:

1. A more stable depth of analgesia, which obviously becomes an important part of pregnant woman satisfaction
2. The possibility of lower blood concentrations of local anesthetic
3. A reduced risk of total spinal block in the presence of an inadvertent injection of local anesthetic in the subarachnoid space
4. Lower blood concentrations of local anesthetic if the catheter is accidentally placed in the vein
5. A lower incidence of hypotension due to the possibility of decreased sympathetic blockade

A loading dose of the local anesthetic is given before the start of the infusion in order to establish an adequate sensory block as well as to confirm correct placement of the epidural catheter. Bupivacaine 0.125% to 0.25% (8 to 10 mL/hr), has been the most popular agent for this purpose; however, other drugs like 1% 2-chloroprocaine and 1% lidocaine have also been used. *One must remember that even with continuous infusion one should frequently check the block to verify uniformity and rule out subarachnoid or intravascular migration of the catheter.* While this method provides adequate analgesia for the first stage of labor, there might be a possibility of *inadequate perineal anesthesia* with the use of the continuous-infusion technique. One might face this problem less frequently if the mother is gradually eased from the horizontal into the reclining position with the progress of labor. A combination of lower concentrations of local anesthetics and narcotics has popularized this technique even further. Different authors have investigated the efficacy of low concentrations of local anesthetics combined with narcotics and have claimed moderate to good success.[14–16] The most popular cocktail at present is the combination of 0.0625% or 0.125% bupivacaine and 2 µg of fentanyl per milliliter infused at the rate of 8 to 10 mL/hr. Alfentanil (5 µg/mL) has been tried in our institution in combination with bupivacaine (0.125% at 8 to 10 mL/hr) with excellent success. However, placental transfer of alfentanil is significant and hence never became popular.

The following materials are needed:

1. An epidural tray (with catheter)
2. Bupivacaine, 0.25% to 0.5%; sterile saline solution; a 50- to 100-mL sterile plastic bag; and a volumetric infusion pump
3. Fentanyl, 1 to 2 ampules (100 to 200 µg)

Once a stable epidural block of at least T10–L1 has been established with 0.125% to 0.25% bupivacaine, continuous infusion can be initiated.

A 50- to 100-mL sterile plastic bag is filled with a 0.0625%, 0.125% to 0.25% solution of bupivacaine and attached to the high-pressure infusion tubing (Luerlock). The tubing, which must be flushed to remove any air, is connected directly to the epidural catheter. All connections must be secured, and the plastic bag must be labeled. The volumetric infusion pump is adjusted to deliver the desired dosage per hour (8 to 10 mL). Ropivacaine 0.1% mixed with fentanyl 2 mcg/ml or levobupivacaine 0.125% mixed with the same amount of fentanyl can also be used.

Parturients should be positioned head-up with left uterine displacement. Patient controlled epidural analgesia has become popular at the present time. Use of background infusion has also been used. This technique has got definite advantage in busy unit as physician's intervention is less compared to continuous infusion technique.

The block must be checked at least hourly to ensure uniformity, rule out subarachnoid or intravascular migration of the catheter, assess the adequacy of analgesia, monitor any changes in fetal well-being, and check the amount of local anesthetic in the reservoir bag. *Notations about the block and vital signs should be made every 1 to 2 hours on the hospital record.*

Possible Problems

Asymmetrical Sensory Block

If a parturient lies continuously on one side, the level of sensory block may become asymmetrical. The situation should be corrected by repositioning the patient, disconnecting the pump, and administering 4 to 6 mL of 0.25% or 8–12 mL of 0.125% bupivacaine mixed with fentanyl 2 mcg/ml solution, (bolus dose) after appropriate aspiration, and then the infusion should be restarted. The patient should be encouraged to turn from side to side to maintain uterine displacement.

Multipore catheter recently has become popular. Inserting 3 cm of catheter in all cases, *one study observed a significantly lower incidence of unilateral block with multiorifice* catheter compared to single-orifice catheter.[17] One recent study found that 5 cm of the multiorifice catheter is optimal for adequate sensory analgesia for labor and delivery.

Diminishing Analgesia

Progressive diminution of the sensory block and loss of the block may be due to a number of factors:

1. The pump on/off switch may be off.
2. The tubing may be disconnected.

3. The reservoir bag may be empty and has been for a while.
4. The catheter may no longer be in the epidural space, and intravascular migration must be ruled out.

The differential diagnosis should consist of rechecking the infusion pump setup and testing to determine the correct position of the catheter. The pump must be disconnected to test for appropriate catheter placement. After aspiration, a 3-mL test dose of 1.5% to 2% lidocaine or 0.25% bupivacaine with 1 : 200,000 epinephrine is injected. The patient is observed for signs of intravascular placement of the catheter, and if there is negative response, an attempt is made to re-establish the block with 3- to 5-mL incremental doses of 0.25% bupivacaine. If the block cannot be re-established or if aspiration and testing indicate intravascular migration of the tip, then the catheter must be removed. Depending on the clinical setting, either a new catheter may be inserted via a second placement, or alternative analgesia may be initiated. *At the above infusion rates, bupivacaine probably will not produce symptoms of intravascular injection.* The only clue may be diminishing or absent analgesia.

Dense Motor Block

Patients given a continuous infusion of 0.0625% to 0.125% bupivacaine usually exhibit mild to moderate motor blockade of the lower extremities. If a progressively dense motor blockade resembling a subarachnoid block ensues, the catheter must be disconnected immediately and careful aspiration performed to rule out subarachnoid migration.

A suspicion of subarachnoid migration after testing mandates withdrawal of the catheter and reinsertion at another site if indicated.

Patchy Block

If a spotty or patchy block occurs, one should attempt to solidify the block by disconnecting the pump, aspirating to determine catheter placement, and injecting 4 to 6 mL of 0.125% to 0.25% bupivacaine. Then the pump is reconnected.

Miscellaneous

If a woman requires an acute change in the character of the block for operative delivery, simply increasing the infusion rate will be inadequate. The parturient must be disconnected from the pump, the catheter placement must be checked, and the woman should then be "topped up" with 0.5% bupivacaine, 2% lidocaine with or without epinephrine, or 3% 2-chloroprocaine to obtain the desired level of sensory anesthesia (to at least a bilateral T4 level).

Often a continuous infusion of bupivacaine does not provide adequate perineal analgesia. At the time of delivery the woman may require an additional increment of 0.25% to 0.5% bupivacaine, 1.5% to 2% lidocaine, or 2% to 3% 2-chloroprocaine to provide sufficient analgesia or anesthesia for forceps delivery or episiotomy. Placing the parturient in the semi-Fowler's position for "pushing" also helps achieve a more complete perineal block.

Local Anesthetic Alone vs. Local Anesthetic and Narcotic Infusion

A "loading dose" of local anesthetic to establish the epidural block by using 0.125% to 0.25% bupivacaine plus a continuous infusion of 0.0625% or 0.125% bupivacaine with fentanyl 2 mcg/ml (8–10 ml/hr) has become an extremely popular technique because of its excellent pain relief during labor with minimal motor blockade. At the time of delivery one must make sure of the presence of adequate perineal analgesia. Bupivacaine 0.0625%, plus narcotic has also been tried with varying success; obviously the lower concentration will be associated with minimal motor blockade, which might benefit the parturients if the sensory analgesia is adequate. Local anesthetic ropivacaine has also been used with success.[17a]

Recently, patient-controlled epidural analgesia (PCEA) has been used for labor and delivery. In the author's institution, a recent study comparing PCEA and CEI observed a significant dosesparing effect associated with PCEA as compared with standard CEI for analgesia during labor and delivery. Background infusion with PCEA has been found to be superior. However, PCEA needs a more sophisticated apparatus.

Contraindications

Besides the usual contraindications for regional anesthesia (e.g., local infection, coagulation problems), continuous infusion should be used carefully in a patient with an accidental dural puncture.

Continuous infusion of a small concentration of local anesthetic mixed with a small amount of a narcotic analgesic has become the standard technique for pain relief in parturients in labor. Although fentanyl is the most commonly used narcotic at the present time, other narcotics are presently being tried. However, there are two important points one should remember when performing this technique: (1) maternal vital signs and the quality of the fetal heart rate must be noted on the anesthetic chart at least every 1½ to 2 hours, and (2) perineal analgesia or anesthesia should be confirmed before delivery, especially if there is a possibility of forceps delivery.

Monitoring Following the Administration of Epidural Analgesia

The blood pressure and pulse rate are routinely noted by the nursing staff before and immediately after the induction of anesthesia. Blood pressure is measured every minute for the first 5 minutes and every 3 to 5 minutes thereafter up to 30 minutes. *If the blood pressure remains stable after 30 minutes,* the nursing staff monitors the blood pressure routinely every 15 minutes throughout labor and delivery. Routine pulse rate measurements are made during the time of blood pressure readings. The use of automatic blood pressure measurement instruments is becoming popular in the obstetric unit. Continuous oxygen saturation measurement may also be an important tool. In many institutions, ECG monitors are used routinely. In most high-risk pregnant women (e.g., diabetic, pre-eclamptic) or if there is any sign of fetal stress, a plastic oxygen mask should be used with high-flow oxygen. Continuous fetal heart rate monitoring becomes absolutely essential after the administration of epidural analgesia. If the parturient complains of ringing, circumoral numbness, a metallic taste, dizziness, high sensory anesthesia, or excessive motor blockade, the nursing staff should immediately inform the anesthesiology team for possible migration of the epidural catheter in either the vascular or subarachnoid space.

Effects of Epidural Anesthesia

Progress of Labor

There exists considerable controversy over the effect of regional anesthesia on the duration of labor and the method of delivery.

The majority of reports show that there is a transient decrease in uterine activity for 10 to 15 minutes following epidural placement.[17] Uterine activity usually returns to normal within 30 minutes. The *intensity of uterine contractions is more affected than the frequency.* Possible suggested mechanisms include (1) associated hypotension, (2) vascular uptake of local anesthetics, (3) vascular uptake of epinephrine if it is used with local anesthetics, and (4) inhibition of the secretion of Pitocin from the posterior pituitary gland and thus a decrease in the intensity of uterine contractions because of acute volume expansion.[18] In most of the studies, it has been shown that the decrease in uterine activity following induction of epidural analgesia is transient and that subsequent injections cause a progressively smaller decrease in activity. Although there is controversy regarding the effects of epidural analgesia on the duration of the first stage of labor, Studies indicate no significant effect on the duration of the first stage of labor.[19,20] However, the second stage has been shown to be prolonged with epidural analgesia in most studies.[20–22] This effect is attributed to laxity of the pelvic musculature and loss of the "bearing-down" reflex. This has been counteracted to a large extent by effective coaching from the labor attendants. Interestingly, there has been shown to be a tendency toward better fetal condition when the second stage was prolonged in the presence of epidural analgesia.[23] This has obviously redefined the concept of a prolonged second stage. At the present time, for a primigravida it is supposed to be greater than 2 hours without epidural analgesia and greater than 3 hours in the presence of epidural analgesia; for a multipara it is greater than 1 hour without epidural analgesia and greater than 2 hours in the presence of epidural analgesia. The incidence of instrumental delivery has been shown to be increased in association with epidural analgesia. Several techniques can be utilized to improve the chances of a spontaneous delivery:

1. Segmental analgesia with low concentrations of local anesthetic. This preserves the reflex urge to push and minimizes laxity of the pelvic musculature. However, one must realize that there is better pain relief with high concentrations of local anesthetic.
2. Low concentrations of local anesthetic mixed with narcotics. In this manner, analgesia can be optimized, the duration of analgesia prolonged, and at the same time the total local anesthetic dose reduced. This technique is also associated with less motor blockade.[15,16]

Although the technique of allowing the epidural analgesia to "wear off" for more effective pushing is advocated by many, this practice is questionable at best. Phillips and Thomas reported a 25% rate of forceps use when the epidural was reinforced as needed and a 43% rate when the epidural analgesia was allowed to wear off.[24] *They concluded that the rate of forceps use was increased because of ineffective pushing in the presence of perineal pain.* Chestnut and colleagues recently performed a randomized double-blind study.[25] Parturients received an infusion of 0.0625% bupivacaine with 0.0002% fentanyl via an epidural catheter during labor. When fully dilated, patients received either bupivacaine with fentanyl or normal saline until delivery. Although the duration of the second stage was prolonged in the presence of bupivacaine and fentanyl, there were no significant differences in the rates of instrumental deliveries between the groups. Recently Thorp et al observed a high incidence of cesarean section when epidural analgesia was provided with cervical dilation of less than 5 cm.[25a] On the other hand, Chestnut et al observed two groups of patients: (1) early epidural group where patients received epidural analgesia before 5 cm of cervical dilation

(3 to 4 cm), and (2) late epidural group where parturients received epidural analgesia after cervical dilation of 5 cm. There was no increase in the incidence of instrumental delivery, cesarean section, or prolongation of second stage in the early group compared to the late group.[25b] Hence there is no consistency in results regarding the epidural analgesia and cesarean section. However, three factors may be important in this regard: (1) concentration of local anesthetic, (2) obstetric practice, and (3) use of oxytocin.

A more recent well-conducted randomized study showed no differences in the cesarean section rate whether or not the mothers received epidural analgesia. A group from Dallas conducted a randomized trial of epidural analgesia versus patient-controlled intravenous meperidine. Using an intent-to-treat basis, there was no difference in the rate of cesarean section.[25c] Another group compared bupivacaine and fentanyl epidural versus intravenous patient-controlled analgesia with butorphanol. They also observed no difference in cesarean delivery rate between the groups.[25d] Finally, a meta-analysis including 2400 cases observed no difference in the risk of cesarean section between epidural or opioid analgesia groups.[25e]

Effect of the Addition of Epinephrine to the Local Anesthetic

The effect of epinephrine on uterine contraction is controversial. Several authors observed decreased uterine activity when an epinephrine-containing solution was used.[26,27] This might be related to a β-mimetic agonist effect on the uterus. On the other hand, when smaller concentrations of epinephrine (1 : 400,000 to 1 : 800,000) were used, no effect on the duration of labor was observed by others.[28,29]

Uteroplacental Perfusion

Maintenance of uterine perfusion is essential for fetal well-being and the progress of labor. The main factors are as follows:

1. The term parturient is very susceptible to hypotension.

2. Uterine vasoconstriction can also result from the high blood levels of local anesthetics that can occur with inadvertent intravascular injections.
3. The effect of epinephrine-containing local anesthetics on uterine blood flow remains controversial. Albright et al measured intervillous blood flow in 12 parturients during labor by using xenon 133. Epidural analgesia was provided with 2-chloroprocaine and epinephrine, 5 ug/mL. There were no significant changes in intervillous blood flow even in the presence of a decrease in mean blood pressure by 11 mm Hg.[30] On the other hand, Hood et al. found that 5 to 20 μg of intravenous epinephrine caused a progressive reduction in uterine blood flow in pregnant ewes (Fig. 11-6).[31]

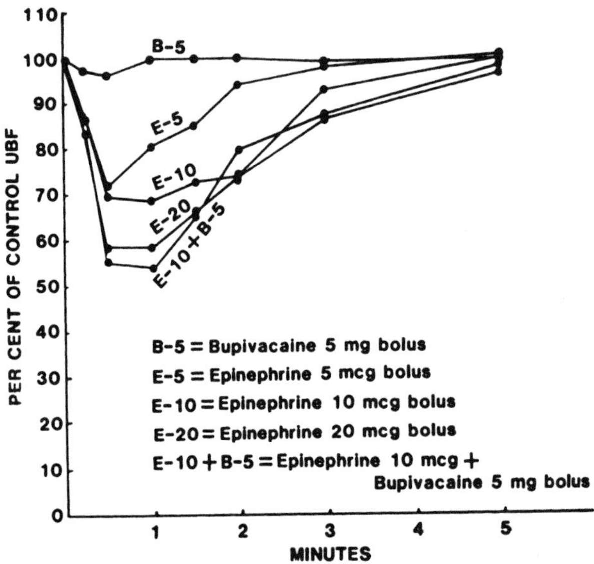

Figure 11-6. Changes in uterine blood flow (*UBF*) in the pregnant ewe following the intravenous administration of various amounts of epinephrine and bupivacaine. (From Hood DD, et al.: *Anesthesiology* 1986; 64:610. Used by permission.)

Fetal Effects

Regional anesthesia can affect the fetus indirectly through alterations in uterine perfusion and directly through placental transfer of drug. All local anesthetics have a molecular weight around 300 daltons, and they cross the placenta by passive diffusion. *Placental transfer of drug is favored by several properties of the drug, including high lipid solubility, decreased protein binding, high concentrations of nonionized drug, and fetal acidosis.* Acidosis results in the conversion of nonionized drug (diffusible form) into the ionized form and hence trapping in the fetus. Due to the rapid metabolism, ester local anesthetics are present in the fetus in much lower concentrations than are amide local anesthetics. When the neurological and adaptive capacity scoring systems are used, it has been shown that none of the clinically used anesthetics are associated with any neonatal problems. The incidence of neonatal retinal hemorrhage has been described to vary from 2.6% to 40%.[32] This finding usually disappears in time. The etiology is controversial; however, Maltau and Egge recently observed less retinal hemorrhage in neonates of mothers who received epidural analgesia when compared with the control group.[33]

Complications of Epidural Analgesia and Anesthesia

One must realize that major anesthesia-related neurological problems are extremely rare; the rate may vary from 1 : 40,000 to 1 : 100,000.[33a] Obstetric-related major complications are much more common, varying between 1 : 2600 to 1 : 6400.[33b]

Paresthesia

The incidence of transient paresthesia varies from 5% to 25% (Table 11-1). If paresthesia persists, the catheter should be removed and reinserted in another space. The incidence of paresthesia lasting for 4 to 6 weeks varies between 5 to 42.3 per 10,000 (see Table 11-1).

Table 11-1. Incidence of Paresthesia After Epidural Anesthesia*

Source	Number of Cases	Incidence per 10,000
Crawford	2,035	14.7
Eisen et al.	9,532	16.8
Abouleish	1,417	42.3
Lund	10,000	5.0
Bonica et al.	3,637	24.7

From Ong BY, Cohen MM, Esmali A: *Anesth Analg* 1987; 66:18. Used by permission.

Accidental Dural Puncture

The incidence varies from institution to institution. The incidence at the Brigham and Women's Hospital is between 1% and 2%. Dural puncture by the epidural catheter is very rare; however, the clinical implication of this is important because of the possibility of total spinal anesthesia. Headache is another complication, with a rate that can vary from 76% to 85%.[34]

Subdural Injection

This involves an injection of local anesthetic between the dura mater and pia-arachnoid; because of the lesser compliance, a higher spread is possible in comparison with epidural anesthesia. The following are characteristics of subdural injection:

1. Incidence, 0.1% to 0.82%
2. Incidence is increased during rotation of the epidural needle after a loss of resistance
3. Incidence is increased in patients with prior back surgery
4. *Widespread sensory anesthesia with the use of a small amount of local anesthetic*
5. *Block usually weak and patchy and spread mainly in a cephalad direction*
6. Delayed onset of 10 to 30 minutes
7. *Hypotension possibly the initial symptom*

8. Faster resolution, in comparison with epidural or subarachnoid blockade

Massive Epidural Analgesia

This represents an excessive segmental spread from a relative overdosage of local anesthetic. This problem is more often seen in massively obese individuals as well as in parturient with severe arteriosclerosis and diabetes. The onset of this problem is more gradual, and very rarely it spreads high enough to produce unconsciousness.

Accidental Intravascular Injection

An accidental intravascular injection of local anesthetic can happen either at the time of induction of epidural analgesia or anesthesia or as a result of subsequent migration of the epidural catheter in the intravascular space. Injection of local anesthetic directly into the epidural vein can give rise to a systemic reaction causing convulsions as well as possible cardiovascular collapse. Initiation of immediate management is important:

1. Provide for left uterine displacement.
2. *Airway patency must be maintained, if necessary, by an endotracheal tube and ventilation with 100% oxygen.*
3. *Convulsions are usually short-lived, but if they continue, one has to use 5 to 10 mg of diazepam or midazolam 1–2 mg or a small amount of thiopental* (50 to 100 mg).
4. *Fetal heart rate monitoring will ultimately govern the next step: if the fetal heart rate is normal, labor can continue for a vaginal delivery, but in the presence of fetal distress, an immediate cesarean section* with general anesthesia should be planned, and active resuscitation of the fetus may be necessary.

Cardiovascular Toxicity of Local Anesthetic

The ratio of the dosage needed to produce convulsions (CNS) to those resulting in cardiovascular collapse (CC) in animals has been found to be narrower for bupivacaine compared with lidocaine, mepivacaine, and ropivacaine. In parturients, ventricular arrhythmias have been observed to be more frequent during the use of bupivacaine. Increased progesterone concentrations during pregnancy may enhance the cardiotoxicity and arrythmogenic potential of bupivacaine;[35] however, this was not observed in the case of lidocaine or ropivacaine.

Backache

This is a frequent problem (30% to 40%) following epidural analgesia in obstetric patients. It may be related to improperly placed retractors and thus unrelated to regional anesthesia. Multiple attempts with needles may increase back pain by causing direct trauma and hemorrhage into the intervertebral ligament and vertebral periosteum. Pre-existing conditions like arthritis or osteoporosis may exacerbate the problem. In a recent study Breen et al observed the incidence of back pain was similar in parturients with or without epidural analgesia (44% vs. 45%).[35a] A study published after Breen and colleagues followed women for up to 1 year. The authors observed no increased risk of back pain in women who had used epidural analgesia compared with those who did not (10% vs. 14%).[35b] Thus, prospective studies observed no correlation between regional analgesia or anesthesia and generalized back pain.

Methemoglobinemia

This condition is associated with *prilocaine especially when the dose exceeds 600 mg. It can also be associated with benzocaine, rarely following a large dose of lidocaine. Treatment includes 1 mg/kg of methylene blue.*

Broken Epidural Catheter

The exact incidence is not known. Most authors advise that a broken catheter be left in place if it is in the lumbar epidural space.[5] Studies in cats showed that implanted epidural catheters were ultimately covered with fibrous tissue after about 3 weeks.

Neurological Complications

Neurological complications in obstetric population must be divided into obstetric causes and anesthesia-related causes.

Obstetric Causes

The incidence of neurological complications related to obstetric causes varied from 1:2,600 to 1:6,400.[36,37] These neurological complications were associated with prolonged labor and forceps delivery. Changes in the obstetric practice of difficult deliveries might have decreased the incidence of major obstetric-related neurological complications.[38] Peripheral nerves that might be involved, apart from regional anesthesia, are as follows:

1. A prolapsed intervertebral disk may happen because of the exertional efforts of labor. This may cause spinal root compression, the incidence of which has been documented to be 1 in 6,000 deliveries.
2. The lumbosacral trunk (L4, L5) may be compressed between the descending fetal head and the ala of the sacrum. It might be associated with the use of mid to high forceps. Clinical findings may include foot drop, hypoesthesia of the lateral aspect of the foot and calf, a slight weakness of hip adductors, and quadriceps weakness.
3. The femoral nerve (L2, L3, L4) can be injured in the lithotomy position because of hyperacute hip flexion as well as the use of retractors during cesarean section. There will be impaired knee extension due to quadriceps paralysis, an absence of the patellar reflex, and hypoesthesia of the anterior portion of the thigh and medial aspect of the calf.
4. The lateral femoral cutaneous nerve (L2, L3) can be injured by retractors during cesarean section or during incorrect lithotomy positioning. There will be transient numbness of the thigh at the anterolateral aspect.
5. The sciatic nerve (L4, L5 and S1, S2, S3) can be injured by incorrect lithotomy positioning along with knee extension and external hip rotation. There will be pain in the gluteal region that radiates to the foot and an inability to flex the leg.

6. The obturator nerve (L2, L3, L4) may be injured due to lithotomy positioning. Acute flexion in the thigh to the groin area, particularly in an obese woman, may lead to compression and cause weakness or paralysis of the thigh adductors.
7. The common peroneal nerve (L4, L5, S1, S2) may be involved in a pressure injury during lithotomy positioning as a result of prolonged compression of the lateral aspect of the knee. The woman will lose the ability to assume an erect position. There will be associated foot drop.
8. The saphenous nerve (L2, L3, L4) can be affected during lithotomy positioning. There will be a loss of sensation over the medial aspect of the foot and anteromedial aspect of the lower portion of the leg.

Table 11-2 lists sensory and motor deficits from obstetric causes of neurological complications.

Anesthesia-Related Causes

Regional anesthesia (epidural and subarachnoid) used for the relief of labor pain or cesarean section is associated with certain neurological problems. The incidence of motor deficits after the epidural technique varies from 0% to 15% (Table 11-3).

Prolonged Neural Blockade. Delayed recovery following epidural analgesia for labor has been described. This was usually associated with the use of tetracaine or bupivacaine in high concentrations. Patchy sensory anesthesia and motor deficit occasionally lasted as long as 10 to 48 hours and ultimately resolved.[39] The etiology of this problem is unknown and may be related to the higher protein binding and lipid solubility of local anesthetics and their prolonged attachment to binding sites in neural and perineural tissues.

Bladder Dysfunction. Overstretching of the bladder due to prolonged continuous epidural blockade can produce this problem. Longer-acting local anesthetics are more often associated with this complication.

Shivering and Shaking. The cause of this is unknown; however, this side effect can be treated with epidural sufentanil or intravenous meperidine.

Table 11-2. Neurological Complications Unrelated to Regional Anesthesia: Obstetric Cause

	Clinical Findings	
Nerve	**Sensory Deficit**	**Motor Deficit**
Lumbosacral trunk (L4, L5)	Hypoesthesia of the lateral aspect of the calf and foot	Weakness of the hip abductor Foot drop Unilateral weakness of the quadriceps
Femoral nerve (L2, L3, L4)	Hypoesthesia of the anterior aspect of the thigh and medial aspect of the calf	Quadriceps paralysis
Lateral femoral cutaneous nerve (L2, L3)	Numbness of the anterolateral aspect of the thigh	
Sciatic nerve (L4, L5, S1, S2, S3)	Pain in posterior gluteal region with radiation to the foot	Inability of flexion of the leg
Obturator nerve (L2, L3, L4)	Decreased sensation over the medial aspect of the thigh	Inability to adduct the leg
Common peroneal nerve (L4, L5, S1, S2)	Sensory deficit over the anterolateral aspect of the calf and dorsum of the foot and toes	Plantar flexion with an inversion deformity
Saphenous nerve (L2, L3, L4)	Loss of sensation over the medial aspect of the foot and anteromedial aspect of the lower portion of the leg	

Horner's Syndrome. The incidence varies from 24% to 75%. *Nerves involved are the upper four thoracic nerves. Symptoms include ptosis, miosis, anhidrosis, enophthalmos, and ecchymosis.*

Trauma to the Nerve Roots. Direct trauma by the needle and catheter to the nerve root is extremely rare, but if it happens, it can give rise to paresthesia with specific distribution. Intraneural injections may create neuritis followed by paresthesia lasting weeks to months.

Cauda Equina Syndrome. This occurs rarely and can give rise to residual numbness, sphincter dysfunction, and various degrees of lower extremity paralysis. Several cases of neurological problems very similar to cauda equina syndrome following the use of 2-chloroprocaine were described in 1980.[40] Gissen and colleagues put forward several factors to explain this problem[41,42]: (1) the large volume of 2-chloroprocaine injected in the epidural space in the presence of an accidental dural puncture can cause maternal hypotension with associated anterior spinal artery syndrome because of increased intraspinal pressure as well as hypotension, and (2) a low pH with a high concentration of bisulfite can cause neural damage. More recently 5% hyperbaric lidocaine via spinal microcatheter has been associated with cauda equina syndrome. The mechanism might be related to high doses of lidocaine that cause nerve damage because of improper mixing with cerebrospinal fluid.[42a]

Epidural Hematoma. This is very rare following regional anesthesia, but it may happen following trauma to epidural blood vessels, especially if the clotting parameters are abnormal because of the use of anticlotting medications or because of associated medical problems (severe preeclampsia, HELLP

Table 11–3. Incidence of Motor Deficits After Epidural Analgesia*

Source	Number of cases	Incidence per 10,000
Dawkins	32,718	Transient, 14.7; permanent, 2.1
Crawford	2,035	0
Abouleish	1,417	14.1
Bonica et al.	3,637	2.7
Lund	10,000	1
Hellman	26,127	0
Moore et al.	6,729	0
Bleyaert	3,000	0

From Ong BY, Cohen MM, Esmali A: *Anesth Analg* 1987; 66:18. Used by permission.

[hemolysis, elevated liver enzymes, and low platelet count] syndrome, etc.). An *immediate diagnosis is necessary, and decompression should be performed within 6 hours.*

Epidural Abscess. Although extremely rare, infection in the spinal canal is usually secondary to infection elsewhere in the body. Four important clinical features include (1) severe back pain, (2) local overlying tenderness, (3) fever, and (4) leukocytosis. One should avoid regional anesthesia, if possible, in the presence of generalized bacteremia or septicemia.

Adhesive Arachnoiditis. This can take place as a result of clinical irritation of the structures in the subarachnoid space, through contamination of spinal needles or solutions. Observed symptoms include headache, nausea and vomiting, nuchal rigidity, fever, and Kernig's sign.

Anterior Spinal Artery Syndrome. *Extremely rare. Anterior part of the spinal cord is more vulnerable because of single arterial supply as well as lack of collateral supply. This can cause ischemic degeneration of the anterior two thirds of the cord with associated motor deficit.*

Anesthesiologists are always requested to consult postpartum women with neurological problems even if these problems are unrelated to regional anesthesia. A clear picture is absolutely necessary to make a proper diagnosis. The following steps will help with the differential diagnosis: history, physical examination, x-ray films, coagulogram, electromyography to possibly define the timing of the lesion (Fig. 11-7), computed tomographic (CT) scans, and magnetic resonance imaging (MRI). The author suggests a neurological consultation for any woman with a complicated neurological deficit that does not resolve within a reasonable period.

A new anesthesia-related neurological problem that had stirred controversy is transient neurological symptoms (TNS) or transient radicular irritation (TRI). This problem, first described by a group from Switzerland, was characterized by (1) aching pain in the buttocks radiating to both dorsolateral sides of the thigh and calves; (2) association with 5% hyperbaric lidocaine; (3) temporary status; and (4) surgery in the lithotomy position.[42b] Subsequent studies by the same group observed that 30% of TNS was associated with 5% hyperbaric lidocaine, 3% with use of 2% hyperbaric prilocaine,

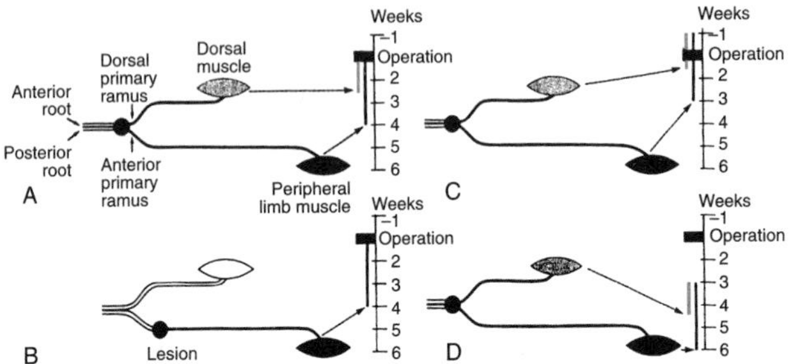

Electromyography in differential diagnosis of postoperative neurological complications. Diagram of spinal roots, dorsal and anterior primary rami, and peripheral nerves.

Symbols:

● = Lesion

= Normal dorsal (paraspinal) muscle

= Denervated dorsal muscle

= Denervated peripheral limb muscle

= Normal nerve

= Damaged nerve distal to lesion

Vertical scale shows elapsed time in weeks from time of lesion to appearance of denervation EMG patterns in muscles.

A, Lesion of spinal roots at time of operation. Dorsal muscles show EMG changes 1½ weeks later. Distal limb muscles show EMG changes three weeks later.

B, Lesion of peripheral nerve at time of operation. No change in dorsal muscle. Distal limb muscles show EMG changes three weeks later.

C, Associated but unrelated lesion of spinal roots one week before operation.

D, Lesion of spinal roots occurring two weeks after operation.

Figure 11–7. Electromyography in the differential diagnosis of postoperative neurological complications. (Adapted from Bromage PR: *Epidural Analgesia.* Philadelphia, WB Saunders Co, 1978, p 703.)

and 0% with 0.5% hyperbaric bupivacaine.[42c] Interestingly, the incidences of TNS increase significantly when the lithotomy position is used compared to the supine position (13% vs. 5%) with 5% hyperbaric or isobaric 2% lidocaine.[42d] The lithotomy position may stretch L5–S1 nerve roots, which remain in the most dorsal position in the spinal canal. Under this condition, blood perfusion of the nerves or a subset of nerve fibers may be hampered and thus increase the vulnerability to injury with 5% hyperbaric lidocaine. More recent studies observed no difference in the concentrations of lidocaine in the manifestation of TNS in patients undergoing surgery in the lithotomy position. Hence TNS is controversial; judicious care is required with the use of drugs that may increase the incidences of TNS.

Treatment of Headache Following Accidental Dural Puncture

The incidence of headache following accidental dural puncture with a 17-gauge needle can be as high as 76% to 85%.[34] Following an accidental dural puncture, the anesthesiologist usually places the epidural catheter in a different space. One has to be very careful while injecting local anesthetic via this newly placed catheter because of direct connection with the dural hole as well as seepage of a small amount of local anesthetic via the dural gap. At the termination of the procedure, several investigators have suggested the use of preservative-free normal saline via the epidural catheter (1) in a single dose (60 mL),[43] (2) every 6 hours (30 to 60 mL),[44] and (3) as a continuous infusion of 1,000 mL over a 24-hour period.[45] The success rate has varied considerably. A prophylactic blood patch has been used with some success.[46] However, the ultimate validity of this technique is controversial. In our institution, the success rate with prophylactic blood patches was less dramatic; hence, the majority of the staff anesthesiologists have abandoned the prophylactic blood patch technique. The women are informed about the occurrence of an accidental dural puncture; however, absolute bed rest is not mandatory (Fig. 11-8). The women are advised to drink plenty of fluids and take analgesic tablets if there is a headache. A therapeutic blood patch is indicated (1) if the headache is postural and does not improve within 48 hours; (2) if there is severe headache without or with associated nausea and vomiting; (3) if there is *blurred vision or diplopia that is related to stretching of the sixth cranial nerve* (*abducens*), *which supplies the*

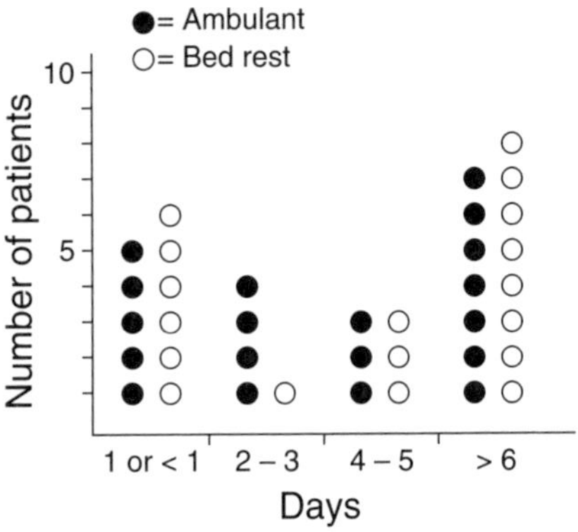

Figure 11-8. Difference in incidence of spinal headache between patients who are ambulatory and on bed rest. (From Carbalt PAT, VanCrevel H: *Lancet* 1981; 2:1133. Used with permission from Elsevier.)

lateral rectus muscle of the eye; and (4) if there is hearing loss following dural puncture, which occurs rarely. Procedures for the use of therapeutic blood patches are as follows:

1. The women must have a postural headache.
2. An intravenous catheter is inserted and acute hydration started.
3. The woman's back is aseptically prepared.
4. If there is only one puncture, then the same interspace is selected; however, if there are multiple punctures, one should use the lowermost interspace because it is easier for epidurally injected blood to spread cephalad than caudad.[47] Loss of resistance by saline should be used to prevent further intensification of the headache by introducing air through the dural hole.
5. Once the epidural needle is positioned properly, *blood should be drawn from a large vein* (20 ml–30 ml) *after proper aseptic care.*
6. Blood should be injected slowly to reduce the intensity of back and neck pain.

7. The woman should lie supine with pillows under the knees for 1 to 2 hours.
8. The woman should be monitored carefully for a few days.

The incidence of success from the first blood patch has been observed to be as high as 70–75%; in a few cases, a second or third blood patch may be necessary. *Main causes of failure of the blood patch are wrong diagnosis and improper placement of the patch.*

If the blood patch fails, one has to re-evaluate the diagnosis, and if necessary, a neurologist should be consulted. *Cortical vein thrombosis, which mimics symptoms after a dural puncture, has to be excluded because a blood patch can make the matter worse. CT scans may confirm the diagnosis.*[48]

Contraindications to Blood Patches

Contraindications to the use of a blood patch include the following:

1. Any coagulation problem
2. Associated temperature of unknown origin
3. Infection of the back

If there is accidental dural puncture with the epidural needle, one can place an epidural catheter in another interspace. In such a situation *one must confirm absence of seepage of local anesthetic via the hole* made by the epidural needle. Then CEI should not be contraindicated. On the other hand, in the presence of accidental dural puncture by the epidural needle one can thread an epidural macrocatheter (19G) via the hole and use continuous spinal anesthesia (CSA). If CSA is used, the following steps are important: (1) the initial dose should consist of 2.5 mg preservative-free isobaric bupivacaine mixed with fentanyl 25 mcg or 10 mcg sufentanil; (2) the parturient should be kept supine with LUD (*the sitting position may be associated with higher sensory anesthesia level*); (3) in the absence of good perenial analgesia or anesthesia at the second stage, a small amount of hyperbaric local anesthesia mixed with opiate will be effective.

Spinal Anesthesia

Spinal anesthesia, indeed, used to have a very limited role in labor and vaginal delivery. Spinal anesthesia will relax the pelvic floor muscle and will thus disturb the integrity of the birth passage; the expulsive powers can also be diminished by blockade of the abdominal segments. Because spinal anesthesia produces an intense motor block of the pelvic floor muscle, it is a desirable technique for forceps delivery. We aim for a T10–S5 block in all forceps deliveries except in the case of a *trial of forceps,* where we aim for a *higher block* (T4). Drugs that can be used are (1) lidocaine, (2) tetracaine, and (3) bupivacaine. Continuous spinal anesthesia can be used if there is an accidental or intentional dural tap. 3 cm of the epidural catheter is inserted in the subarachnoid space. Advantages of the continuous spinal catheter technique include (1) small dose, (2) rapid onset of action, (3) quick recovery because of the small dose, (4) the absence of accidental intravenous injections of large doses of local anesthetic, and (5) the possibility of the use of small doses of intraspinal narcotics for the relief of labor pain in a few special situations.

Combined Spinal/Epidural (CSE)

The CSE technique has become popular since the introduction of neuroxial opioids. The epidural needle is first inserted in the epidural space with loss-of-resistance technique. Then a long pencil-point spinal needle (25- or 27-gauge) is inserted via the epidural needle. This spinal needle is usually 12 mm longer than the tip of the epidural needle. With the appearance of free-flowing CSF, a mixture of lipid-soluble opioid (fentanyl or sufentanil) mixed with isobaric bupivacaine is injected via the spinal needle. At this point the spinal needle is withdrawn, the epidural catheter is inserted, and the epidural needle is removed. Different lipid-soluble opioids have been tried; 10 mcg sufentanil or 25 mcg of fentanyl are most popular. Addition of small doses of morphine or epinephrine with the fentanyl and bupivacaine will prolong the duration of analgesia. The advantages of CSE include (1) faster onset of analgesia; (2) decreased or nonexistent motor blockade; (3) less cardiovascular instability; (4) lower amount of local anesthetic in the systemic circulation; and (5) shorter first stage of labor in nulliparous women compared to CEI technique.[49]

CEI, or patient-controlled epidural analgesia (PCEA), can be started once the expectant mother is comfortable. *If a bolus dose is selected, one must reduce the doses of local anesthetics because of the possible synergistic effect of the local anesthetic and opioid.* Side effects of CSE technique include:

(1) Pruritus, usually mild and short-lasting. If severe, intravenous nalbufine (Nubaine) in 5–10 mg doses can be given. Small doses of nalaxone (40–80 mcg) or propofol (10 mg) also have been used with success. Recently 8 mg ondansetron has been used successfully for spinal opioid-induced pruritus.[50]

(2) Nausea and/or vomiting. Less lipophilic morphine may be associated with higher incidences of this side effect.

(3) Respiratory depression is extremely rare with lipophilic opioid.

(4) Fetal bradycardia may be associated with CSE technique.[51] The mechanism is not understood at present. Postulated mechanisms include:

   1. Decrease in maternal epinephrine concentrations; unopposed norepinephrine effect may be associated with uterine vessel (macro and micro) vasoconstriction and hence increased uterine tone.[52]
   2. Maternal hypotension also may decrease uteroplacental perfusion.
   3. Finally, direct vagotonic effect of the sufentanil on the fetus has been suggested; however, this effect may be just theoretically important.

Treatment should include intravenous ephedrine to increase maternal cardiac output; if the FHR does not improve intravenous terbutaline should be used.

Caudal Anesthesia

The caudal space is the lowermost part of the epidural space and lies in the sacral canal. This technique involves the introduction of a 17-gauge epidural or 19-gauge 3.8- to 7.6-cm needle. A catheter can be introduced for continuous use, or a one-shot technique can be used just before the delivery for perineal analgesia. This technique has become unpopular because of the requirement of higher doses of local anesthetics.

Paracervical Block

This technique involves blocking nerve impulses from the uterine body and cervix by injecting local anesthetics in the paracervical tissues. Usually it is performed during the first stage of labor. A paracervical block does not relieve the perineal pain. A continuous technique has also been tried. This technique is getting less popular at the present time mainly because of its depressant effects on the fetus. *Fetal bradycardia following a paracervical block is mainly due to two factors: (1) constriction of uteroplacental blood vessels by local anesthetic and (2) vascular absorption of a large amount of local anesthetic that will directly depress the fetal myocardium.*

Lumbar Sympathetic Block

This technique is seldom used at present; it is useful *only for the first stage of labor.*

Pudendal Block

A pudendal block is performed by the obstetrician just before the delivery by blocking the pudendal nerves while passing over the ischial spine. This technique will provide analgesia of the perineum. Interestingly, it has been shown that the uptake of local anesthetic from this technique is very similar to that in an epidural block.

Regional anesthesia (epidural, spinal) has become very popular in recent times for the relief of labor pain and delivery. One has to be careful and meticulous in performing these procedures, and all equipment and medications should be available for active maternal resuscitation if necessary. At Brigham and Women's Hospital, most of the equipment and drugs are kept in the epidural cart:

1. Oxygen delivery apparatus
2. Airways: oral, nasal, and endotracheal tubes of different sizes
3. Laryngoscope (short handle) with blades of different sizes and shapes
4. Electrocardiograph
5. Succinylcholine, thiopental, ephedrine
6. Cardiac defibrillator and other resuscitative medications in a crash cart in close vicinity

References

1. Hollmen A, Jouppila R, Jouppila P, et al: Effect of extradural analgesia using bupivacaine and 2-chloroprocaine on intervillous blood flow during normal labor. *Br J Anaesth* 1982; 54:837.
2. Jouppila P, Jouppila R, Hollmen A, et al: Lumbar epidural analgesia to improve intervillous blood flow during labor in severe preeclampsia. *Obstet Gynecol* 1982; 59:158.
3. Shnider SM, Wright RG, Levinson G, et al: Uterine blood flow and plasma norepinephrine changes during maternal stress in the pregnant ewe. *Anesthesiology* 1979; 50:524.
4. Greiss FC, Still JG, Anderson SG: Effects of local anesthetic agents on the uterine vasculatures and myometrium. *Am J Obstet Gynecol* 1976; 124:889.

4a. Hogan H: Epidural anatomy: New observations. *Can J Anaesth* 1998; 45:5 R40–R44.

4b. Beilin Y, Zahn J, Bernstein HH, et al: Treatment of incomplete analgesia after placement of an epidural catheter and administration of local anesthetic for women in labor. *Anesthesiology* 1998; 88:1502.

5. Bromage PR: *Epidural Analgesia.* Philadelphia, WB Saunders Co, 1978, p 57.
6. Moore DC, Batra MS: The components of an effective test dose prior to epidural block. *Anesthesiology* 1981; 55:693.
7. Cartwright PD, McCarroll SM, Antzaka C: Maternal heart rate changes with a plain epidural test dose. *Anesthesiology* 1986; 65:226.

8. Leighton BL, Norris MC, Sosis M: Limitations of an epinephrine epidural anesthesia test dose in laboring patients (abstract). *Anesthesiology* 1986; 65:403.
9. Abraham RA, Harris AP, Maxwell LG: The efficacy of 1.5% lidocaine with 7.5% dextrose and epinephrine as an epidural test dose for obstetrics. *Anesthesiology* 1986; 64:116.
10. Leighton BL, Norris MC, DeSimone CA, et al: The air as a clinically useful indicator of intravenously placed epidural catheters. *Anesthesiology* 1990; 73:610.
11. Popitz-Bergez F, Datta S, Ostheimer GW: Intravascular epinephrine may not increase heart rate in patients receiving metoprolol. *Anesthesiology* 1988; 68:815.
12. Scott DB, Walker LR: Administration of continuous epidural analgesia. *Anaesthesia* 1963; 18:82.
13. Smedstad KG, Morrison DH: A comparative study of continuous and intermittent epidural analgesia for labour and delivery. *Can Anaesth Soc J* 1985; 32:101.
14. Skerman JH, Thompson BA, Goldstein MT: Combined continuous epidural fentanyl and bupivacaine in labour: A randomized study (abstract). *Anesthesiology* 1985; 63:450.
15. Chestnut DH, Owen CL, Bates JN: Continuous infusion epidural analgesia during labor: A randomized, double-blind comparison of 0.0625% bupivacaine/0.0002% fentanyl versus 0.125% bupivacaine. *Anesthesiology* 1988; 68:754.
16. Phillips G: Continuous infusion of epidural analgesia in labor. The effect of adding sufentanil to 0.125% bupivacaine. *Anesth Analg* 1988; 67:462.
17. Raabe N, Belfrage P: Lumbar epidural analgesia in labour. A clinical analysis. *Acta Obstet Gynecol Scand* 1976; 55:125.
18. Cheek TG, Samuels P, Tobin M, et al: Rapid intravenous saline infusion decreases uterine activity in labor. Epidural analgesia does not (abstract). *Anesthesiology* 1989; 71:884.
19. Hall WL: Epidural analgesia and its effect on the normal progress of labor (discussion). *Am J Obstet Gynecol* 1977; 129:316.
20. Crawford JS: The second thousand epidural blocks in an obstetric hospital practice. *Br J Anaesth* 1972; 44:1277.
21. Crawford JS: Lumbar epidural block in labor: A clinical analysis. *Br J Anaesth* 1972; 44:66.
22. Belfrage P, Berlin A, Raabe N, et al: Lumbar epidural analgesia with bupivacaine in labor. Drug concentration in maternal and neonatal blood at birth and during the first day of life. *Am J Obstet Gynecol* 1975; 123:839.
23. Maresh M, et al: Delayed pushing with lumbar epidural analgesia in labour. *Br J Obstet Gynaecol* 1983; 90:623.

24. Phillips KC, Thomas TA: Second stage of labour with or without extradural analgesia. *Anaesthesia* 1983; 38:972.
25. Chestnut DH, Laszewski LJ, Pollack KL, et al: Continuous epidural infusion of 0.0625% bupivacaine–0.0002% fentanyl during the second stage of labor. *Anesthesiology* 1990; 72:613.
25a. Thorp JA, Hu DH, Albin RM, et al: The effect of intrapartum epidural analgesia on nulliparous labor: A randomized, controlled, prospective trial. *Am J Obstet Gynecol* 1993; 169: 851.
25b. Chestnut DH, McGrath JM, Vincent RD, et al: Does early administration of epidural analgesia affect obstetric outcome in nulliparous women who are in spontaneous labor? *Anesthesiology* 1994; 80:1201.
25c. Sharma SK, Sidawi JE, Ramin SH, et al: Cesarean delivery: A randomized trial of epidural versus patient controlled meperidine analgesia during labor. *Anesthesiology* 1997; 87:487.
25d. Bofill JA, Vincent RD, Ross EL, et al: Nulliparous active labor, epidural analgesia, and cesarean delivery for dystocia. *Am J Obstet Gynecol* 1997; 177:1465.
25e. Halpern SH, Leighton BL, Ohlsson A, et al: Effect of epidural vs parenteral opioid analgesia on the progress of labor: A meta analysis. *JAMA* 1998; 280:2105.
26. Craft JB Jr, Epstein BS, Coakley CS: Effect of lidocaine with epinephrine versus lidocaine (plain) on induced labor. *Anesth Analg (Cleve)* 1972; 51:243.
27. Tyack AJ, Parsons RJ, Millar DR, et al: Uterine activity and plasma bupivacaine levels after caudal epidural analgesia. *J Obstet Gynaecol Br Commonw* 1973; 80:896.
28. Bleyaert A, Soetens M, Vaes L, et al: Bupivacaine 0.125%in obstetric epidural analgesia: Experience in three thousand cases. *Anesthesiology* 1979; 51:435.
29. Abboud TK, David S, Nagappala S: Maternal, fetal and neonatal effects of lidocaine with and without epinephrine for epidural anesthesia in obstetrics. *Anesth Analg* 1984; 63:973.
30. Albright GA, Jouppila R, Hollmen AL: Epinephrine does not alter human intervillous blood flow during epidural anesthesia. *Anesthesiology* 1981; 54:131.
31. Hood DD, Dewan DM, Rose JC: Maternal and fetal effects of intravenous epinephrine containing solutions in gravid ewes. *Anesthesiology* 1986; 64:610.
32. Schlaeder G, Gerhard JP, Demot M: Les hemorrhagies retimiennes chez le nouveaune apres accouchmant par ventoose of accouchment spontane. *Gynecol Obstet Paris* 1971; 70:27.

33. Maltau JM, Egge K: Epidural analgesia and perinatal retinal hemorrhages. *Acta Anaesthesiol Scand* 1980; 24:99.

33a. Scott DB, Hibbard BM: Serious non-fatal complications associated with extradural block in obstetric practice. *Br J Anaesth* 1990; 64:537.

33b. Donaldson J: Neurology of Pregnancy, 2nd ed. Philadelphia. W. B. Saunders, 1989.

34. Brownridge P: The management of headache following dural puncture in obstetric patients. *Anaesth Intensive Care* 1983; 11:4.

35. Moller RA, Datta S, Fox J, et al: Effects of progesterone on the cardiac electrophysiologic action of bupivacaine and lidocaine. *Anesthesiology* 1992; 76:604.

35a. Breen TW, Ransil BJ, Groves PA, et al: Factors associated with back pain after childbirth. *Anesthesiology* 1994; 81:29.

35b. MacArthur AJ, Macarthur Colin, Weeks SK: Is epidural anesthesia in labor associated with chronic low back pain? A prospective chart study. *Anesth Analg* 1997; 85:1066.

36. Hill EC: Maternal obstetric paralysis. *Am J Obstet Gynecol* 1962; 83:1452.

37. Cole JT: Maternal obstetric paralysis. *Am J Obstet Gynecol* 1946; 52:372.

38. Ong BY, Cohen MM, Esmali A: Paresthesias and motor dysfunction after labor and delivery. *Anesth Anal* 1987; 66:18.

39. Bromage PR: An evaluation of bupivacaine in epidural analgesia for obstetrics. *Can Anaesth Soc J* 1969; 16:46.

40. Ravindran RS, Bond VK, Tasch MD, et al: Prolonged neural blockade following regional analgesia with 2-chloroprocaine. *Anesth Analg* 1980; 59:447.

41. Gissen AJ, Datta S, Lambert D: The chloroprocaine controversy. I. A hypothesis to explain the neural complications of chloroprocaine epidural. *Reg Anaesth* 1984; 9:124.

42. Gissen AJ, Datta S, Lambert D: The chloroprocaine controversy. II. Is chloroprocaine neurotoxic? *Reg Anaesth* 1984; 9:135.

42a. Rigler ML, Drasner K, Krejcie TC, et al: Cauda equina syndrome after continuous spinal anesthesia. *Anesth Analg* 1991; 72:275.

42b. Schneider M, Ettlin T, Kaufman M, et al: Transient neurologic toxicity after hyperbaric subarachnoid anesthesia with 5% lidocaine. *Anesth Analg* 1993; 76:1154.

42c. Hampl KF, Heinzmann-Weidmer S, Luginbuehl I, et al: Transient neurologic symptoms after spinal anesthesia: A lower incidence with prilocaine and bupivacaine than with lidocaine. *Anesthesiology* 1998; 88:629.

42d. Pollock JE, Neal JM, Stephenson CA: Prospective study of the incidence of transient radicular irritation in patients undergoing spinal anesthesia. *Anesthesiology* 1996; 84:1361.
43. Craft JB, Epstein BS, Coakley CS: Prophylaxis of dural puncture headache with epidural saline. *Anesth Analg* 1973; 52:228.
44. Smith BE: Prophylaxis of epidural wet tap headache (abstract). Presented at the Annual Meeting of the American Society of Anesthesiologists, San Francisco, 1979, p 119.
45. Crawtord JS: The prevention of headache consequent upon dural puncture. *Br J Anaesth* 1972; 44:598.
46. Colona-Romano P, Shapiro BE: Unintentional dural puncture and prophylactic epidural blood patch in obstetrics. *Anesth Analg* 1989; 69:552.
47. Szeinfeld M, Ihmedian IH, Moser MM: Epidural blood patch: Evaluation of the volume and spread of blood injected into the epidural space. *Anesthesiology* 1986; 64:820.
48. Gewirtz EC, Costin M, Marx GF: Cortical vein thrombosis may mimic postdural headache. *Reg Anaesth* 1987; 12:188.
49. Tsen LC, Thue B, Datta S, et al: Is combined spinal-epidural analgesia associated with more rapid cervical dilation in nulliparous patients when compared with conventional epidural analgesia? *Anesthesiology* 1999; 91:920.
50. Borgeat A, Stirnemann HR: Ondansetron is effective to treat spinal or epidural morphine-induced pruritus. *Anesthesiology* 1999; 90:432.
51. Friedlander JD, Fox HE, Cain CF: Fetal bradycardia and uterine hyperactivity following subarachnoid administration of fentanyl during labor. *Reg Anaesth* 1997; 22(4):378.
52. Segal S, Savoy A, Datta S: The tocolytic effect of catecholamines in the gravid rat uterus. *Anesth Analg* 1998; 87:864.

12
Anesthesia for Cesarean Delivery

▼

A cesarean section is defined as the delivery of an infant through incisions in the abdominal and uterine walls.

In recent years, the frequency of cesarean delivery has increased markedly. From an incidence of 3% to 8% 20 years ago, its present utilization is 9% to 30% throughout the United States depending on the geographic region and population characteristics.[1]

Successful anesthesia for cesarean delivery can be accomplished in a number of ways. Common to all is the need for expert technical skills and understanding of maternal and fetal physiology, pathophysiology, and pharmacology. The two major anesthetic approaches are regional and general anesthesia. My discussion of regional anesthesia will include three techniques, spinal, epidural and combined spinal epidural anesthesia since local infiltration and field blocks are rarely used in the United States.

Regional Anesthesia

Spinal Anesthesia (Subarachnoid Block)

The advantages of spinal anesthesia for cesarean delivery are as follows:

1. Simplicity of technique
2. Speed of induction (in contrast to an epidural block)
3. Reliability
4. Minimal fetal exposure to the drug(s)
5. An awake parturient
6. Minimization of the hazards of aspiration

Disadvantages of spinal anesthesia for cesarean delivery include the following:

1. High incidence of hypotension
2. Intrapartum nausea and vomiting
3. Possibility of headaches after dural puncture
4. Limited duration of action (unless a continuous technique is used)

Problems

Hypotension. Following induction of spinal anesthesia for cesarean delivery, the incidence of maternal hypotension, usually defined as a decrease in systolic blood pressure to below 100 mm Hg or a decrease of more than 30 mm Hg from the preanesthetic value, can be as high as 80%. These hemodynamic changes result from a blockade of sympathetic vasomotor activity that is accentuated by compression of the aorta and inferior vena cava by the gravid uterus when the patient is in the supine position.

The higher the segmental sympathetic blockade (especially greater than T4), the greater the risk of hypotension and associated emetic symptoms.[2] The supine position significantly increases the incidence of hypotension. Ueland and colleagues observed an average reduction in blood pressure from 124/72 to 67/38 mm Hg in mothers who were placed in the supine position following the induction of spinal anesthesia, whereas the blood pressure averaged 100/60 mm Hg for mothers in the lateral position[3] (Fig. 12-1).

The significance of maternal hypotension lies in the threat to the well-being of both mother and fetus if the reductions in

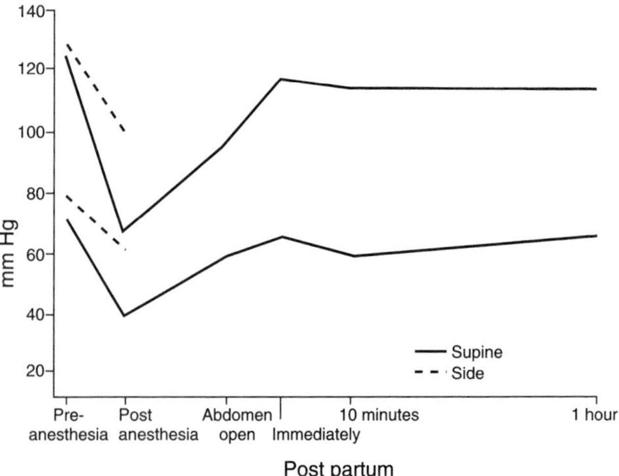

Figure 12-1. Effect of maternal blood pressure during cesarean section under spinal anesthesia. (Adapted from Ueland K, Gills RE, Hansen JM: *Am J Obstet Gynecol* 1968; 100:42.)

the blood pressure and cardiac output are not promptly recognized and corrected. Brief episodes of maternal hypotension have lowered Apgar scores, prolonged the time to sustained respiration, and produced fetal acidosis.[4,5] With short periods of hypotension (not more than 2 minutes), we have observed minimal fetal acidosis but no effect on newborn neurobehavioral findings between 2 to 4 hours of age. With prolonged periods of hypotension Hollmen and associates have shown neurological changes for at least 48 hours in infants born to mothers who had epidural anesthesia for cesarean delivery.[6] Since spinal anesthesia offers major clinical advantages for cesarean delivery, efforts have been directed at preventing maternal hypotension. Prehydration or acute volume expansion (15 to 30 minutes) with 1,000 to 1,500 mL of lactated Ringer's solution has been suggested.[7] Recently, however, this dictum has been challenged. A group from South Africa found no beneficial effect of a predetermined amount of volume expansion before the induction of spinal anesthesia for cesarean section.[7a] Using 10 ml–30 ml/kg of Ringer's lactate for acute volume expansion before induction of spinal anesthesia, no differences in the incidences of maternal hypotension or doses of ephedrine were observed.[7b] Hence a predetermined amount of volume expansion may not be necessary before initiation of cesarean section. Several authors have observed fetal hyperglycemia, acidosis, and ultimately, neonatal hypoglycemia when a dextrose-containing solution was used for acute volume expansion.[8,9] On the other hand, a few authors recommend a small amount of dextrose (1% dextrose in Ringer's lactate solution) to maintain euglycemia.

The use of a small amount of colloid combined with crystalloid did not show consistent results regarding a decrease in the incidence of maternal hypotension.

Vasopressors. The value of the administration of a prophylactic vasopressor is still controversial. We do not routinely use prophylactic ephedrine because it might not be necessary in all cases. Prophylactic ephedrine may produce iatrogenic hypertension if one fails to administer the spinal anesthesia. However, there is general agreement that if hypotension should develop, it should be promptly treated by a combination of a bolus infusion of intravenous crystalloid, further uterine displacement if possible, and the administration of intravenous doses of ephedrine, beginning with 5- to 10-mg increments. In a few situations, tachycardia followed by ephedrine administration may be contraindicated (cardiac problems). In such a situation hypotension may be treated with a small amount of phenylephrine (Neo-Synephrine). Recent studies suggest that intravenous phenylephrine in small doses (40 μg at a time) may be used intraoperatively after the induction of spinal or epidural anesthesia for the treatment of maternal hypotension during cesarean section, without any detrimental effect on the fetus.[10–12] However, it should be stressed that these studies included only healthy parturients who had healthy fetuses and no history of uteroplacental insufficiency.

The incidence of hypotension during spinal anesthesia for cesarean delivery in parturients who have active labor is lower than in pregnant women not in labor.[12] Possible explanations may be (1) the *autotransfusion of approximately 300 mL of blood into the maternal systemic circulation with intermittent uterine contractions,* (2) *a decrease in the size of the uterus secondary to a loss of amniotic fluid if the membranes are ruptured,* and (3) *higher maternal catecholamine concentrations in parturients in labor.*

Nausea and Vomiting. These symptoms commonly accompany spinal anesthesia. The mechanism is unclear but probably involves (1) systemic hypotension, which decreases cerebral blood flow and produces cerebral hypoxia, and (2) traction on the peritoneum or other viscera, which produces a vagal response manifested by a decrease in the heart rate and a resultant decrease in cardiac output. We have evaluated the effectiveness of prompt treatment of any drop in blood pressure on the prevention of nausea and vomiting. Our conclusion was that intravenous ephedrine, when given as soon as any reduction in blood pressure is detected, prevents a further decrease in blood pressure and significantly diminishes the incidence of nausea and vomiting. In addition, acid-base values from the umbilical vessels of newborns whose mothers were so treated were significantly better than in the newborns of mothers who developed frank hypotension.[13] In one study authors observed a reduction of nausea and vomiting when phenylephrine was used in comparison of ephedrine to treat maternal hypotension.

Traction of the uterus and/or peritoneum at the time of surgery may increase the incidence of emetic symptoms in the presence of inadequate regional anesthesia.[14] Visceral pain from traction of the peritoneum or abdominal viscera (e.g., exteriorization of the uterus or stretching of the lower uterine segment) will transmit afferent stimuli via the vagus nerve to stimulate the central vomiting center. Adequate sensory anesthesia can be obtained with appropriate doses of local anesthetic, and this will also decrease the incidence of discomfort in parturients. The addition of intrathecal or epidural opioids will intensify the quality of sensory anesthesia and will decrease the incidence of intraoperative nausea and vomiting.[15,16] Nausea and vomiting following delivery of the baby can be minimized with the administration of a small dose of droperidol or metoclopramide[17,17a,18] (Figs. 12-2 and 12-3).

Headache. Headache as a result of dural puncture (PDPH) is the most troublesome complication of spinal anesthesia in obstetrics. The reported incidence of PDPH varies greatly from institution to institution (0% to 10%). However, recently several interesting techniques have been reported to reduce the incidence of PDPH: (1) the method of insertion of the spinal needle may be an important factor in reducing PDPH. A recent study by Mihic in nonpregnant patients showed a significant reduction in PDPH with parallel insertion of the spinal needle in relation to the dural fibers.[19] (2) Needles of different sizes were tried to observe the incidence of PDPH.[20] When 27-gauge Quincke needles were used, the incidence of PDPH in the author's institution remained 2% to 3%. (3) Configuration of the needles is also important. The long beveled Quincke needle is associated with a higher incidence of headache than are pencil point needles like the Greene, Whitacre, and Sprotte (Fig. 12-4). This might be related to the amount of injury to the dural fibers. Ready and colleagues observed the effect of needle size and angle of dural puncture in relation to the rate of transdural fluid leak.[21] Quincke needles with a 30-degree approach caused a rate of leak across the dura significantly less than those following 60- and 90-degree approaches. An approach perpendicular to the dural fibers was associated with a higher incidence of PDPH.

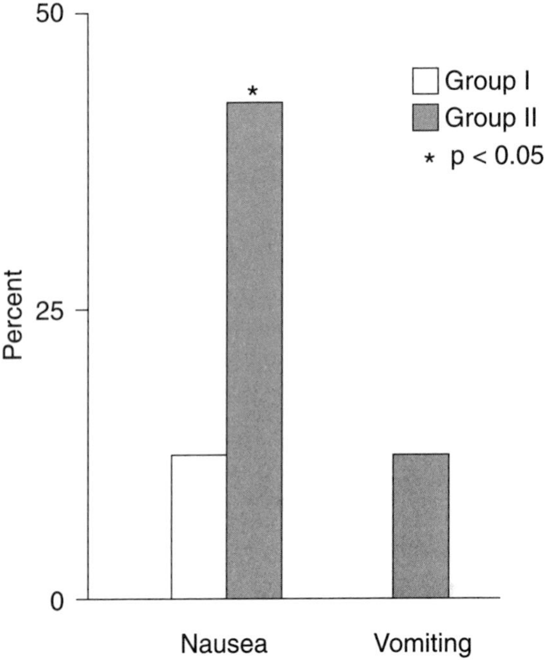

Figure 12-2. Incidence of nausea and vomiting with intravenous droperidol following delivery of the fetus during cesarean section.

The 22-gauge Whitacre needle was also associated with less leak than the 22-gauge Quincke needle. When a 25-gauge Whitacre needle was used, the incidence of headache in the author's institution was about 1%. The majority of headaches are mild and self-limited and resolve without problems. Oral and intravenous caffeine can decrease the incidence of headaches temporarily.[20]

Technical Factors. A sensory level between the fourth and sixth thoracic dermotome is necessary for adequate anesthesia. This level is achieved in the pregnant women with doses of local anesthetic well below those required in nonpregnant

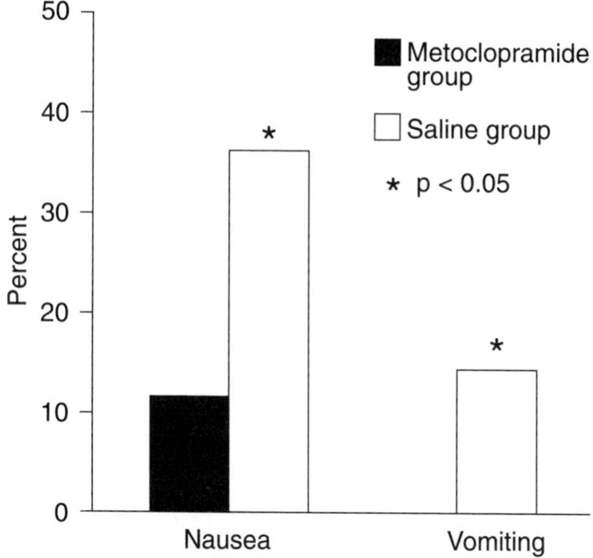

Figure 12–3. Incidence of nausea and vomiting with intravenous metoclopramide following delivery of the fetus during cesarean section. (Adapted from Chestnut DH, Vandewalker GE, Owen CI: *Anesthesiology* 1987; 66:563.)

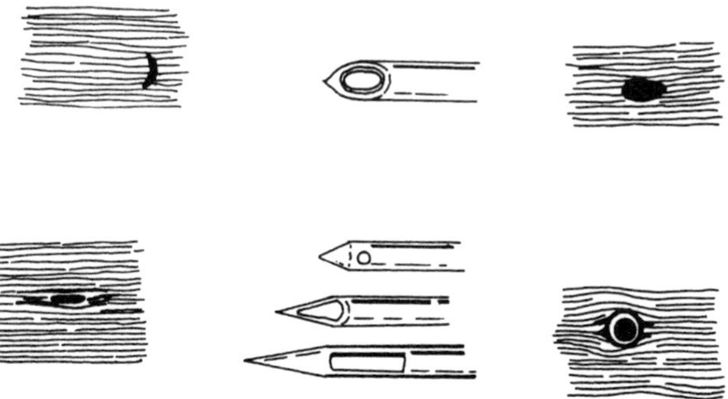

Figure 12–4. Openings made in the dura during and after insertion of pencil point needles (Pajunk, Greene, Whitacre) and beveled needle (Quincke). Small openings are made by pencil point needles.

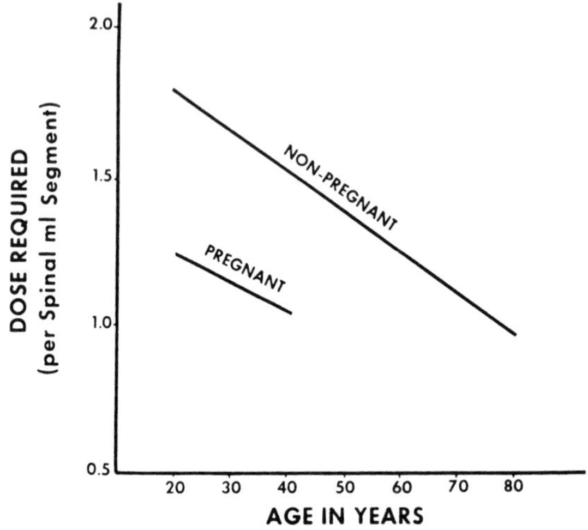

Figure 12–5. Dose required (milliliters of lidocaine per spinal segment) in parturients and nonpregnant patients. (From Bromage PR: *Epidural Analgesia.* Philadelphia, WB Saunders Co, 1978, p 566. Used with permission from Elsevier.)

individuals in both spinal and epidural anesthesia (Fig. 12-5). A hyperbaric solution is preferred for cesarean section because it tends to spread to the thoracic kyphosis at approximately T5–6[22] regardless of the parturients height. Norris recently observed no correlation between the height or weight of parturients and the spread of spinal anesthesia when using a fixed dose (12 mg) of 0.75% hyperbaric bupivacaine in woman between 4′11″ and 5′8″.[23] DeSimone and colleagues, on the other hand, compared a 12-mg with a 15-mg dose of hyperbaric bupivacaine for cesarean section and observed a significantly higher spread with 15 mg.[24] Hartwell and colleagues recently studied the correlation between vertebral length measured from C7 to the level of the iliac crest and to the sacral hiatus and the sensory anesthetic level after the subarachnoid administration of 12 mg of hyperbaric bupivacaine for cesarean section.[25] There was no correlation between patient height, weight, or body mass index and the sensory anesthesia level; however, interestingly, there was a correlation between vertebral length and sensory anesthesia level. Twelve milligrams should be adequate for the majority of parturients.

Sprague showed that in order to avoid placing the patient in the supine position, spinal anesthesia should be induced with the patient in the *right* lateral position. Subsequent placement in the left semilateral position with a wedge under the right hip allows for immediate left uterine displacement and for more even distribution of the hyperbaric local anesthetic through the subarachnoid space.[26]

Medications for Spinal Anesthesia

Table 12-1 lists current medications as well as their durations of action.

Hyperbaric bupivacaine, 0.75%, has become a popular local anesthetic for cesarean section in our hospital in recent years. The addition of 0.2 mg of epinephrine will improve the quality of analgesia.[27] Recently intrathecal narcotics have been administered together with local anesthetics at the time of administration of spinal anesthesia. A combination of local anesthetic and narcotic has been shown to intensify the sensory anesthesia; visceral nociceptive afferents have also been found

Table 12–1. Medications for Spinal Anesthesia

Drugs in Current Use	Duration of Surgical Anesthesia
0.5% tetracaine in 5% dextrose	90–120 minutes
5% lidocaine in 7.5% dextrose in water	45–60 minutes
0.75% bupivacaine in 8.5% dextrose in water	90–120 minutes
0.5% bupivacaine in 8.0% dextrose in water	90–120 minutes but not yet approved by FDA
5% meperidine in 10% dextrose, same volume to make it hyperbaric	45–50 minutes

to be blunted. Fentanyl (6.25 to 12.5 μg) mixed with 0.75% bupivacaine was associated with excellent intraoperative analgesia as well as a few hours of postoperative pain relief.[16] Courtney and colleagues recently observed longer postoperative pain relief with 10 μg of sufentanil as compared with 6.25 μg of fentanyl.[28] Subarachnoid morphine, 0.1 to 0.5 mg, mixed with 0.75% hyperbaric bupivacaine has also been used,[29] with postoperative pain relief lasting between 17 and 27 hours. However, one should be aware of the possibility of delayed respiratory depression with the use of subarachnoid morphine. Addition of small doses of clonidine (30–60 mcg) mixed with fentanyl and morphine will improve postoperative pain relief. Using the dose-response effect of intrathecal morphine, 0.1 mg was observed to be optimal with fewer side effects.[7c] Recently, 0.4 mg of butorphanol mixed with 0.75% hyperbaric bupivacaine was used in the subarachnoid space. Postoperative analgesia lasted as long as 8.2 hours, but this has not become popular at this time.[30] Interestingly, intrathecal meperidine has been used exclusively (1 mg/kg) for cesarean section with success. One study compared 5% hyperbaric lidocaine with 1 mg/kg hyperbaric meperidine for cesarean section. The duration of sensory anesthesia was longer with hyperbaric meperidine.[31] The newer anesthetics levobupivacaine and ropivacaine do not add any great advantage.

Summary of Spinal Anesthesia for Cesarean Section

1. Bicitra, 30 mL, and metoclopramide, 10 mg, intravenously (unless contraindicated)
2. Good intravenous access and use of Ringer's lactate, unless contraindicated
3. Monitoring of pulse, blood pressure, electrocardiogram (ECG), and oxygen saturation
4. Hyperbaric bupivacaine, 0.75% (12 mg), except in extreme heights, mixed with 0.2 mL of fentanyl or 0.1 to 0.2 mg of morphine, depending upon the institution
5. Use of 27-gauge Quincke or 25-gauge Whitacre needles
6. Right lateral position for induction of spinal anesthesia
7. Routine left uterine displacement during surgery until delivery of the baby

8. Treatment of a drop in maternal blood pressure: ephedrine in 5 to 10 mg increments and additional volume expansion; phenylephrine (Neo-Synephrine), 40 µg, in incremental doses, if ephedrine is contraindicated
9. Oxygen by face mask
10. Close monitoring for delayed respiratory depression if subarachnoid morphine is used

Continuous spinal anesthesia can be used in patients with short stature and morbidly obese parturients because one can use small doses to build up the level of sensory anesthesia to reduce the incidence of hypotension and avoid an overly high block.

Contraindications for Single Shot Spinal Anesthesia for Cesarean Section

1. Severe maternal bleeding
2. Severe maternal hypotension
3. Coagulation disorders
4. Some forms of neurological disorders
5. Patient refusal
6. Technical problems
7. Short stature and morbidly obese parturients
8. Sepsis, local in the area of needle insertion or generalized

Continuous spinal anesthesia may be used if there is an accidental dural tap while performing the epidural anesthesia or where intentional dural puncture is made by an epidural needle e.g. in obese parturients. Small doses of local anesthetic 6 mg of bupivacaine mixed 10 mcg of fentanyl and 0.1 mg of morphine can be used for initiation of the block. Further local anesthetic can be given by the catheter if needed.

Epidural Anesthesia

Advantages of epidural anesthesia for cesarean section include the following:

1. Lesser incidence and severity of maternal hypotension
2. Avoidance of dural puncture, which may diminish the incidence of headaches. At this time it is controversial.

3. With a catheter technique, can be used for longer operations and also for postoperative pain relief, either with local anesthetics or epidural narcotics

Disadvantages of epidural analgesia include the following:

1. Increased complexity of the technique with a greater chance of failure. (This has *not* been the case in our institution.)
2. Slower onset of anesthesia, so not useful in urgent situations; this may be avoided to a certain extent by adding bicarbonate to the local anesthetic.
3. Need for larger amounts of local anesthetic agent

Problems

Cardiovascular Effects. There are substantial differences between the cardiovascular effects of lumbar epidural anesthesia and spinal anesthesia for cesarean delivery. A reduction in arterial blood pressure is usually less in epidural anesthesia because of the slower onset of the block.

Local anesthetic containing epinephrine (1:200,000), when used for cesarean section, may contain epinephrine from 100 to 125 μg when injected into the epidural space. Systemic absorption of epinephrine can cause a decrease in maternal blood pressure because of its β-mimetic effect.[32]

Technical Factors. Maternal position affects both the adequacy of anesthesia and fetal outcome. We found that placing the mother in the lateral position during induction of a lumbar epidural block for cesarean delivery did not affect the adequacy of the block and resulted in improved acid-base values in umbilical cord blood.[33] Higher concentrations of bupivacaine *were found in the umbilical cord blood of the more acidotic fetuses delivered to mothers who had been supine. This is probably the result of "ion trapping" of the weakly basic local anesthetic in the more highly acidic fetal blood.* However, none of the newborns in this study demonstrated any untoward effects as a result of the higher level of bupivacaine. We routinely keep our parturients in the semisitting position during induction of anesthesia. With this technique, one can ensure an adequate block of the sacral nerves in order to block pelvic pain during delivery and during traction of the vagina and peritoneal structures. An additional advantage of this maneuver may lie in the higher cardiac output in the pregnant woman while in the sitting position as compared with the supine position.

Complications

1. Unintentional intravascular injection of local anesthetic through the epidural catheter occurs in approximately 2.3% of patients.
2. The incidence of dural puncture varies between 0.2% and 20%, depending on the experience of the anesthesiologist. The incidence of PDPH with a 17-gauge needle may be as high as 76%.
3. The incidence of venous air embolism during cesarean delivery has been reported to be between 9.5% and 65%,[34,35] and this can happen during epidural, spinal, and general anesthesia. Air emboli in the pulmonary circulation may cause a ventilation/perfusion mismatch and can lower oxygen saturation.[36] Chest pain and dyspnea may be associated with venous air embolism, and ECC changes have also been observed. *The majority of changes have been noted with uterine incision and delivery*[34] *as well as at the time of uterine exteriorization.*[37] *Hence, oxygen saturation, blood pressure, and pulse should be closely monitored during delivery and immediately postpartum.*
4. The incidence of shivering after induction of epidural anesthesia has been observed to vary from 14% to 68%. The peak onset of shivering usually takes place 10 minutes after induction of epidural anesthesia.[38] The mechanism of shivering is not known; however, the incidence can be decreased by epidural fentanyl[39] or sufentanil[40] or by intravenous meperidine.

Contraindications

1. Severe maternal hypotension
2. Coagulation disorders
3. Some forms of neurological disorders
4. Patient refusal

5. Technical problems
6. Sepsis, local in the area of needle insertion or generalized

Local Anesthetics for Cesarean Delivery

Table 12-2 lists current medications as well as their durations of action.

Unless contraindicated, 2% lidocaine with epinephrine is my drug of choice because of its excellent sensory and motor anesthesia and its long duration of action. The lower concentration of bupivacaine (0.5%) provides a slower onset of action; hence, there is a lesser incidence of hypotension. Recently both 0.5% ropivacaine and 0.5% levobupivacaine have been compared with 0.5% bupivacaine for cesarean section.[41,42] Ropivacaine was associated with a lesser degree and shorter duration of motor block. There were no differences between bupivacaine and levobupivacaine. The addition of 50 to 100 μg of fentanyl can improve the intensity of sensory anesthesia[41] and thus can reduce the requirements of added analgesics and tranquilizers during the operation. *2-Chloroprocaine is an ideal local anesthetic in the presence of fetal distress. Its short maternal half-life as well as fetal plasma half-life will be beneficial in such a situation.* The onset of the block can be hastened by adding 8.4 mEq of bicarb to the local anesthetic. This will not only make the block faster but also improve the quality of the block. One of the disadvantages of chloroprocaine for cesarean section is the poor quality and shorter duration of analgesia when epidural μ-agonist narcotics are used following the use of this local anesthetic. The mechanism of this is not known at the present time. However, 2-chloroprocaine or its metabolite chloroaminobenzoic acid

Table 12-2. Local Anesthetics for Cesarean Delivery

Drugs in Current Use	Duration of Surgical Anesthesia
Bupivacaine 0.5%	75–90 minutes
Ropivacaine 0.5%	75–90 minutes
Levobupivacaine 0.5%	75–90 minutes
Lidocaine with epinephrine 2%	75–90 minutes
2-chloroprocaine 3%	25–35 minutes

can act as a μ-antagonist. When the κ-agonist butorphanol, 2 mg, was used epidurally, we observed effective pain relief following the use of 2-chloroprocaine.[42] Morphine, 5 to 10 mg, has been used extensively for postoperative pain relief following epidural anesthesia, and its effect can last between 12 and 24 hours.[29] A more recent trend is to use a smaller amount of epidural morphine (3 mg).

Summary of Epidural Anesthesia for Cesarean Section

1. Bicitra and metoclopramide, 10 mg intravenously (unless contraindicated).
2. Acute volume expansion with a nondextrose solution (2,000 mL) unless contraindicated.
3. Monitoring of pulse and blood pressure, ECG, oxygen saturation, and fetal heart rate tracing during induction of anesthesia.
4. Two percent lidocaine with epinephrine, 0.5% bupivacaine, 5% ropivacaine, 0.5% levobupivacaine, or 3% 2-chloroprocaine. Continuous-infusion epidural analgesia with a low concentration of local anesthetic has become very popular at the present time for labor and delivery. One should note that larger amounts of a higher concentration of local anesthetic will be necessary for surgical anesthesia if cesarean section is contemplated in such a situation.
5. Routine left uterine displacement.
6. Treatment of decreases in maternal blood pressure with ephedrine (5 to 10 mg at a time) and further volume expansion. Phenylephrine (Neo-Synephrine) (40 μg) may be used in incremental doses if ephedrine is contraindicated.
7. Oxygen by face mask (6 to 8 L/min) (Fig. 12-6) to maintain better maternal and fetal acid-base values.
8. Close monitoring for delayed respiratory depression if epidural morphine is used.

Cardiovascular Complications of Bupivacaine and Neurological Complications of 2-Chloroprocaine

Albright in a 1979 editorial in *Anesthesiology* pointed out the higher incidence of cardiac arrest associated with highly

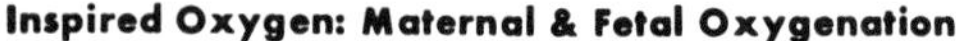

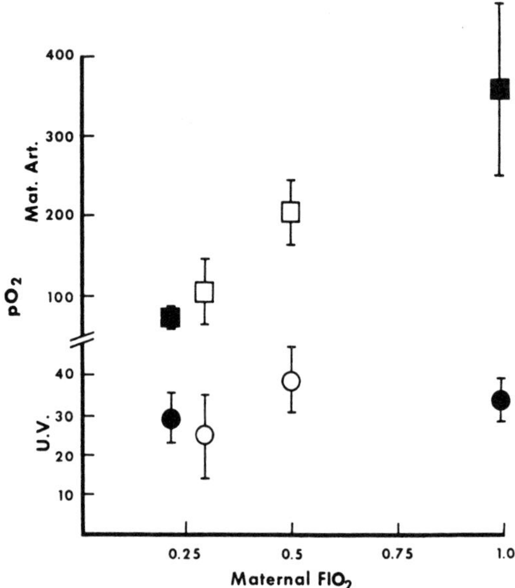

Figure 12-6. Influence of maternal inspired oxygen on maternal and fetal oxygenation at birth during cesarean section under epidural and general anesthesia. *Filled circles* (fetal) and *filled squares* (maternal) indicate epidural analgesia, whereas *open circles* and *squares* indicate a light general anesthesia plus relaxant. (From Bromage PR: *Epidural Analgesia.* Philadelphia, WB Saunders Co, 1978, p 578. Used with permission from Elsevier.)

lipid-soluble and protein-bound drugs like etidocaine and mainly bupivacaine.[43] The incidence of cardiac arrhythmias and cardiac arrest was higher in parturients receiving 0.75% bupivacaine; in 1980 the FDA banned the use of 0.75% bupivacaine in obstetric patients. Numerous animal studies were performed following Albright's report regarding the central nervous system (CNS) and cardiovascular system toxicity of different clinically used local anesthetics, and these can be summarized as follows:

1. The CC/CNS ratio (CC toxicity, cardiovascular collapse; CNS toxicity, convulsion) was lower for bupivacaine and etidocaine when compared with lidocaine.
2. Ventricular arrhythmias, fatal ventricular fibrillation, and cardiac arrest occurred after the rapid intravenous injection of bupivacaine.
3. *Pregnant animals were found to be more sensitive than nonpregnant animals to the cardiotoxic effects of bupivacaine.*
4. *Cardiac resuscitation following bupivacaine toxicity was much more difficult* than in the case of lidocaine. Hypoxia and acidosis were important factors for this problem.

As a rule, the cardiovascular system is more resistant than the CNS to local anesthetic. The CC/CNS ratio of lidocaine in adult sheep was 7.1 ± 1.1, whereas with bupivacaine and etidocaine it was 3.7 ± 0.5 and 4.4 ± 0.9, respectively.[44,45] The same group of observers also noticed a higher sensitivity of the myocardium to bupivacaine in pregnant animals than in nonpregnant animals. The CC/CNS ratio for nonpregnant animals was 3.7 ± 0.5 as compared with 2.7 ± 0.4 in pregnant animals.[46a] In a subsequent study, the authors did not observe any enhancement of systemic toxicity of ropivacaine or bupivacaine during pregnancy. The exact mechanism for this difference in sensitivity in pregnant animals is not known; however, the authors speculated that the lower protein binding in pregnancy may be responsible for this increased sensitivity. Using an in vitro model, Moller and colleagues observed a significantly higher depression of V_{max} of ventricular muscles obtained from progesterone-treated animals as compared with controls.[46b] It is possible that progesterone and its metabolites can interfere with sodium, potassium, or calcium channels. A study using B-estradiol in a rabbit ventricular muscle and Purkinjee fibers model observed depression of V_{max}.[46c] Higher degree of depression of Vmax in case of bupivacaine. Clarkson and Hondeghem, observing the sodium channel blocking effect of bupivacaine, suggested that in high concentrations lidocaine blocked sodium channels in a fast-in–fast-out manner, bupivacaine in low concentrations blocked sodium channels in a slow-in–slow-out manner, whereas in high concentrations the block was of the fast-in—slow-out type.[47] The practical implication of this phenomenon is important: this might be one of the reasons for the longer resuscitation time required for bupivacaine cardiotoxicity. Kasten and Martin showed successful cardiovascular resuscitation after a massive intravenous bupivacaine overdosage in dogs by (1) ventilation with 100% O_2, (2) open heart massage, (3) *bretylium for ventricular tachycardia; unless circulation is present, cardioversion will be necessary,* and (4) *epinephrine and atropine for electromechanical dissociation and bradycardia.*[48]

The following is a summary of the cardiovascular complications of bupivacaine:

1. Bupivacaine is more cardiotoxic than is lidocaine.
2. *Parturients may be more susceptible than nonpregnant patients to bupivacaine cardiotoxicity,* but the mechanism is unknown.
3. *The resuscitation time following bupivacaine administration may be longer, and one must remember to relieve aortocaval compression by proper left uterine displacement.*
4. *Epinephrine and atropine may be necessary in high doses.*
5. *Amiodarone should be the drug of choice for the treatment of ventricular tachyarrhythmias.*
6. The treatment of hypoxia and acidosis should be prompt. 2-Chloroprocaine neurotoxicity has been discussed in Chapter 11.
7. Amrinone may be the drug of choice to treat bupivacaine induced myocardial depression.
8. If necessary woman can be resuscitated in a heart lung machine.

Differences Between Spinal and Epidural Anesthesia for Cesarean Delivery

Table 12-3 lists the differences between spinal and epidural anesthesia for cesarean delivery.

Table 12-3. Differences Between the Spinal and Epidural Anesthesia for Cesarean Delivery

Spinal Anesthesia	Epidural Anesthesia
Advantages	
Simple, rapid, reliable	Lesser incidence of hypotension
Prolonged recovery room stay	Prolonged recovery room stay
Minimal drug exposure	Avoidance of dural puncture
An awake mother	With a catheter, it can be used for a longer operation and for postoperative pain relief
Disadvantages	
Hypotension	More complex
Nausea and vomiting	Longer onset time
Headache	Large amount of local anesthetic required
Limited duration of action unless a continuous technique is utilized	
Combined spinal and epidural anestheia	
Advantages Shortened recovery room stay if small amount of local anesthetic used for spinal block	

Combined Spinal Epidural (CSE) Technique

The CSE technique has been popularized by a group from Sweden.[49] The authors suggested the following advantages of CSE technique: 1) Speed of onset 2) Superior surgical analgesia and muscular relaxation 3) Lesser need for supplementary analgesics, sedatives, and antiemetics 4) Lower incidences of hypotension 5) Lower dose of local anesthetics in the mother and fetus 6) Blocking of sacral nerve roots due to use of hyperbaric local anesthetic 7) CSE block appears to combine the reliability of spinal block and the versatility of epidural block. If properly done, the epidural technique may be associated with all of the advantages as mentioned by the author. Davies et al, conducted a randomized blind study comparing CSE technique with the epidural procedure. Their conclusions were, both epidural anesthesia and CSE were associated with lower failure rates, with good operative conditions, and it also conferred high levels of maternal satisfaction. Maternal advantages with CSE technique included greater satisfaction after block placement before surgery and reduced pain during delivery of the fetus.[49a] One can use a small amount of local anesthetic for the spinal part of the CSE block. This will be associated with short recovery room stay.[50] One can always activate the epidural catheter when necessary.

General Anesthesia

The practice of general anesthesia for cesarean delivery has undergone considerable change in the past three decades, with abandonment of the flammable anesthetics ether and cyclopropane.

The *advantages* of general anesthesia are as follows:

1. Speed of induction
2. Reliability
3. Reproducibility
4. Controllability
5. Avoidance of hypotension

The following are *disadvantages* of general anesthesia:

1. Possibility of maternal aspiration
2. Problems of airway management
3. Narcotization of the newborn
4. Maternal awareness during light general anesthesia

Complications of General Anesthesia

Maternal Aspiration

Since Mendelson recognized the importance of gastric pH in maternal aspiration, the necessity of neutralizing this acid has become apparent.[49a] Roberts and Shirley reported the aspiration of gastric contents during anesthesia for cesarean delivery despite the previous administration of particulate antacids.[50a] Another disturbing factor is the demonstration, in animals, that particulate antacids, if aspirated, may cause physiological and structural alterations in the lung. *Nonparticulate antacids* (0.3M *sodium citrate or Bicitra*) *avoid this problem.*[51] Dewan and colleagues demonstrated the effectiveness of 30mL of *0.3M* sodium citrate administered within an hour of induction of cesarean .section. None of the parturients given sodium citrate had gastric aspirates at risk ($pH < 2.5$) of acid aspiration.[52] Proper mixing of antacid with the gastric contents is important.

Anticholinergics. Glycopyrrolate (Robinul), an anticholinergic, has been advocated because of its ability to decrease gastric secretions. *However, it can relax the gastroesophageal sphincter.* Hypothetically, this action might increase the risk of regurgitation and aspiration.

Other Pharmacological Agents. The histamine (H_2) receptor antagonists cimetidine and ranitidine have recently been used to inhibit basal gastric acid secretion in order to increase the gastric pH and decrease gastric volume.[53] *Metoclopramide, which increases gastric motility as well as esophageal sphincter tone, is a commonly used medication, especially for parturients undergoing cesarean section under general anesthesia.*[54] Metoclopramide also has a central antiemetic property related to its antidopaminergic action on the chemoreceptor trigger zone (CTZ).[55]

Airway Management

Parturients decrease arterial oxygen saturation faster than nonpregnant women (*Table 12-4*), *and this is related to increased oxygen consumption and decreased functional residual capacity.* Preoxygenation with 100% oxygen is absolutely essential before the induction of anesthesia. *Norris and Dewan*[56] *compared two methods of preoxygenation: 100% oxygen for 3 minutes vs. four maximal deep breaths in 30 seconds. The mean* Pa_{O_2} *was not different between the groups. Hence in a situation of acute fetal distress, four deep breaths of 100% oxygen may suffice.* Rapid-sequence induction utilizing cricoid pressure (Sellick's maneuver) followed by endotracheal intubation is the routine induction procedure. *Routine* O_2 *and* CO_2 *monitoring devices should be used.*

An additional hazard of general anesthesia could be a difficulty or impossibility of endotracheal intubation following the intravenous induction of anesthesia. It may be possible to continue administering inhalation anesthesia by mask, or it may be necessary to discontinue the procedure and have the women recover to allow time for reassessment and the adoption of an alternative anesthetic strategy. A means of instituting transtracheal ventilation should be immediately available in every obstetric suite. Recently Patel described a system for delivering transtracheal ventilation. It consists of a 12- or 14-gauge intravenous catheter that will connect easily to the adapter of a 3-mm endotracheal tube. The end of this system can be attached easily to any bag-valve device for ventilation.

Recently, laryngeal mask airway has been used in parturients difficult to ventilate with success[57]; however, the possibility of aspiration in such cases remains the major problem.

A difficult or failed intubation drill is extremely important, and every institution should have a plan before the situation arises (Table 12-5). When a difficult intubation is suspected, close communication with the obstetrician and the woman is absolutely vital to make the final decision.

Table 12-4. Maternal Oxygen Tension in Pregnant and Nonpregnant Patients Following Apnea

	Parturient Women		Gynecological Patients	
Parameter	Before Apnea	After Apnea (1 min)	Before Apnea	After Apnea (1 min)
Pa_{O_2} (mm Hg)	473 ± 34*†	334 ± 43*†	507 ± 38	449 ± 40
Pa_{CO_2} (mm Hg)	31.4 ± 2.4	40.4 ± 2.7	35.6 ± 1.8	44.3 ± 1.1
pH	7.41 ± 0.02	7.33 ± 0.01	7.45 ± 0.02	7.35 ± 0.01

From Archer GW, et al: *Br J Anaesth* 1974; 46:358 © The Board of Management and Trustees of the British Journal of Anaesthesia. Reproduced by permission of Oxford University Press/British Journal of Anaesthesia.

†$P < 0.05$.

Table 12–5. Steps in a Drill When Intubation is Difficult During Cesarean Section

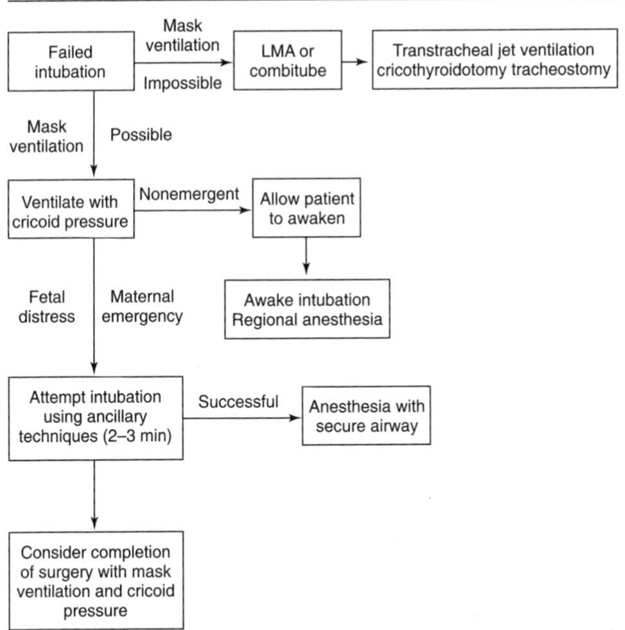

Adapted from Malan TP, Johnson MO: *J Clin Anesth* 1988;1:104.

Comparison of Regional and General Anesthesia

Regional Anesthesia

Many anesthesiologists will prefer either epidural or a continuous spinal technique in such a situation as mentioned above (difficult airway), and these should be instituted if possible before the onset of active labor.

The *advantages* of regional anesthesia include the following:

1. They can be used for an acute fetal distress situation without facing difficult intubation and thus promoting further fetal compromise.

2. The woman is awake, and thus there is less chance of gastric aspiration.
3. The continuous spinal technique can be induced in a very short time and can be used for fetal distress if the catheter is not already in position.

If regional anesthesia is elected, meticulous technique is absolutely essential to avoid accidental intravascular or subarachnoid injection. The continuous spinal technique has one major advantage in that a small amount of local anesthetic can be used to build the level up gradually.

Disadvantages of regional anesthesia include the following:

1. *Accidental intravascular injection with a possibility of convulsion, cardiovascular collapse, and aspiration.*
2. *Accidental subarachnoid injection causing total spinal anesthesia with the possibility of severe hypotension, unconsciousness, and aspiration. Obviously, in both these situations, ventilation with 100% oxygen will be absolutely essential. These will be the main reasons to avoid regional anesthesia.*

General Anesthesia

The *advantages* of general anesthesia include the following:

1. *One obviously will be able to secure the airway. Awake intubation by using either a laryngoscope or fiber-optic technique after anesthetizing the oral cavity with local anesthetic will be the method of choice.*
2. *One can avoid the complications of regional anesthesia (accidental intravascular or subarachnoid injection).*

The following are *disadvantages* of general anesthesia:

1. It might take a longer time; hence, it may not be ideal in acute fetal distress situations.
2. Maternal discomfort.

Neonatal Depression

Causes of neonatal depression under general anesthesia can be classified as follows:

I. Physiological causes
   A. Maternal hypoventilation

B. Maternal hyperventilation
C. Reduced uteroplacental perfusion due to aortocaval compression

II. Pharmacological causes
A. Induction agents
B. Neuromuscular blockers
C. Low oxygen concentration
D. Nitrous oxide and other inhalational agents
E. Effect of prolonged induction-delivery and uterine incision-delivery intervals

Physiological Causes

The physiological changes of pregnancy render the parturient more susceptible to rapid changes in blood gas tension. Hypoventilation will reduce the oxygen tension in the mother and in turn will cause neonatal acid-base alterations or biochemical depression. *Maternal hyperventilation may also impose potential harm to the fetus during general anesthesia by decreasing fetal oxygen tension. Mechanisms (Fig. 12-7) that have been invoked to explain this phenome-*

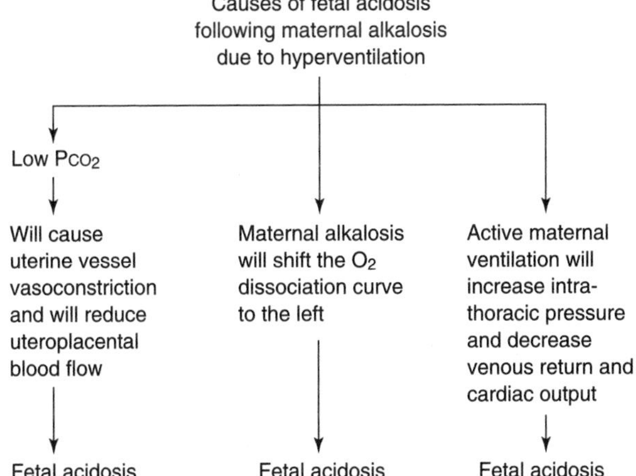

Figure 12-7. Causes of fetal acidosis following maternal alkalosis due to hyperventilation.

non[58] *include* (*1*) *vasoconstriction of umbilical vessels secondary to maternal hypocarbia,* (*2*) *altered maternal hemodynamics secondary to increased intrathoracic pressure during hyperventilation that causes a reduction in aortic and uterine blood flow, and* (*3*) *a shift of the maternal oxyhemoglobin dissociation curve to the left* (Fig. 12-8). A minute

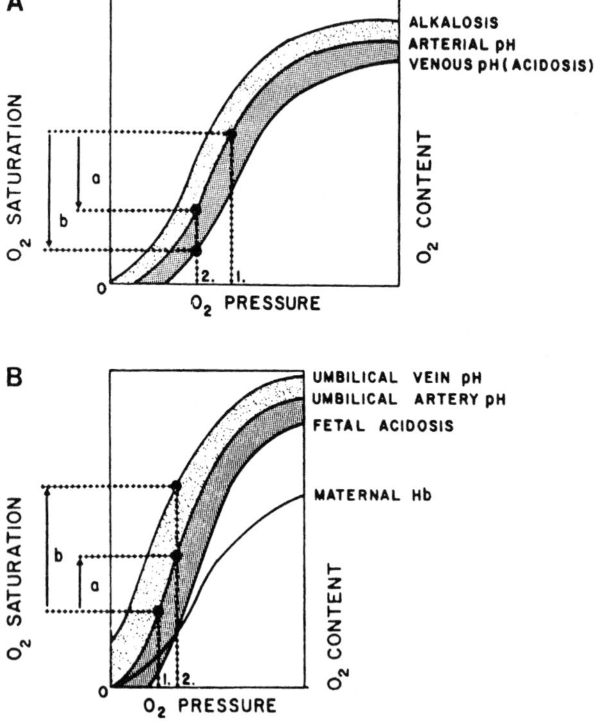

Figure 12-8. Hemoglobin dissociation curves of mother and fetus at the intervillous space and the importance of maternal P_{CO_2}. A lower maternal P_{CO_2} will shift the curve to the left. (From Abouleish E: The placenta and placental transfer of drugs of term, in *Pain Control in Obstetrics.* Philadelphia. JB Lippincott, 1977, p 4. Used by permission.)

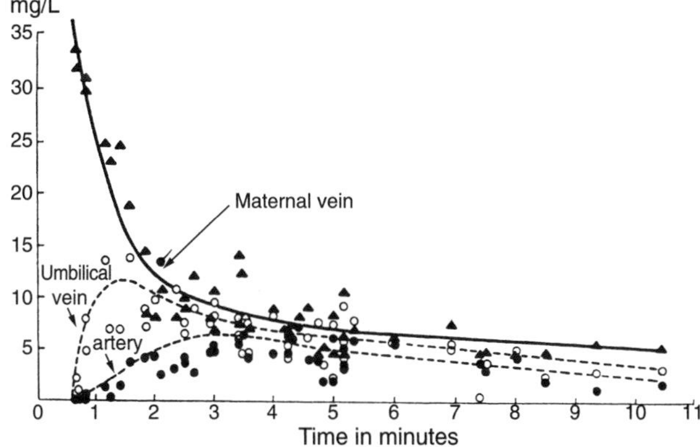

Figure 12–9. Thiamylal concentrations in the maternal vein, umbilical vein, and umbilical artery. (From Kosaka Y, Takahashi T, Mark LC: *Anesthesiology* 1969; 31:489. Used by permission.)

volume in excess of 10 mL/kg/min should be avoided during general anesthesia.

Aortocaval compression becomes more important when abdominal delivery is undertaken for suspected or documented fetal asphyxia. The imposition of a further increment in asphyxia by permitting the patient to be supine will be highly detrimental to the fetus. Better fetal outcomes result from avoiding aortocaval compression.

Pharmacological Causes

Induction Agents. Standard practice is induction of anesthesia with an intravenous injection of thiobarbiturate, usually thiopental. The recommended dose is 4 mg/kg pregnant body weight. Thiobarbiturates cross the placenta rapidly and are detected in fetal blood within seconds of their administration to the mother (Fig. 12-9). *The concentration of umbilical vein blood remains lower than that of maternal vein blood; the concentration of umbilical artery blood is lower than that of umbilical vein blood*[59] *These gradients result from (1) a rapid* *decline in concentration of thiobarbiturate in maternal blood secondary to rapid redistribution,* (2) *nonhomogeneous distribution in the intervillous space,* (3) *extraction of thiobarbiturate from umbilical vein blood by the fetal liver, and* (4) *progressive dilution through shunting in the fetal circulation.* Ketamine (1 to 1.5 mg/kg) may be the induction agent of choice in the presence of hemorrhage. The recently approved nonbarbiturate induction agent propofol (2 to 2.5 mg/kg) did not show any significant advantage for cesarean section.[60] Etomidate (0.3 mg/kg) has been associated with less myocardial depression and greater hemodynamic stability (hypovolemic patient) when compared with thiopental. A summary of induction agents is shown in Table 12-6.

Neuromuscular Blockers. Neuromuscular blockers are highly ionizable, and except in unusual circumstances, there is little observable effect on the newborn that can be attributed to muscle relaxants. Studies of *d*-tubocurarine, pancuronium, metocurine, and succinylcholine suggest that after a volume injection small quantities of these drugs may cross the placenta but maternal paralyzing doses do not affect the fetus. However, prolonged maternal and newborn neuromuscular blockade has been reported after the administration of succinylcholine to the mother.[61] This was due to the presence of atypical pseudocholinesterase in both the mother and newborn. Many authors recommend the administration of a small dosage of a nondepolarizing muscle relaxant *before the use of succinylcholine to prevent fasciculations and an associated increase in intragastric pressure.*[62] This concept is not agreed upon universally; opponents will not use any nondepolarizing muscle relaxants prior to the use of succinylcholine because (1) *parturients rarely undergo fasciculations after succinylcholine*[63]; (2) *succinylcholine produces inconsistent and unpredictable elevations in intragastric pressure*[64]; (3) *succinylcholine tends to increase lower esophageal sphincter pressure in association with increased intragastric pressure, and thus the barrier pressure remains essentially unchanged*[65]; (4) *intubation may be difficult if a nondepolarizing muscle relaxant is used prior to succinylcholine;* and (5) muscle pain after succinylcholine administration is negligible following cesarean section. There is a report of only one case of prolonged neonatal paralysis after the use of *d*-tubocurarine; here a total dose of 245 mg was used over a period of 10 hours to control maternal convulsions. Atracurium is a short-acting drug, and the placental transfer has been observed to be only 5% to 20%.

Oxygenation. Fetal oxygenation is also affected by maternal inspired oxygen concentrations. A higher maternal inspired oxygen concentration will increase both maternal and fetal oxygen tensions and will improve the fetal condition at birth. A maternal inspired oxygen concentration of 65% to 70% appears to yield optimal results. *Contrary to earlier reports, maternal hyperoxygenation does not result in fetal acidosis.* A significant amount of oxygen is extracted by the placenta.

Nitrous Oxide. *Nitrous oxide* crosses the placenta rapidly and attains a fetal umbilical artery/umbilical vein concentration ratio of 0.8 after 15 minutes. The prolonged administration of nitrous oxide in high concentrations may result in low Apgar scores, possibly caused by direct CNS depression and diffusion hypoxia. Our current practice is not to exceed a nitrous oxide concentration of 50%. Mankowitz and his associates[66] have demonstrated that newborns whose mothers received nitrous oxide (50% oxygen and 50% N_2O with 0.6% to 1.0% enflurane) for cesarean delivery were largely unaffected at birth. However, they recommend (as does the author) that all infants born to mothers who have received nitrous oxide before delivery receive oxygen or oxygen-enriched air, especially when the induction-to-delivery interval is prolonged, to further aid the infants to make the adaptation from intrauterine to extrauterine life.

Various inhalational agents have been used in combination with nitrous oxide, including halothane (Fluothane), methoxyflurane (Penthrane), trichloroethylene (Trilene), enflurane (Ethrane), and isoflurane (Forane). All are reported to produce satisfactory anesthesia with few side effects. The two new inhalation anesthetics sevoflurane and desflurane have been used for cesarean sections without any problems.

Effect of Induction-Delivery and Uterine Incision-Delivery Intervals. There is a difference of opinion about the optimal time for delivery of the infant when general anesthesia is used for cesarean delivery. Several authors found a better neonatal status when the induction-delivery interval was less than 10 minutes. More recently, Crawford et al. emphasized that if aortocaval compression is avoided, the inspired oxygen concentration is 65% to 70%, and there is no hypotension, then an induction-delivery interval as long as 30 minutes has no significant effect on the acid-base status of the newborn infants.[67] When we used 50% nitrous oxide/50% oxygen and a small concentration of a volatile agent to produce amnesia, we found no significant effect on the acid-base values and Apgar scores when babies were delivered within 10 minutes.

Another important factor related to the induction-delivery interval that may have considerable influence on the infant's condition is the duration of the uterine incision delivery interval. In the absence of hypotension during spinal anesthesia, the length of the induction-delivery interval is not a factor in regard to neonatal outcome as measured by Apgar scores and neonatal acid-base values. However, uterine incision delivery intervals longer than 180 seconds are associated with low Apgar scores as well as acidotic babies. During general anesthesia when induction-delivery intervals were greater than 8 minutes or uterine incision-delivery intervals were greater than or equal to 180 seconds, lower 1-minute Apgar scores (less than 7) and neonatal umbilical artery acidosis were present.[68] Recently, we observed that prolonged uterine incision-delivery intervals during regional anesthesia resulted in elevated fetal umbilical artery norepinephrine concentrations and associated fetal acidosis.[69] An adverse outcome with prolonged uterine incision–delivery intervals may be the result of (1) the effects of uterine manipulations on uteroplacental and umbilical blood flows, (2) pressure of the uterus with accentuation of aortocaval compression, (3) compression of the fetal head during a difficult delivery, or (4) inhalation of amniotic fluid as a result of gasping respirations by the fetus in utero. The presence of increased norepinephrine concentrations in the fetus may be a sign of fetal hypoxia.

Maternal Awareness

A major problem with general anesthesia for cesarean delivery is the incidence of maternal awareness and unpleasant recall associated with the use of small doses and low concentrations of anesthetics to minimize neonatal effects. Incidences of recall have been reported to range from 17% to 36%. The use of low concentrations of potent volatile anesthetic agents will successfully prevent awareness and recall without adverse neonatal effect or excessive uterine bleeding.[70]

Summary of General Anesthesia for Cesarean Delivery

1. Premedication with metoclopramide, 10 mg intravenously, and nonparticulate antacid (30mL of a 0.3*M* sodium citrate solution)
2. Monitoring of blood pressure, pulse, ECC, O_2 saturation, capnometer, temperature, blockade monitor
3. Left uterine displacement
4. Preoxygenation with 100% oxygen
5. Defasciculating dose of nondepolarizing muscle relaxant?
6. Induction with thiopental/ketamine/propofol and succinylcholine while maintaining cricoid pressure
7. Cuffed endotracheal tube
8. Fifty percent O_2, 50% N_2O with a small amount of isoflurane (0.75%), enflurane (1%), desflurane (4%)[70a] or sevoflurane (1.5%)[70b] unless contraindicated
9. Avoidance of hypoventilation or hyperventilation
10. Muscle relaxants: either a 0.1% succinylcholine drip or nondepolarizing muscle relaxants with the use of a blockade monitor
11. Desufflation of the stomach by a gastric tube
12. Minimization of the induction–delivery interval
13. Minimization of the uterine incision–delivery interval
14. Use of narcotics in the mother after delivery of the baby
15. Extubation performed when the mother is wide awake

Postoperative Pain Relief

Patient-controlled analgesia (PCA) has become extremely popular for postoperative pain relief following general anesthesia for cesarean section. Morphine remains the drug of choice for this purpose.[71] Sinatra and colleagues compared morphine, meperidine, and oxymorphone for PCA and observed a rapid onset and less sedation, nausea, vomiting, and pruritus with meperidine.[72] Recently, in a very interesting study the same group reported neonates whose mothers received meperidine for PCA scored lower in the neurobehavioral scoring system than did the morphine-treated group.[73] A significant amount of normeperidine was found in the breast milk of the mothers who received meperidine. The authors concluded that PCA with morphine for pain relief following cesarean section provided equivalent maternal analgesia and overall satisfaction to that provided by PCA with meperidine, but with significantly less neurobehavioral depression among breast-fed neonates on the third day of life. One should not expect such problems if meperidine PCA is not used for more than 24 hours.

Conclusion

Our understanding of the physiology, pharmacology, and clinical management of anesthesia for cesarean delivery has greatly advanced in recent years. If one meticulously follows the criteria for the various anesthetic techniques, one should expect an excellent maternal and fetal outcome with either general or regional anesthesia in the normal parturient.

References

1. Nageotte M: How we can lower the cesarean section rate. *Contemp Obstet Gynecol* 1990; 63:74.
2. Crocker JS, Vandam LD: Concerning nausea and vomiting during spinal anesthesia. *Anesthesiology* 1959; 20:589.
3. Ueland K, Gills RE, Hansen JM: Maternal cardiovascular dynamics. I. Cesarean section under subarachnoid block anesthesia. *Am J Obstet Gynecol* 1968; 100:42.
4. Cosmi EV, Marx GF: Acid-base status of the fetus and clinical condition of the newborn following cesarean section. *Am J Obstet Gynecol* 1968; 102:378.
5. Corke BC, Datta S, Ostheimer GW, et al: Spinal anesthesia for cesarean section: The influence of hypotension on neonatal outcome. *Anesthesiology* 1982; 37:658–662.

6. Hollmen AI, Joupilla R, Koivisto M, et al: Neurologic activity of infants following anesthesia for cesarean section. *Anesthesiology* 1978; 48:350–356.
7. Marx GF, Cosmi EV, Wollman SB: Biochemical status and clinical condition of mother and infant at cesarean section. *Anesth Analg* 1969; 48:968.
7a. Rout CC, Rocke DA, Levin J, et al: A reevaluation of the role of crystalloid preload in the prevention of hypotension associated with spinal anesthesia for effective cesarean section. *Anesthesiology* 1993; 79:262.
7b. Park GE, Hauch MA, Curlin F, Datta S, Bader A: The effects of varying volume preload before cesarean delivery on maternal hemodynamics and colloid osmotic pressure. *Anesth Analg* 1996; 83:299.
7c. Palmer CM, Emerson S, Volgoropolus, et al: Dose-response relationship of intrathecal morphine of postcesarean analgesia. *Anesthesiology* 1999; 90:437.
8. Kenepp NB, Shelley WC, Gabbe SC, et al: Fetal and neonatal hazards of maternal hydration with 5% dextrose before cesarean section. *Lancet* 1982; 1:1150.
9. Philipson EH, Kalhan SC, Riha MM, et al: Effects of maternal glucose infusion on fetal acid-base status in human pregnancy. *Am J Obstet Gynecol* 1987; 157:866.
10. Ramanathan S, Grant GJ: Vasopressor therapy for hypotension due to epidural anesthesia for cesarean section. *Acta Anaesthesiol Scand* 1988; 32:559.
11. Moran DH, Perillo M, LaPorta RF, et al: Phenylephrine in the prevention of hypotension following spinal anesthesia for cesarean delivery. *J Clin Anesth* 1991; 3:301.
12. Clark RB, Thompson DS, Thompson CH: Prevention of spinal hypotension with cesarean section. *Anesthesiology* 1976; 45:670.
13. Datta S, Alper MH, Ostheimer CW, et al: Method of ephedrine administration and nausea and hypotension during spinal anesthesia for cesarean section. *Anesthesiology* 1982; 56:68–70.
14. Bonica JJ, Crepps W, Monk B: Postanesthetic nausea, retching and vomiting. *Anesthesiology* 1958; 19:532.
15. Ackerman WE, Juneja MM, Colclough GW: Epidural fentanyl significantly decreases nausea and vomiting during uterine manipulation in awake patients undergoing cesarean section (abstract). *Anesthesiology* 1988; 69:679.
16. Hunt CO, Naulty S, Bader AM, et al: Perioperative analgesia with subarachnoid fentanyl-bupivacaine for cesarean delivery. *Anesthesiology* 1989; 71:535.

17. Santos A, Datta S: Prophylactic use of droperidol for control of nausea and vomiting during spinal anesthesia for cesarean section. *Anesth Analg* 1984; 63:85–87.
17a. Meister GC, D'Angelo R, Owen M, et al: A comparison of epidural analgesia with 0.125% ropivacaine with fentanyl versus 0.125% bupivacaine with fentanyl during labor. *Anesth Analg* 2000; 90:632.
18. Chestnut DH, Vandewalker CE, Owen CI: Administration of metoclopramide for prevention of nausea and vomiting during epidural anesthesia for elective cesarean section. *Anesthesiology* 1987; 66:563–566.
19. Bafill JA, Vincent RD, Ross EL, et al: Nulliparous active labor, epidural analgesia, and cesarean delivery for dystocia. *Am J Obstet Gynecol* 1997; 177:1465.
20. Chestnut DH, McGrath JM, Vincent RD, et al: Does early administration of epidural analgesia affect obstetric outcome in nulliparous women who are in spontaneous labor? *Anesthesiology* 1994; 80:1201.
21. Ready LB, Cuplin S, Haschke RH: Spinal needle determinants of rate of transdural fluid leak. *Anesth Analg* 1989; 69:457.
22. Kitahara T, Kuri S, Yoshida J: The spread of drugs used for spinal anesthesia. *Anesthesiology* 1956; 17:205.
23. Norris MC: Height, weight and the spread of subarachnoid hyperbaric bupivacaine in the term parturient. *Anesth Analg* 1988; 67:555.
24. DeSimone CA, Norris MC, Leighton B, et al: Spinal anesthesia with hyperbaric bupivacaine for cesarean section: A comparison of two doses (abstract). *Anesthesiology* 1988; 69:670.
25. Hartwell B, Aglio LS, Hauch MA, et al: Vertebral column length and spread of hyperbaric subarachnoid bupivacaine in the term parturient. *Reg Anaesth* 1991; 16:17.
26. Sprague DH: Effects of position and uterine displacement on spinal anesthesia for cesarean section. *Anesthesiology* 1974; 44: 164–166.
27. Abouleish EI: Epinephrine improves the quality of spinal hyperbaric bupivacaine for cesarean section. *Anesth Analg* 1987; 66: 395–400.
28. Courtney M. Bader AM, Hartwell BL, et al: Perioperative analgesia with subarachnoid sufentanil-bupivacaine (abstract). *Anesthesiology* 1990; 73:994.
29. Chadwick HS, Ready LB: Intrathecal and epidural morphine sulfate for postcesarean analgesia—A clinical comparison. *Anesthesiology* 1988; 68:925.

30. Gould DB, Singer SB, Smeltzer JS: Dose-response of subarachnoid butorphanol analgesia concurrent with bupivacaine for cesarean section. *Reg Anaesth* 1991; 15:46.
31. Kalfe SK: Intrathecal meperidine for elective Caesarean section: A comparison with lidocaine. *Can J Anaesth* 1993; 40:718.
32. Bonica JJ, Akamatsu TJ, Berges MU: Circulatory effect of peridural block. II. Effects of epinephrine. *Anesthesiology* 1971; 34:514.
33. Datta S, Alper MH, Ostheimer GW, et al: Effects of maternal position on epidural anesthesia for cesarean section, acid-base status, and bupivacaine concentrations at delivery. *Anesthesiology* 1979; 50:205–209.
34. Malinow AM, Naulty JS, Hunt CO, et al: Precordial ultrasonic monitoring during cesarean delivery. *Anesthesiology* 1987; 66:816.
35. Fong J, Gadalla F, Pierri MK: Are Doppler-detected venous air emboli during cesarean section air embolism? *Anesth Analg* 1990; 71:254.
36. Vartikar JV, Johnson MD, Datta S: Precordial Doppler monitoring and pulse oximetry during cesarean delivery: Detection of venous air embolism. *Reg Anaesth* 1989; 14:145.
37. Handler JS, Bromage PR: Venous air embolism during cesarean delivery. *Reg Anesth* 1990; 15:170.
38. Chan VWS, Morley-Forster PK, Vosu HA: Temperature changes and shivering after epidural anesthesia for cesarean section. *Reg Anaesth* 1989; 14:48.
39. Shebai Y, Gatt S, Buckman T: Effect of adrenaline, fentanyl and warming of injectate on shivering following extradural analgesia in labour. *Anaesth Intensive Care* 1990; 18:31.
40. Sevarino FB, Johnson MD, Lema MJ, et al: The effect of epidural sufentanil on shivering and body temperature in parturient. *Anesth Analg* 1989; 68:520.
41a. Gaffud MP, Bansal P, Lawton C: Surgical analgesia for cesarean delivery and epidural bupivacaine and fentanyl. *Anesthesiology* 1986; 65:331–334.
42a. Camann WR, Hartigan PM, Gilbertson LI, et al: Chloroprocaine antagonism of epidural opioid analgesia: A receptor-specific phenomenon? *Anesthesiology* 1990; 78:860.
43. Albright GA: Cardiac arrest following regional anesthesia with etidocaine and bupivacaine. *Anesthesiology* 1979; 51:285.
44. Morishima HO, Pedersen H, Finster M, et al: Is bupivacaine more cardiotoxic than lidocaine? (abstract). *Anesthesiology* 1983; 59:409.

45. Morishima HO, Pedersen H, Finster M, et al: Is etidocaine more cardiotoxic than lidocaine (abstract)? *Anesthesiology* 1982; 57:401.
46a. Morishima HO, Pedersen H, Finster M, et al: Bupivacaine toxicity in pregnant and nonpregnant ewes. *Anesthesiology* 1985; 63:134.
46b. Moller RA, Datta S, Fox J, et al: Progesterone-induced increase in cardiac sensitivity to bupivacaine. *Anesthesiology* 1988; 69:A675.
46c. Moller RA, Datta S, Strichartz GR: B-Estradiol acutely potentiates the depression of cardiac excitability by lidocaine and bupivacaine. J Cardiovasc Pharm 1999; 34:718.
47. Clarkson CW, Hondeghem LM: Mechanism for bupivacaine depression of cardiac conduction: Fast block of sodium channels during the action potential with slow recovery from block during diastole. *Anesthesiology* 1985; 62:396.
48. Kasten GW, Martin ST: Successful cardiovascular resuscitation after massive intravenous bupivacaine overdosage in anesthetized dogs. *Anesth Analg* 1985; 64:491.
49. Rawal N: Epidural versus combined spinal-epidural block for cesarean section. *Acta Anaesthesiol* Scand 1988; 31:61.
49a. Davies SJ, Paech MJ, Welch H, et al: Maternal experience during epidural or combined spinal-epidural anesthesia for cesarean section: A prospective, randomized trial. *Anesth Analg* 1997; 85:607.
50. Vercauteren MP, Coppejans HC, Hoffman VL, et al: Small-dose hyperbaric vs plain bupivacaine during spinal anesthesia for cesarean section. *Anesth Analg* 1998; 86:989
50a. Roberts RB, Shirley MA: Reducing the risk of acid aspiration during cesarean section. *Anesth Analg* 1974; 53:859.
51. Gibbs CP, Schwartz DJ, Wynne JW, et al: Antacid pulmonary aspiration in the dog. *Anesthesiology* 1979; 51:380.
52. Dewan DM, Floyd HM, Thistlewood JM, et al: Sodium citrate pretreatment in elective cesarean section patients. *Anesth Analg* 1985; 64:34.
53. Okasha AS, Motaweh MM, Bali A: Cimetidine-antacid combination as premedication for elective caesarean section. *Can Anaesth Soc J* 1983; 30:593.
54. Howard FA, Sharp DS: Effect of metoclopramide on gastric emptying during labour. *Br Med J* 1973; 1:446.
55. Harrington RA, Hamilton CW, Brogden RN, et al: Metoclopramide: An updated review of its pharmacological properties and clinical use. *Drugs* 1983; 24:451.

56. Norris MC, Dewan DM: Preoxygenation for cesarean section: A comparison of two techniques. *Anesthesiology* 1985; 62:827.
57. Hasham FM, et al: The laryngeal mask airway facilitates intubation at cesarean section: A case report of difficult intubation. *Int J Obstet Anesthesia* 1993; 2:185.
58. Levinson G, Shnider SM, deLorimier AA, et al: Effects of maternal hyperventilation on uterine blood flow and fetal oxygenation and acid-base status. *Anesthesiology* 1974; 40:340.
59. Kosaka Y, Takahashi T, Mark LC: Intravenous thiobarbiturate anesthesia for cesarean section. *Anesthesiology* 1969; 31:489.
60. Dailland P, Cockshott ID, Lirzin JD, et al: Intravenous propofol during cesarean section: Placental transter, concentration in breast milk and neonatal effects. A preliminary study. *Anesthesiology* 1989; 71:827.
61. Wiessman DB, Ehrenwerth J: Prolonged neuromuscular blockade in a parturient associated with succinylcholine. *Anesth Analg* 1983; 62:444.
62. Roe RB: The effect of suxamethonium on intragastric pressure. *Anaesthesia* 1962; 17:179.
63. Crawford JS: Suxamethonium muscle pains and pregnancy. *Br J Anaesth* 1971; 43:677.
64. Miller RD, Way L: Inhibition of succinylcholine induced increased intragastric pressure by nondepolarizing muscle relaxants and lidocaine. *Anesthesiology* 1971; 34:185.
65. Cotton BR, Smith G: The lower oesophageal sphincter and anaesthesia. *Br J Anaesth* 1984; 56:37.
66. Mankowitz E, Brock-Utne JG, Downing JW: Nitrous oxide elimination by the newborn. *Anaesthesia* 1981; 36:1014.
67. Crawford JS, James FJ, Crawley M: A further study of general anaesthesia for caesarean section. *Br J Anaesth* 1976; 48:661.
68. Datta S, Ostheimer GW, Weiss JB, et al: Neonatal effects of prolonged anesthetic induction for cesarean section. *Obstet Gynecol* 1981; 58:331.
69. Bader AM, Datta S, Arthur GR, et al: Maternal and fetal catecholamines and uterine incision-to-delivery interval during elective cesarean section. *Obstet Gynecol* 1990; 75:600.
70. Warren TM, Datta S, Ostheimer GW, et al: Comparison of the maternal and neonatal effects of halothane, enflurane, and isoflurane for cesarean delivery. *Anesth Analg* 1983; 62:516.
70a. Abboud TK, Zhu J, Richardson M, et al: Desflurane a new volatile anesthetic for cesarean section. Maternal and neonatal effects. *Acta Anaesthesiol Scand* 1995; 39(6):723.

70b. Gambling DR, Sharma SK, White PF, et al: Use of sevoflurane during elective cesarean birth: a comparison with isoflurane and spinal anesthesia. *Anesth Analg* 1995; 81(1):90.
71. Harrison DM, Sinatra RS, Morgese L, et al: Epidural narcotics and PCA for post-cesarean section pain relief. *Anesthesiology* 1988; 68:454.
72. Sinatra RS, Lodge K, Sibert K, et al: A comparison of morphine, meperidine and oxymorphone as utilized in PCA following cesarean delivery. *Anesthesiology* 1989; 70:585.
73. Wittels B, Scott DT, Sinatra RS: Exogenous opioids in human breast milk and acute neonatal neurobehavior: A preliminary study. *Anesthesiology* 1990; 73:864.

13
High–Risk Pregnancy

Neurological Problems
Paraplegia
Cerebrovascular accidents
Multiple sclerosis
Space-occupying lesions (brain tumors)
Epilepsy
Myasthenia gravis

Renal Disorders
Physiological changes
Anesthetic management

Hematological Disorders
Anesthetic management
Sickle cell disease
Idiopathic thrombocytopenia

Hypercoaguable States

Factor V Leiden Mutation

Endocrine Disorders
Hyperthyroidism
Pheochromocytoma

Problems Because of Miscellaneous Factors
Prematurity
Postmaturity

Autoimmune Disease
Rheumatoid arthritis
Systemic lupus erythematosus

Breech Presentation
Multiple gestation
Anesthetic management

Maternal Addiction
Alcohol
Amphetamines
Cocaine

Infectious Diseases
Genital herpes
Infection with the human immunodeficiency virus

Emboli in Pregnancy
Thrombotic embolism
Amniotic fluid embolism
Venous air embolism

Psychiatric Disorders
Clinical implications

Malignant Hyperthermia
Anesthetic management

A parturient is designated as "high risk" because of the various problems that might arise in the antenatal or peripartum periods. Anesthetic management—both in choice and technique—should be based on a thorough understanding of the physiology of pregnancy and also on the pathophysiology of the problems that made the parturients "high risk." Any high-risk parturient can be a potential candidate for an obstetric emergency. Hence, continuous vigilance and constant communication with the obstetric team is mandatory.

Classification

I. Maternal
   A. Problems related to pregnancy, labor, and delivery:
      1. Antepartum hemorrhage—placenta previa, abruptio placentae
      2. Hypertensive disorders of pregnancy
   B. Problems unrelated to pregnancy:
      1. Diabetes mellitus
      2. Cardiac disorders
      3. Respiratory disorders
      4. Neurological disorders
      5. Renal disorders
      6. Hematological disorders
      7. Endocrinological disorders
      8. Maternal addiction, history of malignant hyperthermia, obesity

   9. Autoimmune disease
   10. Embolic problems
   11. Psychological problems

II. Fetal
   A. Problems related to pregnancy, labor, and delivery:
      1. Prematurity
      2. Postmaturity
      3. Multiple gestations
      4. Abnormal presentations
      5. Intrauterine growth retardation
      6. Prolapsed cord
      7. Placental insufficiency
      8. Preeclampsia
      9. Diabetes mellitus

Techniques of Anesthesia (Keys to Successful Management)

Subarachnoid Block

1. A large-bore intravenous catheter (16-gauge or larger is preferred) should be used unless contraindicated. A predetermined amount of intravenous volume expansion has recently been challenged. Monitoring should include pulse and blood pressure, electrocardiogram (ECG), O_2 saturation, and precordial sounds.
2. Avoid the supine position to prevent aortocaval compression.
3. Use a small needle (27-gauge Quincke or 25-gauge Whitacre) to reduce the incidence of post-dural puncture headache (PDPH).
4. Tetracaine, lidocaine, or bupivacaine (most popular) local anesthetic.
5. Prompt treatment of hypotension with a bolus infusion of crystalloid and increments of ephedrine, 5 to 10 mg intravenously as needed, and phenylephrine (Neo-Synephrine), 40 μg at a time if necessary.
6. Oxygen by face mask (6 or more L/min).
7. Minimize the induction delivery interval.
8. Minimize the uterine incision delivery interval.

During general anesthesia, prolonged induction-delivery and uterine incision–delivery intervals were associated with a higher incidence of low Apgar scores and acidotic babies. On the other hand, with spinal anesthesia in the absence of hypotension, a longer induction–delivery interval did not alter either the Apgar score or the acid-base values of the neonates. However, a uterine incision delivery interval of more than 180 seconds was associated with a high incidence of low Apgar scores and acidotic infants; this might be related to reduced placental circulation.

Epidural Block

1. Proper selection of the local anesthetic—bupivacaine, ropivacaine, levobupivacaine, lidocaine, or 2-chloroprocaine.
2. Adequate prehydration (approximately 1,500 to 2,000 mL of Ringer's lactate solution) before initiation of blockade via a large-bore cannula (16 gauge or larger is preferred) and monitoring as for the spinal technique.
3. Avoid the supine position to prevent aortocaval compression.
4. Prompt treatment of hypotension with a bolus infusion of crystalloid or increments of ephedrine, 5 to 10 mg intravenously as needed, or if indicated with phenylephrine (Neo-Synephrine) in 40-μg increments.
5. Oxygen by face mask (6 or more L/min).
6. Minimize the induction-delivery interval.
7. Minimize the uterine incision—delivery interval.

Combined spinal epidural anesthesia (CSE) also can be used. The epidural catheter gives flexibility in duration of surgery. On the other hand, if the epidural catheter is not confirmed from the beginning the CSE technique is relatively contraindicated in parturients with difficult airways.

General Anesthesia

1. Use of antacids (nonparticulate) and metoclopramide, 10 mg intravenously
2. Avoid the supine position to prevent aortocaval compression

3. Preoxygenation for 3 to 5 minutes or four deep breaths and rapid-sequence induction. Monitoring should include pulse and blood pressure, ECG, O_2 saturation, capnogram, temperature, and neuromuscular block.
4. Limit the thiopental dosage to a bolus of 4 mg/kg pregnant body weight.
5. Succinylcholine, 1.0 to 1.5 mg/kg pregnant body weight.
6. Minimal inspired oxygen concentration of 50%; N_2O 50%; and small concentration of inhalation anesthetic.
7. Avoid hypoventilation or hyperventilation.
8. Minimize the induction–delivery interval.
9. Minimize the uterine incision–delivery interval.
10. Depolarizing or nondepolarizing muscle relaxants to continue the operation, and narcotics after delivery of the baby.
11. Deflation of the stomach by a gastric tube.
12. Extubation is performed when the patient is wide awake.

Specific Problems

Antepartum Hemorrhage

Antepartum hemorrhage is the major cause of maternal mortality in the obstetric patient. Severe bleeding during the antepartum period is usually due to placenta previa or abruptio placentae.

Placenta Previa

Placenta previa is classified into three groups[1] (Fig. 13-1):

1. *Complete Previa (37%)*—The internal os is completely covered.
2. *Partial Previa (27%)*—The internal os is partially covered.
3. *Marginal Previa*—Part of the internal os is encroached on by the placenta.

The incidence varies between 0.1% and 1%. Bleeding is caused by tearing of the placenta and its detachment from the decidua.

Anesthetic Management. ***Actively Bleeding.*** If the parturient is actively bleeding, emergency cesarean delivery

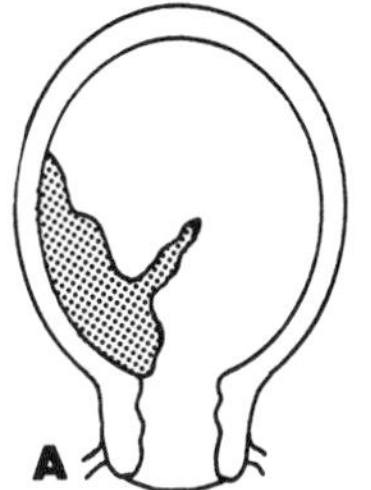

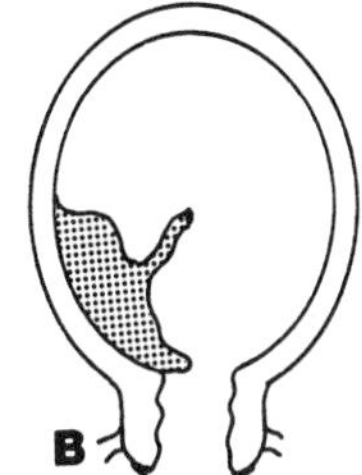

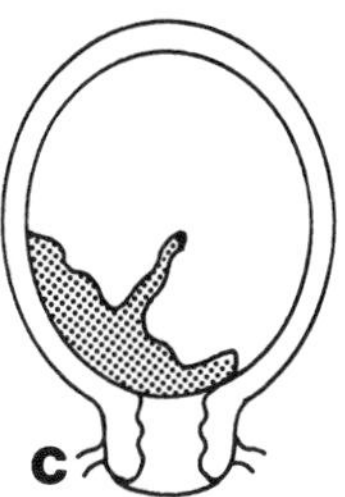

Figure 13-1. Classification of placenta previa. **(A)** Low-lying placenta. **(B)** Incomplete placenta previa. **(C)** Complete placenta previa. (From Bonica JJ, Johnson WL: *Principles and Practice of Obstetric Analgesia and Anesthesia*, vol 2. Philadelphia, F.A. Davis. Used with permission.)

should be performed under general anesthesia. Blood, plasma, and crystalloids should be infused as rapidly as possible as determined by the blood pressure, central venous pressure (CVP), and urine output. Induction of anesthesia should include a small dose of etomidate and/or ketamine if there is significant hypotension. Because of the higher percentage of repeat cesarean sections, the incidence of placenta accreta, increta, and percreta has gone up. *Placenta accreta* includes adherence of placenta to the uterine wall, *placenta increta* involves the invasion of placenta inside the myometrium, and *placenta percreta* includes the placenta invading through the myometrium. A significant number of these women might end up having gravid hysterectomies. Parturients with previous caesarean sections associated with placenta previa should be treated more carefully: a large-bore intravenous line, a warming blanket, and blood for a quick transfusion should be ready. Clark and colleagues observed the relationship between the number of previous caesarean sections and the subsequent occurrence of placenta accreta.[2] The incidence of placenta accreta from placenta previa with one prior cesarean section was 24%, whereas it was as high as 67% with four or more previous cesarean sections. The ideal anesthetic technique for this procedure is controversial, but the following outline lists the advantages and disadvantages of regional versus general anesthesia:

I. Regional anesthesia
   A. Advantages
      1. Less blood loss.[3]
      2. Awake patient with less chance of aspiration; parturient will be able to experience delivery of baby.
   B. Disadvantages
      1. Peripheral vasodilation may exacerbate hypotension.
      2. General anesthesia may be necessary for patient's comfort if a gravid hysterectomy is necessary. *Recently Chestnut and colleagues[4] reported on 12 parturients out of 46 who underwent gravid hysterectomy under epidural anesthesia, none of whom needed general anesthesia.* The rest of the patients (34) received general anesthesia from start of operation.

II. General anesthesia
   A. Advantages
      1. Hemodynamic stability.
      2. Security of the airway from the onset of surgery.
      3. Comfortable patient.
   B. Disadvantages
      1. Chance of a difficult intubation, inability to intubate, and possible gastric aspiration.
      2. Unconscious patient.

Not Bleeding. Major regional anesthesia (subarachnoid or epidural block) may be used if the parturient so desires, provided that there is no evidence of hypovolemia. Epidural or combined spinal epidural anesthesia is preferable, because it will provide flexibility for the duration of the operation. To minimize blood transfusions, these new techniques have been used: Blood transfusions from blood bank. (1) Autologus blood transfusion is not a popular technique (2) Acute hemodilution – in this technique about 750–1000 ml of blood is taken away from the parturient before the cesarean section and replaced by equal volume of 10% pentastarch. Fetal heart rate monitoring is done routinely. The collected blood is then transfused either during or completion of the surgery.[4a] (3) Various studies have observed that cell saver technique can filter away tissue factor, lamellar bodies, fetal squamous cells and alpha fetoprotein. A few studies have shown success of this method with no increased incidences of adult respiratory distress syndrome, amniotic fluid embolism, disseminated intravascular coagulation, infection or length of hospital stay.[4b] This may be a method of choice in pregnant women who refuses homologous blood transfusion. (4) Selective arterial embolization is getting popular to control obstetric hemorrhage. It has a high success rate and the uterus is saved for subsequent pregnancy. The procedure is done by interventional radiologist under fluoroscopic guidance. Depending upon the indications, it can be done using regional, general anesthesia or conscious sedation.[4c]

Abruptio Placentae

Abruptio placentae is a premature separation of a normally implanted placenta from the decidua basalis (incidence, 0.2% to 2%)[1] (Fig. 13-2). It is classified as mild, moderate, or severe. Bleeding might be concealed, with the blood retained behind the placenta, or else revealed, with the blood flowing externally. *Severe abdominal pain with fetal distress may be the*

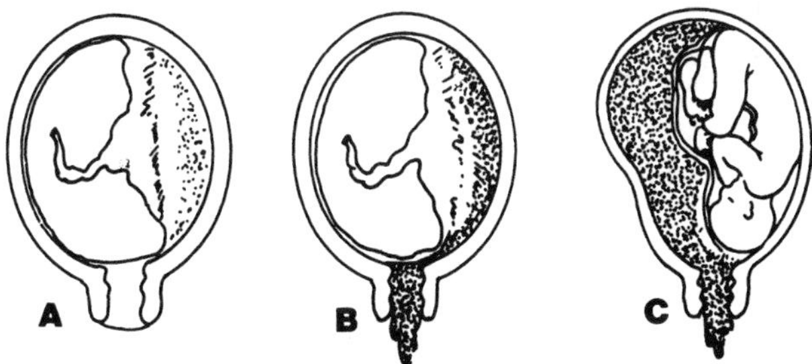

Figure 13-2. Classification of abruptio placentae. **A,** Concealed hemorrhage. **B,** External hemorrhage. **C,** External hemorrhage with prolapse of the placenta. (From Bonica JJ, Johnson WL: *Principles and Practice of Obstetric Analgesia and Anesthesia,* vol 2. Philadelphia, F.A. Davis. Used with permission.)

initial clinical findings. Use of cocaine or crack may be associated with abruptio placentae.

Anesthetic Management. If there is active bleeding, repeat as for placenta previa.

Abruptio placentae may be associated with blood coagulation defects and is the most common cause of coagulopathy in pregnancy. Diagnostic tests include hemoglobin/hematocrit, platelet count, fibrinogen level, prothrombin time (PT), and partial thromboplastin time (PTT). *If there is no evidence of maternal hypovolemia or uteroplacental insufficiency and if the clotting studies are normal, continuous epidural anesthesia may be used for labor and vaginal delivery.* In severe abruption, emergency delivery should be performed under general anesthesia. A massive and rapid blood transfusion might be necessary.

If the infant is alive at delivery, active resuscitation is usually required because of the maternal and fetal hypovolemia resulting in neonatal shock.

Table 13-1 compares placenta previa and abruptio placentae.

Besides the clinical features, *confirmation of the diagnosis is made at the present time by ultrasound; however, occasionally a double setup may be necessary to confirm low-lying placenta previa.* Anesthetic management for a double setup should include the following:

1. Availability of general anesthesia (the parturient should be prepared as such)
2. Crossmatching of at least 2 units of blood
3. Two or more large-bore intravenous lines

Table 13–1. Differential Diagnosis (Placenta Previa vs. Abruptio Placentae)

Clinical Features	Placenta Previa	Abruptio Placentae
Bleeding	Painless	Painful
Blood	Fresh	Dark, old, mixed with clots
Clotting problems	Uncommon	Common
Sudden fetal distress	Uncommon	Common

4. CVP and arterial lines if necessary
5. Preoxygenation

Postpartum Hemorrhage

Four main causes of postpartum hemorrhage are retained placenta, uterine inversion, laceration, and uterine rupture.

Retained Placenta

Retention of the placenta or placental fragment is the third most frequent cause of postpartum hemorrhage.

Anesthetic management will depend upon the severity of bleeding and cardiovascular stability. In the presence of severe bleeding the following steps are necessary:

1. Two large-bore intravenous lines are immediately inserted.
2. Two units of ABO Rh type-specific blood should be immediately asked for, and the blood bank should be alerted about the situation.
3. Intravenous Ringer's lactate and 5% albumin or hespan should be used rapidly, depending upon the situation.
4. Vasopressors may be necessary.

Anesthetic Techniques. ***Epidural Anesthesia.*** If possible, reestablishment of ongoing epidural anesthesia is the choice in the author's institution.

Subarachnoid Block. If the parturient does not already have epidural anesthesia instituted, then subarachnoid anesthesia may be used, depending upon the condition of the woman.

General Anesthesia. If the cardiovascular situation prevents the use of regional anesthesia, then general anesthesia using an endotracheal tube should be used. Induction agents should include, depending on the situation, a small amount of etomidate, or a small amount of ketamine.

Inhalation anesthetic may be necessary to relax the uterus. However, the anesthetic should be shut off as soon as possible to prevent uterine relaxation and hemorrhage.

Recently intravenous nitroglycerin up to 500 μg has been used for uterine relaxation with great success.[5] The author prefers to use 50 to 100 μg of nitroglycerin in the first instance after proper volume replacement. A small amount of diazepam

(2.5–5 mg), midazolam (1–2 mg) and fentanyl (50 to 100 μg) may be necessary and will help in extracting the placenta by providing pain relief.

Uterine Inversion

Uterine inversion is a rare complication that can be associated with massive hemorrhage (Fig. 13-3). Hemorrhage and shock are common findings. For acute inversion, ongoing epidural or spinal anesthesia can be used provided that the patient is cardiovascularly stable; however, in the presence of subacute or chronic inversion, uterine relaxation with inhalation anesthetic may be necessary, and general anesthesia will

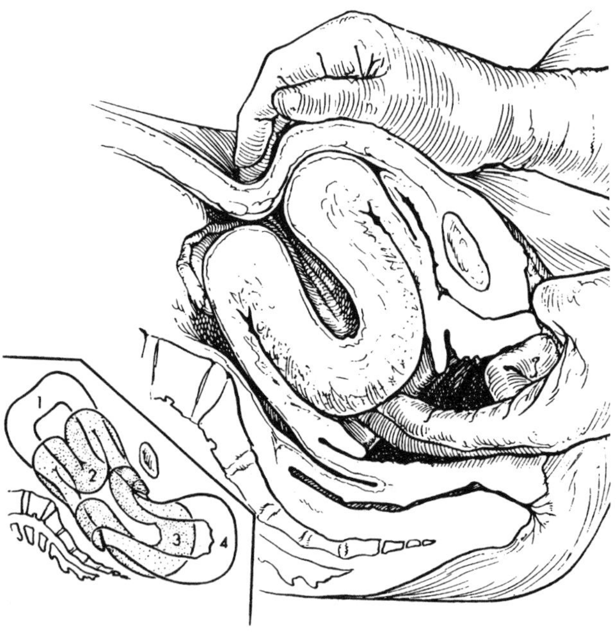

Figure 13-3. Incomplete inversion of the uterus. (From Cunningham FG et al: *Williams Obstetrics, 20th ed.* East Norwalk, CN, Appleton-Lange, Crofts, 1997. Reproduced with permission from The McGraw-Hill Companies.)

become essential. Nitroglycerin may also be used to relax the uterus; however, the blood pressure should be closely monitored. Shah-Hosseini and Evrad have published the incidence of uterine inversion that occurred between 1978 and 1988 in the Women and Infants' Hospital of Providence, Rhode Island.[6] Out of 70,481 deliveries, 11 women had uterine inversion (1 in 6,407), and 73% of the parturients were nulliparous. The overall calculated blood loss varied from 150 to 4,300 mL. Anesthetic techniques included (1) local anesthesia, (2) epidural anesthesia, and (3) general anesthesia using thiopental, ketamine, thiopental and ketamine, and in a few cases halothane for uterine relaxation. *In one case, surgery was necessary to reduce the inversion.* The authors concluded that early diagnosis, adequate volume therapy, and immediate correction of inversion are absolutely necessary for a good outcome.

Lacerations

Lacerations of the cervix, vagina, and perineum are the second most common cause of postpartum hemorrhage. Proper resuscitation of the woman is important.

Uterine Rupture

Uterine rupture most commonly occurs from a previous uterine scar from either cesarean section or uterine surgery. Trophoblastic invasion of the uterus can also be an important factor in uterine rupture. Gravid hysterectomy may be indicated on a few occasions. Thus parturients undergoing vaginal delivery after previous cesarean section or following uterine surgery should be closely followed.

Vaginal Birth after Cesarean Section. This has become extremely popular in recent times following the recommendation of the American College of Obstetricians and Gynecologists (ACOG).[7] The adequacy of a hospital setup with the capability of performing emergency cesarean section within 30 minutes remains the most important issue in taking care of these parturients.

Anesthetic Management. The chance of uterine rupture because of the uterine scar remains the major problem.

Epidural analgesia for labor and delivery was relatively contraindicated for two main reasons: (1) masking of pain from uterine rupture because of epidural blockade and (2) blunting of sympathetic responses because of ongoing epidural analgesia.[8] A few studies using 0.25% to 0.37% bupivacaine showed that these concentrations of local anesthetic did not relieve the continuous pain of a ruptured uterus.[9,10] Crawford concluded that pain from a ruptured uterus should "break through" a previously established epidural anesthetic. However, further studies showed that *abdominal pain and tenderness may not be specific and sensitive signs of uterine scar separation:* Golan and colleagues observed that uterine or uterine scar tenderness was an infrequent presentation of uterine rupture.[11] *Fetal distress as well as stoppage of uterine activity are more reliable signs for separation of a uterine scar. The majority of anesthesiologists as well as ACOG do not consider epidural analgesia to be contraindicated for vaginal birth after cesarean section. On the contrary, Demianczuk and colleagues suggested a few advantages of epidural analgesia during this procedure*[12]*: (1) palpation of the scar during labor and (2) bimanual examination of the uterus to examine the scar after delivery. In summary, epidural analgesia may be used for vaginal birth after cesarean section; however, continuous fetal heart rate monitoring and an intrauterine pressure catheter to measure the intensity of uterine contractions should be used,* and a low concentration of local anesthetic for epidural analgesia may also be beneficial.

Recently several different procedures have been proposed to minimize bleeding and blood transfusion or to avoid gravid hysterectomy. Examples include autologous blood transfusion,[12a] hemodilution technique,[12b] cell saver, and arterial embolization.[12d]

Pregnancy-Induced Hypertension

Hypertension during pregnancy is a common medical problem that occurs in approximately 250,000 American women every year. This disease is associated with a higher incidence of maternal, fetal, and neonatal mortality and mor-

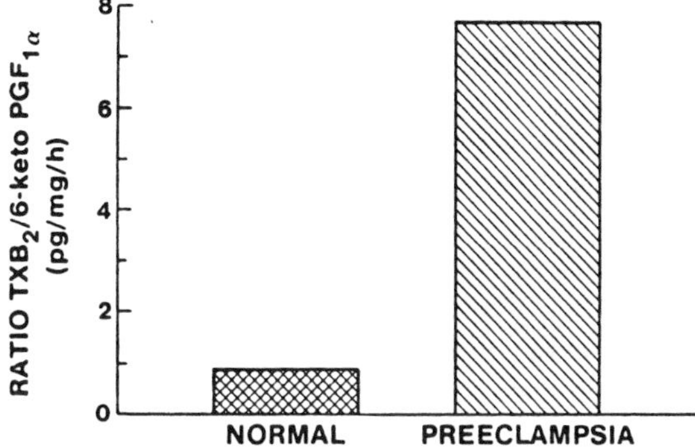

Figure 13–4. Ratio of the placental production rates of thromboxane to prostacyclin in normal and pre-eclamptic pregnancies. (From Walsh SW: *Am J Obstet Gynecol* 1985; 152:335. Used with permission from Elsevier.)

bidity. The ACOG classifies hypertension during pregnancy into four subgroups:

1. Pre-eclampsia, eclampsia
2. Chronic hypertension
3. Chronic hypertension with superimposed pre-eclampsia (or eclampsia)
4. Gestational hypertension

Recently the American College of Obstetrics and Gynecology (ACOG) has changed the definition of hypertension related to preeclampsia. Hypertension is defined as a sustained blood pressure increase to levels of 140 mmHg systolic or 90 mmHg diastolic. Blood pressure should be measured in sitting position. In pre-eclampsia, a parturient should have two clinical findings; (1) hypertension (2) proteinuria. These should occur after the 20th week of gestation. If the pre-eclampsia is associated with convulsions, then the term is changed to eclampsia. *It usually occurs in very young or elderly primigravidas. Parturients will be included in the category of severe pre-eclampsia if they have the following clinical findings:* (1) systolic blood pressure of 160 mm Hg or more, (2) diastolic blood pressure of 110 mm Hg or more, (3) proteinuria of

Table 13-2. Clinical Effects of Prostacyclin vs. Thromboxane

Prostacyclin	Thromboxane
Vasoconstriction↓	Vasoconstriction↑
Platelet aggregation↓	Platelet aggregation↑
Uterine activity↓	Uterine activity↑
Uteroplacental blood flow↑	Uteroplacental blood flow↓

5 g/24 hr or more, (4) oliguria with 500 mL or less of urine output in 24 hours, (5) cerebra] and visual disturbances, (6) epigastric pain, (7) pulmonary edema or cyanosis, and (8) HELLP syndrome (hemolysis, elevated liver enzymes, and low platelet count). The main causes of maternal mortality are (1) cerebral hemorrhage (30% to 40%), (2) pulmonary edema

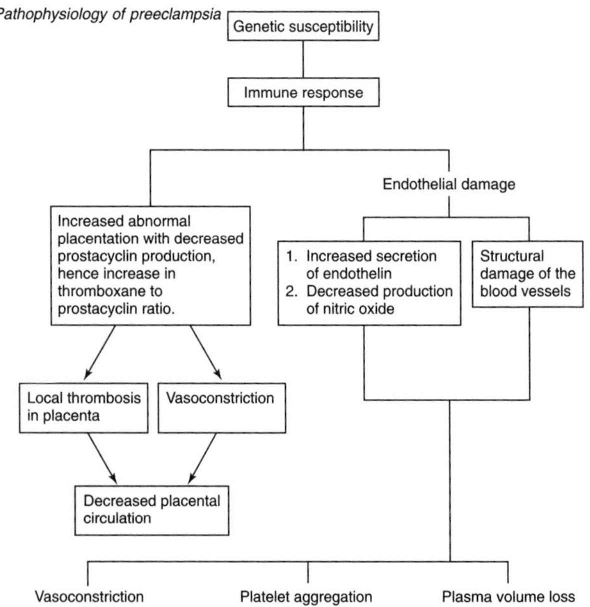

(30% to 38%), (3) renal failure (10%), (4) cerebral edema (19%), (5) disseminated intravascular coagulation (9%), and (6) airway obstruction (6%).

The intravascular volume and protein content are markedly lower in severe pre-eclampsia than in normal pregnancy. There is associated vasoconstriction, possibly caused by increased circulating levels of renin, angiotensin, aldosterone, and catecholamines. Thromboxane, endothelin. *These circulating vasoactive substances make pre-eclamptic—eclamptic patients extremely sensitive to vasoconstricting drugs, and thus drugs like ephedrine should be used cautiously.* An interesting observation regarding the P_{50} values of normal parturients and pre-eclamptic women was made by Kambam et al[15] (Table 13-3). The authors concluded that in normal pregnant women there was a significant shift of P_{50} to the right as compared with non-pregnant women and that the extent of the shift to the right was directly related to the duration of pregnancy. However, the pre-eclamptic parturients showed a significant shift of P_{50} to the left when compared with normal pregnant women at term (Table 13-3). The hypovolemia will decrease placental perfusion, and this together with the impaired placental function and shifting of the maternal P_{50} to the left can cause a decrease in the

Table 13–3. P_{50} Values of Nonpregnant, Pregnant, and Pre-eclamptic Subjects

Subjects		P_{50} (mm Hg)	
Status	***n***	**Mean**	**SEM**
Nonpregnant†	10	26.7	0.11
Pregnant			
1st trimester†	10	27.8	0.08
2nd trimester†	10	28.8	0.17
At or near term†	24	30.4	0.20
Pre-eclamptic‡	14	25.1	0.38

From Kambam JR, Handte RE, Brown WU, et al: *Anesthesiology* 1986; 65:426. Used by permission.

†All means are significantly different from one another ($p < 0.01$), Newman-Keul's test.

‡Significant level of difference between pregnant at term and pre-eclamptic at term ($p < 0.001$).

transplacental exchange of respiratory gases. This disease process can involve multiple organs. Liver involvement can cause disseminated intravascular coagulation, and kidney involvement will cause oliguria and azotemia. *Severe vasospasm of retinal vessels may be associated with visual disturbances. Examination of fundi may not show any signs of increased intracranial pressure. Magnesium sulfate or hypotensive medications may relieve this clinical feature.* On the other hand, there may be associated cerebral edema and increased intracranial pressure. The laryngeal edema of normal pregnancy can be aggravated to the point of airway obstruction. In 1999, a study from Japan showed an increased amount of catecholamines in these women. The authors observed two groups of parturients with severe pre-eclampsia: (1) Those with coninuous epidural from 28 weeks, (2) Those on conventional therapy. The epidural group had lowered blood pressure, decreased proteinuria, increased urine output, increased fetal weight, and increased platelet count.

Magnesium Therapy

In the United States, parenterally administered magnesium is considered the drug of choice in controlling pre-eclampsia and eclampsia. *The normal plasma magnesium level is 1.5 to 2.0 mEq/L. The therapeutic range occurs at 4 to 8 mEq/L. A loss of tendon reflexes happens at 10 mEq/L, ECC changes (prolonged PQ, widened QRS complex) appear at 5 to 10 mEq/L, respiratory paralysis happens at 15 mEq/L, and ultimately cardiac arrest can occur at 25 mEq/L (Table 13-4). Magnesium sulfate therapy can potentiate both depolarizing and nondepolarizing muscle relaxant activity.*[16] Magnesium is now accepted as a specific medication for the prevention of recurrent convulsion (eclampsia).[17] The beneficial effect of magnesium sulfate for this pathology is multifactoral. It has an inhibitory effect at the neuromuscular junction. Both in vivo and in vitro studies found magnesium to increase production of endothelial vasodilator prostacyclin. Magnesium also can protect against ischemic damage of the cells by substitution of calcium and also prevents the entry of calcium ions into ischemic cells. Finally magnesium may be anticonvulsant

Table 13-4. Effects of Increasing Plasma Magnesium Levels

Plasma Mg (mEq/L)	Effects
1.5-2.0	Normal plasma level
4.0-8.0	Therapeutic range
5.0-10	Electrocardiographic changes (PQ interval prolonged, QRS complex widens)
10	Loss of deep tendon reflexes
15	Sinoatrial and atrioventricular block
15	Respiratory paralysis
25	Cardiac arrest

From Shnider SM, Levinson G: *Anesthesia for Obstetrics.* Baltimore, Williams & Wilkins, 1987. Used by permission.

by acting as a N-methyl-D-asparate (NMDA) receptor antagonist.[18]

Anesthetic Management

For vaginal delivery epidural analgesia has the distinct advantage of relieving labor pain. Epidural analgesia will decrease maternal blood pressure (Fig. 13-5) and can indirectly increase placental perfusion[17] by decreasing circulating catecholamine levels. Epidural analgesia may also improve both uteroplacental and renal blood flow. However, one must make sure that the clotting parameters are normal before using epidural analgesia. Although the incidence of frank disseminated intravascular coagulation is not high in parturients with pre-eclampsia, coagulation abnormalities can occur in the presence of decreased platelet counts, increased fibrin split products, and slightly prolonged PTT values. Kelton et al[18] in a recent study observed thrombocytopenia in 34% of 26 pre-eclamptic patients. Five of these women had a prolonged bleeding time. However, the most interesting observation was that 4 parturients with normal platelet counts had prolonged bleeding times (more than 10 minutes). *The authors concluded that a significant proportion of women with pre-eclampsia develop an acquired defect of platelet function that could contribute to prolonged bleeding time. However bleeding time is not performed at the present time.*

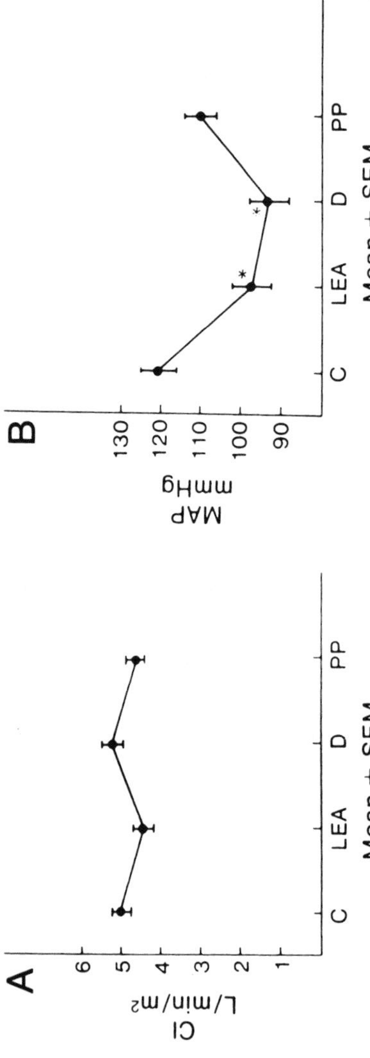

Figure 13–5. Effect on mean maternal artery blood pressure (*MAP*) following epidural anesthesia in severe pre-eclamptic patients. (From Newsome LR, Bramwell RS, Curling PE: *Anesth Analg* 1986; 65:31–36. Used by permission.)

There is controversy regarding clotting parameters and use of regional anesthesia. If the platelet count is just less than 100,000mL with no history of abnormal bleeding conditions and with normal PT and aPTT, regional anesthesia can be used both for labor, delivery and cesarean section. If the platelet count is less than 75,000mm^3 DeBoer and colleagues reported laboratory evidence of coagulopathy in 10% of preeclamptic women and 30% of severely preeclamptic parturients.[19] Clinically significant coagulopathy has been observed in 5% of mildly preeclamptic women and in 15% of severely preeclamptic parturients. The clotting parameter that is becoming popular is thromboelastography (TEG). Figure 13-6 shows a normal TEG, whereas figure 13-7 describes parturients with normal as well as abnormal bleeding conditions.[19a] In a recent study, Sharma and colleagues observed hypocoagulable tracing in parturients with severe preeclampsia especially when platelet count was less than 75,000 mm^3 compared to mild preeclamptic and healthy pregnant women.[20] The risk-benefit ratio will ultimately dictate the anesthetic technique in a borderline case. The postpartum women should be closely followed for any signs of epidural hematoma if regional analgesia or anesthesia is used in borderline cases.

Previously, spinal anesthesia was contraindicated for cesarean section in parturients with severe preeclampsia. This is because of the possibility of severe hypotension in volume contracted individuals as well as parturients who are receiving hypotensive medications. However, several well conducted studies argued against this dictum.[20ab] In two studies, no differences in blood pressure were observed between spinal and epidural anesthesia while undergoing cesarean section. The requirements of ephedrine were also similar. When compared with healthy parturients, women with severe preeclampsia developed less hypotension following spinal anesthesia.[21] However in another study, significant maternal hypotension was observed following spinal anesthesia in severe preeclamptic parturients.[21a] Women were treated with fluid and ephedrine. Because of the possibility of hypotension in volume contracted parturients with severe preeclampsia undergoing cesarean section with spinal anesthesia, there is a

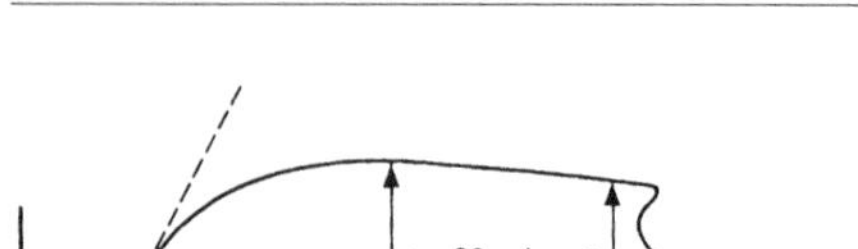

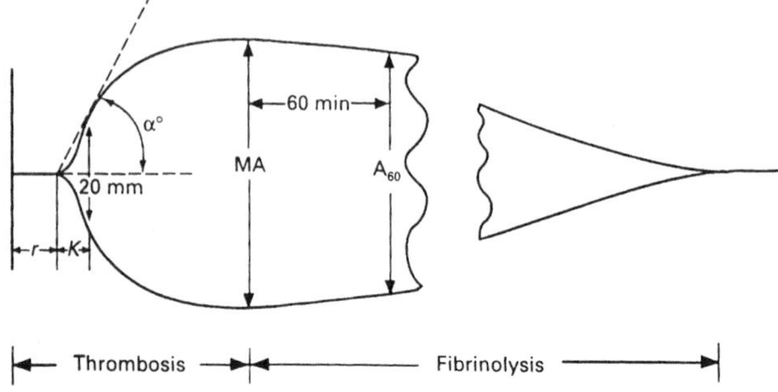

Figure 13-6. Analysis of thromboelastograph (TEG). (1) r = reaction time (normal range = 6 to 8 min). This represents the rate of initial fibrin formation and is related functionally to plasma clotting factor. (2) K = clot formation time (normal range = 3 to 6 min). The coagulation time represents the time taken for a fixed degree of viscoelasticity to be achieved by the forming clot as a result of fibrin build-up and cross-linking. It is affected by the activity of intrinsic clotting factors, fibrinogen, and platelets. (3) (α° (normal range = 50 to 60°) is the angle formed by the slope of the TEG tracing from the r to the K value. It denotes the speed at which solid clot forms. (4) The maximum amplitude (MA) (normal range = 50 to 60 mm) is the greatest amplitude on the TEG trace and is a reflection of the absolute strength of the fibrin clot. It is a direct function of the maximum dynamic properties of fibrin and platelets. (5) A_{60} (normal range = MA – 5 mm) is the amplitude of the tracing 60 min after MA has been achieved. It is a measurement of clot lysis or retraction. (From Mallet SV, Cox DJA: *Br J Anaesth* 69:307–313, 1992. © The Board of Management and Trustees of the British Journal of Anaesthesia. Reproduced by permission of Oxford University Press/British Journal of Anaesthesia.)

tendency to give a larger amount of fluid in this population. Many prefer colloid for volume expansion in parturients with severe preeclampsia.[22] Some pregnant women with severe preeclampsia may present with an increased afterload, normal CVP, and isolated left ventricular dysfunction. Aggressive volume expansion in these women may lead to pulmonary edema (Fig. 13-8). Reduction of the afterload with

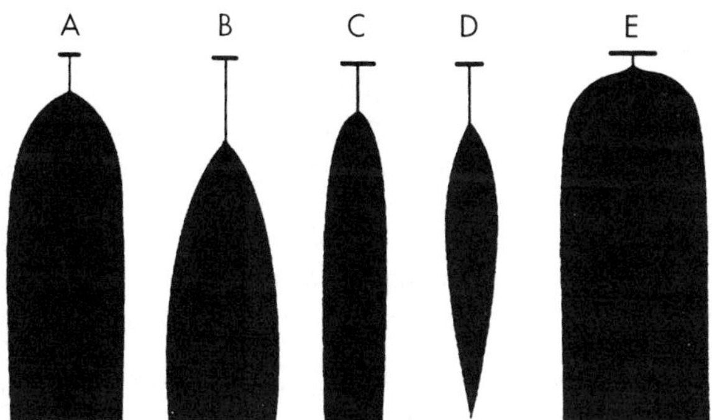

Figure 13–7. Specific hemostatic defects produce a characteristic TEG. **A,** Normal trace. **B,** Hemophilia: marked prolongation of *r* and *K* times; decreased α angle. **C,** Thrombocytopenia: normal *r* and *rK* times: decreased MA (>40 mm). **D,** Fibrinolysis. **E,** Hypercoagulability: short *r* time; increased MA and steep clot formation rate. (**A** to **E** from Mallet SV, Cox DJA: *Br J Anaesth* 69:307–313, 1992. © The Board of Management and Trustees of the British Journal of Anaesthesia. Reproduced by permission of Oxford University Press/British Journal of Anaesthesia.)

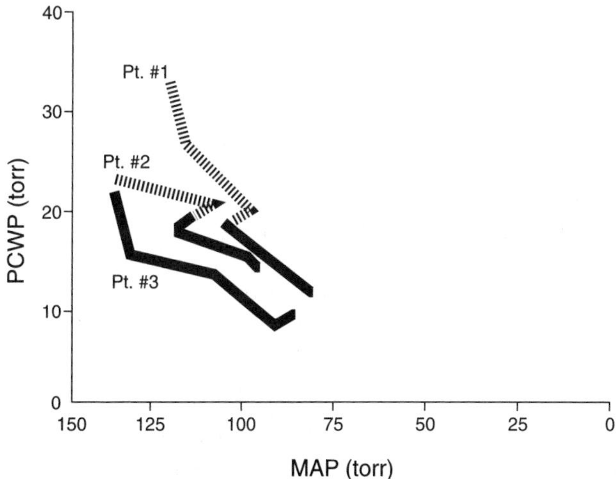

Figure 13–8. Correlation between pulmonary capillary wedge pressure (*PCWP*) and mean arterial pressure (*MAP*) during vasodilator therapy. *Interrupted line,* before cesarean section; *solid line,* after cesarean section. (Adapted from Strauss RG, et al: *Obstetric Gynecol* 1980; 55:170.)

arteriolar vasodilators should be the initial treatment in such cases. Hemodynamically severe preeclampsia has a variable expression, and thus not all parturients with the diagnosis of severe preeclampsia should be classified under one diagnostic "umbrella." One of the major fears expressed by obstetricians concerning hydrating these women with either colloid or crystalloid is the risk of maternal pulmonary edema.

Recently Benedetti et al[23] reported the etiology of pulmonary edema in severely preeclamptic parturients, 20% of whom had left ventricular dysfunction as shown by an increased pulmonary artery wedge pressure associated with a low ventricular stroke work index. Thirty percent of the cases of pulmonary edema were due to altered capillary permeability, and the diagnosis was made by observing a normal pulmonary artery wedge pressure and a normal or elevated left ventricular stroke work index (normal left ventricular stroke work index, 55 to 85 g/min/m^2). Finally, 50% of the cases of pulmonary edema were due to low hydrostatic-oncotic forces diagnosed by the normal left ventricular stroke work index and the elevated pulmonary artery wedge pressure. *Normal colloidal oncotic pressure during pregnancy is 22 mm Hg;* colloidal oncotic pressure can be reduced significantly in parturients with pregnancy-induced hypertension. A clinically useful estimate of the net intravascular fluid filtration pressure can be obtained by simply subtracting the pulmonary capillary wedge pressure from the plasma colloidal oncotic pressure. The normal gradient in nonpregnant individuals ranges from 9 to 17 mm Hg. A decrease in the gradient to below 5 mm Hg either by an increase in the pulmonary capillary wedge pressure or a decrease in the colloidal oncotic pressure can result in pulmonary edema. Thus in women in whom colloidal oncotic pressure is low, colloid may be used for intravenous volume expansion with proper monitoring. In conclusion, volume loading with crystalloid and colloid prior to the induction of spinal, combined spinal epidural or epidural anesthesia might be necessary, and when this is expertly done with adequate monitoring of vascular pressure, it is safe for both the fetus and the mother. Another major concern in these women is the increased incidence of oliguria. Recently Clark and colleagues[24] classified the etiology of oliguria in severely preeclamptic women (Fig. 13-9) into three classes. Parturients exhibiting oliguria received a fluid challenge consisting of 300 to 500 mL of lactated Ringer's solution or half-normal saline solution administered over a

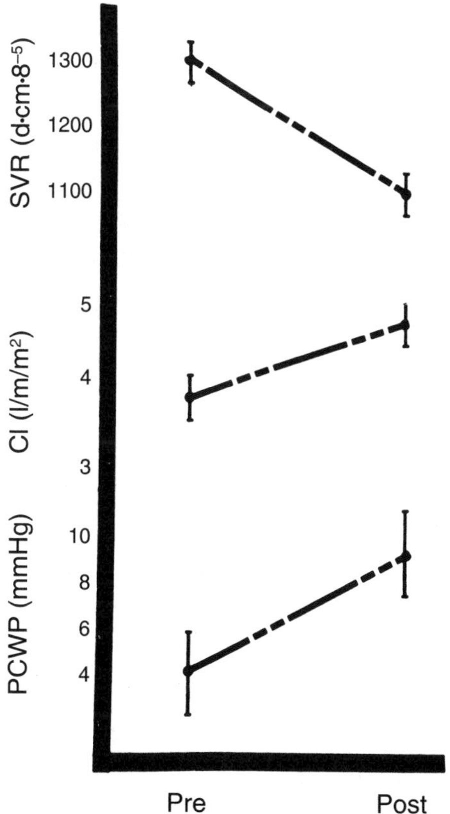

Figure 13-9. Hemodynamic changes following volume expansion. *PCWP* = pulmonary capillary wedge pressure; *SVR* = systemic vascular resistance. (Adapted from Clark SI, Greenspoon JS, Aldahn D, et al: *Am J Obstet Gynecol* 1986; 154:490.)

period of 20 minutes. In category I, the hemodynamic profile was one of hyperdynamic left ventricular function, low to low-normal pulmonary capillary wedge pressure, and only a moderate increase in systemic vascular resistance. Oliguria in these population appeared to be on the basis of a relative intravascular volume depletion in the face of systemic arteriospasm. In category II, persistent oliguria with concentrated urine in the presence of essentially normal systemic vascular resistance suggested renal hypoperfusion caused by a selective degree of renal arteriospasm beyond that reflected in the measurement of systemic vascular resistance. The administration of hydralazine and, in parturients with normal pulmonary capillary wedge pressure, cautious fluid administration resulted in resolution of the oliguric phase. In category III, women exhibited a hemodynamic picture of depressed left ventricular function (low left ventricular stroke work index), elevated pulmonary capillary wedge pressure, and marked elevation of systemic vascular resistance. Oliguria appeared to be on the basis of decreased renal perfusion secondary to intense vasospasm and diminished cardiac output. In such parturients, fluid restriction with aggressive afterload reduction is indicated.

The final controversy that may exist regarding the treatment of these individuals is related to invasive monitoring. Monitoring of severely pre-eclamptic parturients can be subdivided into the following categories:

A. *Noninvasive*
   a. Oxygen saturation monitoring (not controversial)
   b. Automatic blood pressure and pulse monitoring
   c. Foley's catheter *for urine output* (*becomes more important if the patient is receiving magnesium sulfate*)
   d. Fetal heart rate monitoring

B. *Invasive monitoring*
   a. *Arterial line*
      1. Morbidly obese woman
      2. Refractory hypertension where sodium nitroprusside is necessary because other hypotensive agents were not effective
      3. Pulmonary edema where serial blood gas measurements may be necessary

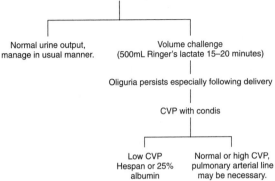

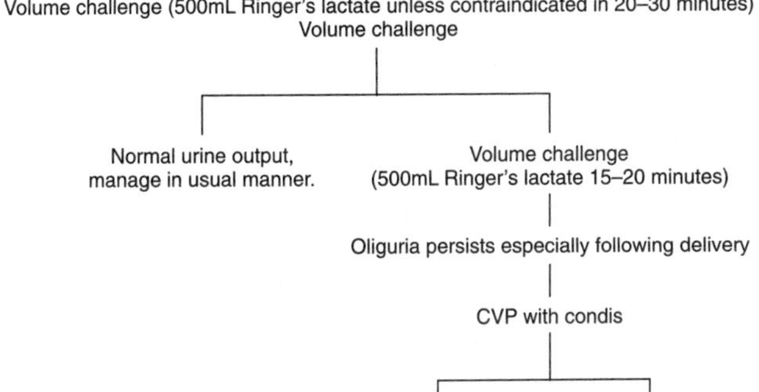
Volume challenge (500mL Ringer's lactate unless contraindicated in 20–30 minutes)
Volume challenge
Normal urine output, manage in usual manner.
Volume challenge (500mL Ringer's lactate 15–20 minutes)
Oliguria persists especially following delivery
CVP with condis
Low CVP Hespan or 25% albumin
Normal or high CVP, pulmonary arterial line may be necessary.

C. *Central venous pressure (CVP) monitoring*
Severe pre-eclampsia with oliguria (urine output > 25 mL/hr
Pulmonary arterial (PA) line
1. If the initial CVP reading is high (8 or above)
2. Oliguria persists even with normal CVP
3. Pulmonary edema
4. Cardiovascular collapse

Summary of Regional Anesthesia.
1. Spinal. One shot spinal or continuous spinal anesthesia can be used. Hypotension should be treated aggressively with a small amount of ephedrine unless contraindicated.
2. Combined spinal epidural technique is preferable over one-shot spinal anesthesia if surgery is expected to be prolonged.
3. Some authors believe that epidural anesthesia is associated with more stable maternal hemodynamics and hence placental perfusion. This may be the ideal anesthetic for parturients with severe preeclampsia.
4. Blood should be drawn for a determination of the hematocrit and all clotting parameters. The hematocrit may be very high in parturients with severe preeclampsia; this may be related to volume constriction.
5. A CVP monitor may be necessary in some cases with severe preeclampsia.

6. A pulmonary artery pressure line may be used when indicated.
7. Urine output should be routinely measured.
8. 2% lidocaine with epinephrine may be the drug of choice for elective cases where as 3% 2-chloroprocaine mixed with bicarbonate can be used for fetal distress situation if an epidural catheter is already has been placed. Fifty microgram of fentanyl will intensify the sensory anesthesia.
9. Continuous fetal heart rate monitoring should be performed during induction of anesthesia.
10. Postoperative analgesia may be maintained by using epidural morphine or a continuous infusion of narcotics or local anesthetics (small concentration) and narcotics combined.

General Anesthesia. For general anesthesia one has to prevent reflex hypertension (especially a systolic blood pressure over 200 mm Hg) during induction under light general anesthesia. The hypotensive drugs that can be used prior to induction are as follows:

1. *Hydralazine*—It has been suggested that hydralazine can increase uterine perfusion; however, a longer time of onset makes this drug impractical for use in urgent situations.
2. *Nitroglycerin*—Nitroglycerin is a fast-acting drug but comparatively unpredictable.
3. *Nitroprusside*—Nitroprusside has a fast onset of action. *However, one should remember the remote theoretical possibility of fetal cyanide intoxication.*
4. *Trimethaphan* (*Arfonad*)—Its large molecule and short half-life (destroyed by cholinesterase) make trimethaphan less transferable via the placenta. Theoretically it will cause the least increase in intracranial pressure. Disadvantages include *drug interaction with succinylcholine* (*both are destroyed by cholinesterase*) *and pupillary dilatation, which might make it difficult to diagnose changes in intracranial pressure.*
5. *Labetalol*—Recent work has shown that labetalol (1 mg/kg) will decrease the maternal blood pressure without affecting the intervillous and fetal blood flow.[25]
6. *Calcium-channel blockers* (*nifedipine*) have become popular in recent years. These have the following advan-

tageous properties: 1) they act as vasodilators, 2) they are uterine muscle relaxants, and 3) they increase renal blood flow. In severely pre-eclamptic parturients, nifedipine was associated with lowering of maternal blood pressure as well as prolongation of pregnancy and improvement of fetal oxygenation.[26] *Recently, however, cardiovascular collapse has been reported after use of nifedipine in presence of magnesium sulfate.*

Intravenous narcotics have also been used preoperatively to prevent reflex hypertension. Lawes and colleagues used 200 μg of fentanyl and 5 mg of droperidol intravenously prior to induction of general anesthesia with success.[27]

Several problems may be encountered when using general anesthesia in severely preeclamptic parturient

1. *Severe airway edema may be encountered in these women*[28]*; hence small endotracheal tubes may be necessary for intubation.*
2. A hypertensive response to light general anesthesia always remains a major problem. *Moore and colleagues encountered a 50% increase in mean arterial pressure during laryngoscopy in pre-eclamptic women even after the preinduction use of nitroprusside.*[29]
3. Drug interactions are common in this population: *Arfonad will interact with succinylcholine, and magnesium sulfate can interact with depolarizing and nondepolarizing muscle relaxants.*

Summary of General Anesthesia for Cesarean Section in Pre-Eclamptic Patients

1. Monitor the pulse and blood pressure, ECG, O_2 saturation, P_{CO_2}, temperature, neuromuscular block, CVP, and pulmonary artery lines, if necessary.
2. Nonparticulate antacid and *metoclopramide should be used cautiously.*
3. Drugs should be used to counter hypertension during induction and extubation, if necessary.
4. Thiopental and succinylcholine are used for induction (the author does not decrease the induction dose of succinylcholine even if the parturient is receiving magnesium

sulfate); *a defasciculating dose of nondepolarizing muscle relaxant is not used during induction.*

5. Further muscle relaxants should be used cautiously in the presence of magnesium sulfate.

HELLP Syndrome

Weinstein originally described a *symptom complex consisting of (1) hemolysis, (2) elevated liver enzyme levels, and (3) low platelet count* and included this syndrome as a severe consequence of pregnancy-induced hypertension.[30] Interestingly, laboratory evidence of the HELLP syndrome may occur before the development of hypertension and proteinuria. Clinical features may include fatigue and right upper quadrant pain. *Serum transaminase levels must be elevated to make the diagnosis of liver dysfunction.* Anesthetic management will depend on the clotting parameters. In the case of severe thrombocytopenia, general anesthesia may be indicated; otherwise, regional anesthesia is usually the author's choice as a technique. *Occasionally we have inserted the epidural catheter before there was a significant drop in platelet count.* Withdrawal of the catheter in the presence of thrombocytopenia is controversial. Advocates of withdrawal point to the possibility of catheter migration in the blood vessels and the risk of epidural hematoma. Opponents of withdrawal fear clot dislodgment and risk of epidural hematoma. In both situations, parturients must be *followed for any signs of epidural hematoma.*

A differential diagnosis may be difficult because thrombotic thrombocytopenic purpura (TTP), postpartum hemolytic-uremic syndrome (HUS), and fatty liver of pregnancy are associated with similar features (Table 13-5).

Eclampsia

Convulsion treatment should include *intravenous magnesium sulfate, adequate protection of the airway, prevention of aspiration,* and treatment of hypertension. Although magnesium sulfate is the drug of choice[31,32] for the treatment of eclamptic seizures, diazepam, midazolam phenytoin, or phenobarbital have been used to stop the convulsions. A diagnosis of eclampsia does not contraindicate the use of epidural

Table 13-5. Differential Diagnosis of HELLP Syndrome, Thrombotic Thrombocytic Purpura, Hemolytic-Uremic Syndrome, and Fatty Liver of Pregnancy

Disorder	HELLP	TTP	HUS	Fatty Liver of Pregnancy
Microangiopathic hemolytic anemia	+	+	+	−
Thrombocytopenic bleeding	+	+	+	+
Neurological dysfunction	+	++	±	±
Renal dysfunction	±	+	+++	+

analgesia/anesthesia; however, clotting parameters should be determined.

Approximately 30% of pre-eclamptic mothers may develop eclampsia in the postpartum period. Parturients remain at risk for eclampsia for at least 48 hours and for as long as one week. *An important clinical implication is performing blood patch for postdural puncture headache.* Blood pressure must be monitored before performing the blood patch, which *should be avoided if the diagnosis of postpartum pre-eclampsia is made*[32a].

Diabetes Mellitus

The major problems encountered in diabetic pregnancy are as follows:

1. Placental insufficiency
2. Superimposed pre-eclampsia
3. Diabetic nephropathy
4. Diabetic ketoacidosis, the main factor in the increased incidence of perinatal morbidity and mortality. Evidence exists that ketones can readily cross the placenta, and this can significantly decrease fetal Pao_2. Biochemical findings include a plasma glucose level greater than 300 mg/dL, plasma HCO_3 less than 15 mEq/L, arterial pH less than 7.30, and serum acetone positive at 1:2. The treatment of

diabetic ketoacidosis should include enough insulin to correct the acidosis and to carefully balance the fluid and electrolyte levels. Continuous fetal heart rate monitoring should be instituted for fetal surveillance.

Pathophysiological Changes

The anesthetic management of diabetic parturients should be based on the understanding of pathophysiological changes associated with diabetic pregnancy.

Deranged Uteroplacental Blood Flow. Maternal diabetes is associated with placental abnormalities even in the case of mild, well-controlled gestational diabetes. The uteroplacental blood flow index was reduced 35% to 45% in diabetic parturients. The blood flow index tended to be further impaired in those diabetic women who had higher blood glucose values.[33]

Impairment of Oxygen Transport in Diabetes. HbA_{1C} (a minor variant of hemoglobin A) levels are two to three times higher in insulin-treated diabetics than in control subjects. In contrast to hemoglobin A, the oxygen affinity of HbA_{1c} is little affected by the in vitro addition of 2,3-diphosphoglycerate (2,3-DPG). It has been observed that red blood cell oxygen transport, saturation, and tension are impaired in insulin-dependent diabetic subjects. *In poorly regulated women, in whom the concentrations of HbA_{1C} are higher and the concentrations of 2,3-DPG tend to be lower, the blood oxygen release at the tissue level may be more impaired*[34] (Figs. 13-10 and 13-11). Recently it has been shown that insulin could cross the placenta from the maternal to the fetal circulation as insulin-antiinsulin antibody complexes.

Deranged Buffering Capacity in Infants of Diabetic Mothers. Recently we observed an interesting phenomenon suggesting that infants of diabetic mothers have a decreased buffering capacity and a different response to an increased acid load. There is an increased affinity of hemoglobin to oxygen in infants of diabetic mothers. The P_{50} (torr) values were significantly less in infants of diabetic mothers when compared with control infants (17.9 vs. 22.6).

This multiplicity of problems makes infants of diabetic mothers more vulnerable, and hence careful anesthetic management is mandatory in these cases.

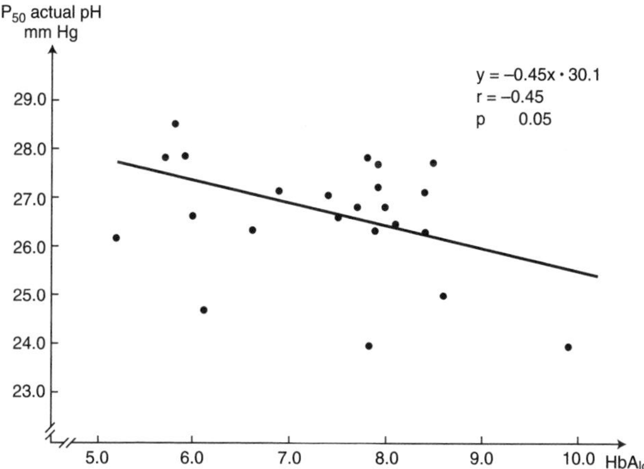

Figure 13–10. Correlation between HbA_{1c} and P_{50} at actual pH in diabetic women. (Adapted from Madsen H, Ditzel J: *Am J Obstet Gynecol* 1982; 143:421-424.)

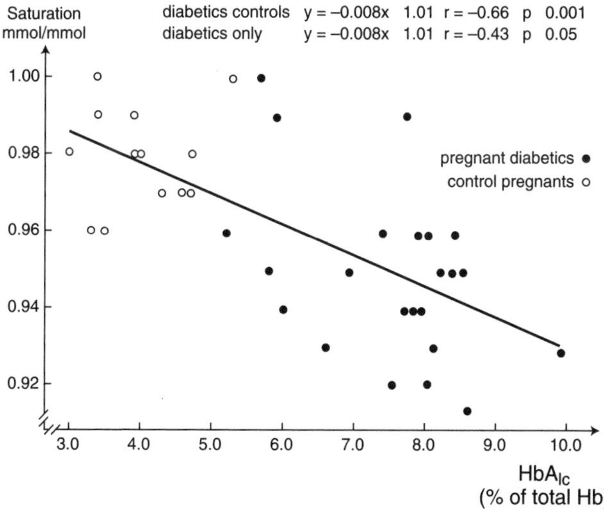

Figure 13–11. Correlation between HbA_{1C} and arterial oxygen saturation in diabetic women. (Adapted from Datta S, Greene MF: The diabetic parturient, in Datta S (ed): *Anesthetic and Obstetric Management of High Risk Pregnancy, 2nd ed.* St Louis, Mosby, 1996.)

Anesthetic Management

Labor and Delivery. For labor and vaginal delivery moderate pain relief can be obtained by administering small doses of narcotics early in the first stage. A lumbar epidural block can provide excellent pain relief for both labor and delivery. It has been noted that the fetus commenced the second stage in a less acidotic state when mothers received epidural analgesia than did fetuses whose mothers did not receive any analgesia.[35] The acidosis was metabolic in origin and was related to high lactate concentrations. A recent report suggested that epidural analgesia will reduce the level of maternal endogenous catecholamines during labor, and this might benefit placental perfusion, a factor possibly more important in this special group of parturients.[36]

Spinal anesthesia can also be used if required at the time of delivery. *One should use a separate intravenous line for the rapid infusion of non–dextrose-containing solutions if necessary to treat hypotension without producing hyperglycemia.* It is also important to realize that the fetus of a diabetic mother might be quite susceptible to hypoxia secondary to maternal hypotension.

Anesthesia for Cesarean Section. The incidence of cardiovascular depression is higher during regional anesthesia for cesarean section and is related to a higher sympathetic blockade accentuated by compression of the inferior vena cava and aorta by the gravid uterus.

In 1977 we compared spinal and general anesthesia for abdominal delivery in healthy mothers and diabetic parturients (Table 13-6). We found that infants of diabetic mothers receiving spinal anesthesia were more acidotic than were infants of diabetic mothers receiving general anesthesia.[37] The acidosis appeared to be related to both maternal diabetes and maternal hypotension. Subsequently, maternal and neonatal acid-base values were also examined after administering epidural anesthesia. We noticed a 60% incidence of neonatal acidosis (umbilical artery pH of 7.20 or less) during epidural anesthesia.[38] The fetal acidosis was related to both the degree and the presence of maternal hypotension. The umbilical artery pH was always greater than 7.20 in the

Table 13–6. Effect of Hypotension in Infants of Diabetic Mothers Following Spinal or Epidural Anesthesia for Cesarean Section

Anesthesia	No Hypotension	Hypotension
Spinal anesthesia (*N* = 15)		
Umbilical artery		
pH	7.24 ± 0.02†	7.16 ± 0.01‡
P_{O_2} (mm Hg)	19 ± 2	16 ± 2
P_{CO_2} (mm Hg)	65 ± 3	71 ± 4‡
Base deficit (mEq/L)	4.35 ± 0.88	8.25 ± 1.74‡
	n = 9	*n* = 6
Epidural anesthesia (*N* = 16)		
Umbilical artery		
pH	7.26 ± 0.02	7.16 ± 0.01‡
P_{O_2} (mm Hg)	25 ± 2.5	18 ± 1.3‡
P_{CO_2} (mm Hg)	52 ± 2	65 ± 3†
Base deficit (mEq/L)	5 ± 1.2	10 ± 0.6‡
	n = 6	*n* = 10

Data from Datta S, Brown WU: *Anesthesiology* 1977: 47:272; and Datta S, Brown WU, Ostheimer GW, et al: *Anesth Analg* 1981; 60:574.

†Mean ± SE.

‡*p* , 0.05.

absence of maternal hypotension. We used 5% dextrose with lactated Ringer's solution for acute volume expansion in both studies.

The genesis of the fetal acidosis in pregnant diabetic parturients appears to be complex, and several factors might be involved: (1) the human placenta produces lactate in vitro, especially under conditions of hypoxia or increased glycogen deposition as in maternal diabetes, and (2) *fetal lactic acidemia might occur due to hypoxia (secondary to maternal hypotension) in the presence of hyperglycemia following acute volume loading with dextrose-containing solutions. An additional risk of maternal and fetal hyperglycemia accompanying acute volume expansion with dextrose-containing solutions before cesarean section in diabetic parturients is the occurrence of neonatal hypoglycemia. (3) Finally, it has been observed that chronic infusion of insulin directly into the sheep fetus increased fetal glucose uptake, increased oxidative utilization of glucose by the fetus, and surprisingly, reduced the fetal arterial oxygen content.*[39] Hyperinsulinemia may increase oxygen consumption. Fetal hyperglycemia and hyperinsulinemia might result in reduced fetal oxygenation in pregnancies complicated by uncontrolled diabetes (Fig. 13-12).

We recently re-evaluated the acid-base status (Table 13-7) of ten rigidly controlled insulin-dependent diabetic mothers and ten healthy nondiabetic control women having spinal anesthesia for cesarean section.[40]

The parturients were all well controlled, dextrose-free intravenous solutions were used for volume expansion before induction of anesthesia, and hypotension was prevented in all cases by prompt treatment with ephedrine. There were no significant differences in the acid-base values between the diabetic and nondiabetic mothers and the infants of the diabetic and control groups. We concluded that (1) if maternal diabetes is well controlled, (2) if dextrose-containing solutions are not used for maternal intravascular volume expansion before delivery, and (3) if maternal hypotension is avoided, regional anesthesia can be used safely for diabetic mothers having cesarean section.[41] If general anesthesia is used, metoclopramide should be used preoperatively because the incidence

Table 13-7. Acid-Base Values in Infants of Diabetic Mothers With Rigid Glucose Control, Non-Dextrose-Containing Solution for Volume Expansion, and Prevention of Maternal Hypotension

Umbilical Artery (n = 20)	**No Hypotension (Diabetic) (n = 10)**	**No Hypotension (Control) (n = 10)**
pH	7.27 ± 0.01[†]	7.30 ± 0.01
P_{O_2} (mm Hg)	20 ± 2	22 ± 2
P_{CO_2} (mm Hg)	56 ± 2	50 ± 2.5
Base deficit (mEq/L)	4 ± 1	3 ± 0.7

From Datta S, Kitzmiller JL, Naulty JS, et al: *Anesth Analg* 1982; 61:662. Used by permission.

[†]Values represent mean ± SE.

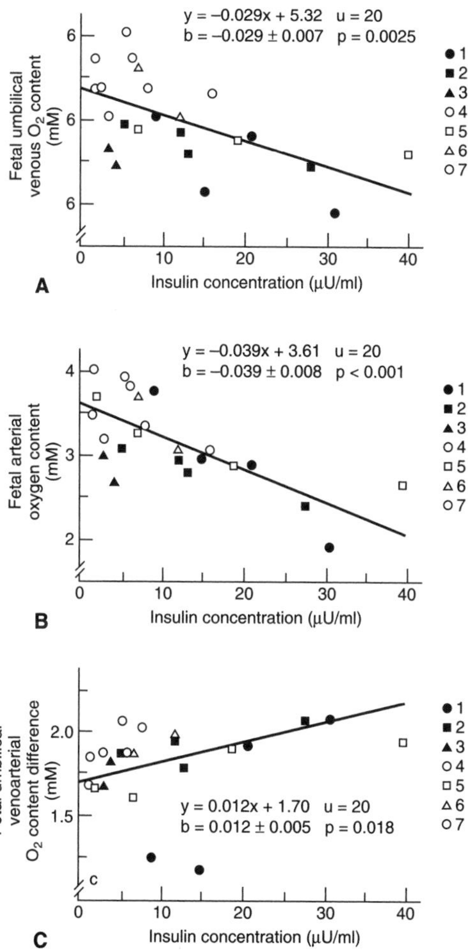

Figure 13–12. Relationship between fetal plasma insulin concentration and **(A)** fetal arterial oxygen content, **(B)** fetal venous oxygen content, and **(C)** fetal umbilical venoarterial oxygen content difference. (From Milley JR, Rosenberg AA, Phillips AF, et al: *Am J Obstet Gynecol* 1984; 149:673. Used with permission from Elsevier.)

of gastric stasis is very high in this group of women. Finally, one should also remember the significant drop in insulin requirement immediately after delivery.[42] *Recently impaired counterregulatory hormone responses to hypoglycemia during sleep have been observed in diabetic subjects.*[43] Although no clinical study exists, one should speculate that the IDDM parturients may benefit from cesarean section under regional rather than general anesthesia.

Summary of Anesthesia for Cesarean Section Diabetic Parturients

1. Hydration is conducted with non—dextrose-containing solutions (separate intravenous line if necessary).
2. Routine left uterine displacement is used
3. Hypotension is promptly treated with intravenous ephedrine.
4. A well-conducted general anesthesia can be used if necessary with good neonatal outcome.

Cardiac Disease

Rheumatic fever-related acquired heart problems have decreased dramatically in recent years, and with better surgical technique, the future population will become pregnant with fewer congenital cardiac problems. The incidence of heart disease during pregnancy varies from 0.4% to 4.1%. Major cardiac problems can be divided into acquired and congenital disease:

I. *Acquired* cardiac disease
   A. Mitral stenosis
   B. Mitral insufficiency
   C. Mitral valve prolapse
   D. Aortic stenosis
   E. Aortic insufficiency
II. *Congenital* cardiac disease
   A. *Left-to-right shunt*
      1. *Ventricular septal defect*
      2. Atrial septal defect
      3. *Patent ductus arteriosus*

B. *Right-to-left shunt*
   1. *Tetralogy of Fallot*
   2. *Eisenmenger's syndrome*

Patients with cardiac disease would be affected by some of the important physiological changes during pregnancy as well as during labor and delivery. An increase in cardiac output is the most important physiological change. *Cardiac output maximally increases during pregnancy at 28 to 32 weeks of gestation, and labor and delivery can impose further stress. During the first stage of labor, cardiac output increases 15% to 30% because of autotransfusion (300 to 500 mL) during each uterine contraction, and an increase in the heart rate and systemic vascular resistance due to the effect of catecholamines will also increase the cardiac output. During the second stage, cardiac output can increase further, and the highest cardiac output is observed immediately after delivery (potentially up to 80% above normal)* (Fig. 13-13).

Treatment

Anticoagulants can be used for specific treatment as well as for prophylaxis of systemic embolism. *Heparin is usually the drug of choice* (*does not cross placenta*), but oral anticoagulant therapy should be discontinued before the time of delivery to avoid potential fetal bleeding caused by the trauma of delivery.

Anesthetic Management

Heparin treatment should be stopped before induction of labor or elective cesarean section, and the aPTT should be measured if regional analgesia/anesthesia is to be used. Anesthetic management of cardiac disease in pregnancy can be summarized as shown in the outline below.

I. Acquired heart diseases:
   A. Labor and delivery:
      1. Relief of stress and apprehension should be accomplished during labor by the administration of tranquilizers.

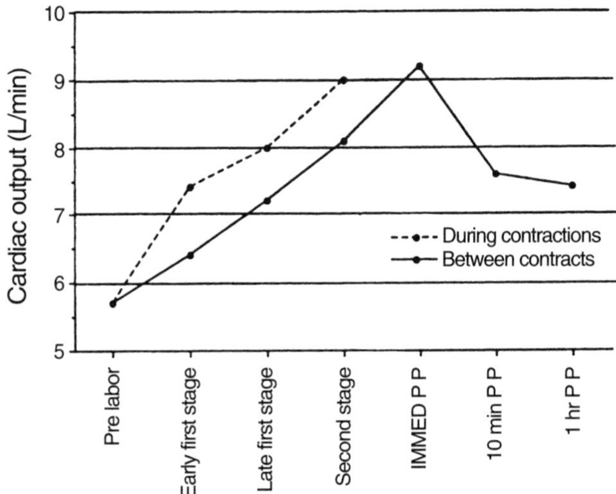

Figure 13-13. Changes in cardiac output during the first and second stages of labor. (From Datta S (ed): *Anesthetic and Obstetric Management of High Risk Pregnancy,* 2nd ed. St Louis, Mosby, 1996. Used with permission from Elsevier.)

2. For relief of pain, epidural analgesia should be considered.
3. Hypotension should be avoided by the judicious administration of local anesthetic doses and the prevention and treatment of aortocaval compression. If there is hypotension, *phenylephrine in dilute solution is preferable to ephedrine because ephedrine can increase the heart rate and thus the work of the heart.*

B. Cesarean section:
1. Parturients with aortic insufficiency and mitral insufficiency can tolerate epidural anesthesia or the continuous spinal technique.
2. Pregnant women with severe aortic stenosis or mitral stenosis need close and careful attention. Both regional anesthesia (epidural) and general anesthesia

have been used. If general anesthesia is selected, then a highdose narcotic technique is preferable.

II. Congenital heart lesions:
   A. Labor and delivery:
      1. *Hypotension will reverse the left-to-right shunt. For this reason, high spinal anesthesia should always be avoided.*
      2. Epidural analgesia with proper invasive monitoring can be used for labor and delivery. This will be beneficial for complete relief of pain and abolition of bearing down, which might further increase the right atrial, right ventricular, and pulmonary pressures. Hypotension should be treated with small doses of phenylephrine. Recently, intraspinal narcotics have been used for maintaining cardiovascular stability.
      3. A combination of systemic analgesics and tranquilizers during the early first stage with a paracervical block during the active phase and a bilateral pudendal block during delivery can also be used. *One must be aware of the problems associated with paracervical blocks, and continuous fetal monitoring is mandatory.*
      4. Regional anesthesia is contraindicated if anticoagulant treatment must be continued for any reason.
   B. Cesarean section:
      1. Epidural anesthesia has been used with invasive monitoring; postoperative analgesia can be used by the epidural route.
      2. General anesthesia can be used with the high-dose narcotic technique. The newborn can be resuscitated accordingly.
      3. A dilute oxytocin solution should be infused to prevent postpartum uterine relaxation and needless blood loss. *A bolus intravenous injection of oxytocin may cause serious hypotension, while intramuscular ergonovine preparations may produce severe peripheral vasoconstriction followed by hypertension. Both these drugs should be used carefully during this situation.*

4. Parturients receiving propranolol are always at "high risk" because anesthesiologists may face problems related to a reduction in cardiac output and maternal myocardial reserve, as well as decreased responsiveness to β-adrenergic–stimulating drugs in the presence of hypotension. Parturients receiving high doses of propranolol may not be candidates for major regional anesthesia for cesarean delivery. *The effects of the chronic administration of propranolol on the fetus include intrauterine growth retardation, fetal bradycardia, and neonatal hypoglycemia, so babies need careful postpartum attention in such cases.*

The anesthetic management for severe cardiac disease (severe mitral stenosis, aortic stenosis) can be summarized as follows:

A. The pregnant woman should be consulted at 24–32 weeks' gestation because cardiac output is highest at this stage. The parturients can be classified into four groups according to New York Heart classification (Table 13-8).
B. Depending on the NYAA classification, one can decide the monitoring of the parturients:
   a. Invasive monitoring should include arterial line, CVP line with cordis, and PA catheter (controversial).
C. Anesthetic management for labor and delivery may include early epidural analgesia. Sensory analgesia levels should be increased gradually, observing the CVP pressure as well as maternal arterial pressure. A drop in blood pressure should be treated with a judicious volume of fluid and vasopressors.

Table 13-8. New York Heart Association Functional Classification

Class I	Asymptomatic
Class II	Symptomatic with exertion
Class III	Symptomatic with normal activities
Class IV	Symptomatic at rest

Neo-Synephrine in small doses (50–100 mcg) should be used unless contraindicated, in which case ephedrine may be the drug of choice. Sensory levels should be maintained to T_6. For the second stage perineal anesthesia should be dense (cardiac delivery) to prevent the urge to push. Forceps or vacuum extraction is usually used. If emergency cesarean section is necessary, the surgical anesthesia can be obtained using either with 2% plain lidocaine or 0.5% ropivacaine mixed with opioids (fentanyl or sufentaril). If general anesthesia is necessary, induction with opioids or mixed with etomidate will be ideal.

Respiratory Problems

Bronchial Asthma

Bronchial asthma might be expected to improve during pregnancy due to the bronchiolar relaxing effect of progesterone. However, it has been shown that pregnancy has no consistent effect on the course of asthma.

Medical therapy for respiratory problems is the same as in nonpregnant women.

For labor and delivery, one should use a continuous epidural block.

Cesarean Section. The possibility of drug interactions should be borne in mind when taking care of pregnant women with a history of bronchial asthma. Different medications that have been used are (1) methylxanthines, e.g., theophylline, aminophylline; (2) β-mimetic drugs, e.g., metaproterenol, albuterol (salbutamol), terbutaline, fenoterol, inhaled β-mimetic agonists (the primary medications for the treatment of acute asthma at the present time); and (3) corticosteroids.

Regional Anesthesia. Studies have suggested that although regional anesthesia has minor effects on inspiratory effort,[45] its effect on expiratory function can be significant. *Spinal anesthesia, because of its more intense motor block, can affect abdominal muscle function as well as cough strength, thus affecting expiratory function considerably.* Severe bronchoconstriction following spinal anesthesia in a parturient with severe asthma has been reported.[46] The author suggested that diminished epinephrine secretion from the adrenal medulla because of sympathectomy might have triggered the bronchospasm. The author prefers epidural anesthesia over spinal anesthesia as the regional anesthetic of choice in a parturient with severe asthma. An interesting study observed less dense intercostal motor block with 0.5% bupivacaine compared to 2% lidocaine with epinephrine (this should be true for 0.5% ropivacaine)[46a].

General Anesthesia. General anesthesia should be avoided in parturients with respiratory problems if possible because the endotracheal tube can trigger severe bronchospasm. However, if it is absolutely essential, several precautions involving premedication should be taken: (1) H_2-receptor blockers like cimetidine and ranitidine should be avoided because the H_2-receptor blockade can increase the sensitivity to histamine-induced bronchoconstriction[47]; (2) a nonparticulate antacid, 0.3 *M* sodium citrate, 30 mL, should be used routinely; and (3) atropine and glycopyrrolate can reduce oral secretions and will also cause broncodilatation; hence some anesthesiologists will use these drugs as a premedicant. *However, these drugs can reduce gastroesophageal sphincter tone.*

Induction Agents. Ketamine should be the drug of choice because it can relax the bronchial muscles through central catecholamine release (Fig. 13-14). Succinylcholine can be used for intubation. Of the nondepolarizing muscle relaxants, vecuronium may be safer than others.

Inhalation Agents. Halothane, enflurane, and isoflurane all provide bronchodilatation. *However, ventricular tachycardia and arrhythmias can occur if halothane is used in the presence of aminophylline or β-mimetic drugs.* Recently sevoflurane has been suggested as an alternative to halothane and isoflurane. *Inhalation anesthetics can cause uterine muscle relaxation and predispose to obstetric hemorrhage. Intraoperative bronchoconstriction can be effectively treated with β-mimetic drugs administered from a metered-dose inhaler.*

Extubation also needs careful attention.

Cystic Fibrosis

Pregnant women with cystic fibrosis should be followed closely in regard to their lung function. These parturients are

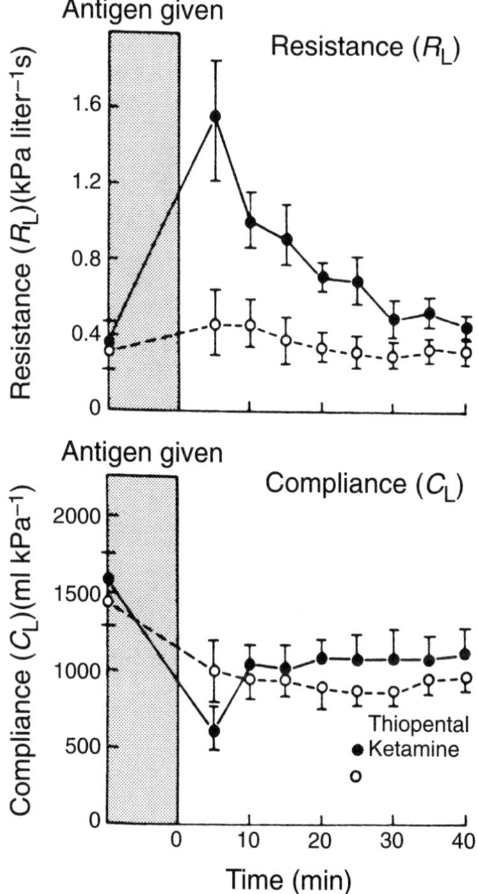

Figure 13–14. Changes in pulmonary resistance in sensitized dogs anesthetized with ketamine or thiopental. (From Hirshman CA, Downes H, Farbood A, et al: *Br J Anaesth* 1979; 51:713–717. © The Board of Management and Trustees of the British Journal of Anaesthesia. Reproduced by permission of Oxford University Press/British Journal of Anaesthesia.)

often associated with severe pulmonary obstruction and respiratory impairment. *For labor and delivery, epidural analgesia should be the ideal choice.* For cesarean section, the anesthetic technique will depend on the condition of the pregnant woman. Epidural anesthesia should be used whenever possible. This technique is associated with fewer pulmonary complications and can also be utilized for excellent postoperative pain relief. Parturients with severe respiratory impairment may need general anesthesia.

Neurological Problems

Neurological problems are uncommon during the childbearing age. Regional anesthesia is contraindicated in the presence of active inflammatory disease in the spinal canal, acute meningitis, or superficial infection at the site of the lumbar puncture. However, regional anesthesia may not be contraindicated in old inflammatory problems, e.g., a parturient with a history of poliomyelitis.

Paraplegia

The unique phenomenon experienced by paraplegics and quadraplegics is called autonomic hyperflexia or mass reflex. Interestingly, the syndrome is not found if the lesion is below T7. It occurs in 85% of cases with lesions above T7 (Fig. 13-15).

Stimulation of the skin below the level of the lesion, the presence of distension, or contraction of a hollow viscus like urinary bladder, uterus, or gut might precipitate the mass reflex. This might present in the form of pilomotor erection, sweating, facial flushing, severe headache, bradycardia, and severe hypertension leading to convulsions, loss of consciousness, and possible subarachnoid or cerebral hemorrhage. Eleven percent of paraplegic patients may develop severe hypertension during pregnancy due to mass reflex. *The incidence of premature labor is high among paraplegics.*

Anesthetic Management. ***Labor and Delivery.*** Epidural analgesia should be used as soon as the patient goes into labor to prevent autonomic hyperreflexia and mass reflex. We have used continuous epidural infusion with 0.125% bupivacaine

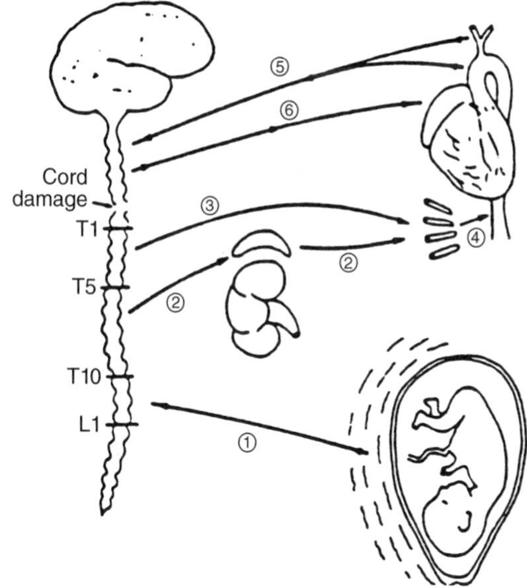

Figure 13-15. Mechanism of autonomic hyperreflexia in paraplegic and quadriplegic patients. (From Abouleish EI, Hanley ES, Palmer SM. Can epidural Fentanyl control automatic hyperreflexia in a quadriplegic parturient? Anesth Analg 1989; 68:523-526.)

and 2 μg fentanyl per milliliter (10 mL/hr) with excellent outcome. Epidural meperidine has been used in one case with success.[48] The main advantage of epidural opioids is sparing of the resting sympathetic tone, which may already be impaired following cord transection.

Cesarean Section. Epidural anesthesia is preferable to spinal anesthesia because the chance of hypotension is less. If general anesthesia is essential, one should avoid succinylcholine administration because of the possibility of hyperkalemia.

Cerebrovascular Accidents

Arterial or venous thrombosis is not common. Cerebral hemorrhage can be seen in association with severe eclampsia. Subarachnoid hemorrhage can occur during pregnancy due to a leaking aneurysm or arteriovenous malformation. Cardiovascular stresses during pregnancy, labor, delivery, and the immediate postpartum period can precipitate a subarachnoid hemorrhage.

Anesthetic Management. For labor and delivery a continuous epidural block is advisable. The use of forceps is indicated to shorten the second stage. In the immediate postpartum period, one should be prepared to treat hypertension aggressively if it occurs. For cesarean delivery, an epidural block is the anesthesia of choice; however, if there is fetal distress or if general anesthesia is indicated for some other reason, one has to be careful about the hypertensive response following endotracheal intubation.

Multiple Sclerosis

This disease is characterized by demyelination of the brain and spinal cord. The course is associated with remissions and exacerbations, and is unpredictable in nature. *However, the relapse rate during the first 3 months postpartum is known to be about three times higher than that in nonpregnant individuals.*[48a]

Anesthetic Management. Bader and colleagues observed the relationship of anesthetic techniques and the type and amount of anesthetic agent used with the postpartum relapse rate of multiple sclerosis at Brigham and Women's Hospital between 1982 and 1987.[49] Postpartum relapses occurred in 9 of the 32 pregnancies during the first 3 months. Seven women had vaginal delivery, whereas 2 parturients underwent cesarean section (Tables 13-9 to 13-11). Pregnant women who had epidural anesthesia for vaginal delivery did not have a significantly higher incidence of postpartum relapse than did parturients who received either pudendal or local infiltration. Interestingly, in the relapsed population, all women received a higher concentration of local anesthetic for a prolonged period (>0.25% bupivacaine). The authors suggested (1) that there is no absolute contraindication to the use of regional analgesia for labor and delivery, (2) that the parturient should be informed beforehand about the possibility of postpartum relapse not related to anesthesia, and

Table 13-9. Relapse Rate of Multiple Sclerosis in the First 3 Months Postpartum

Type of Anesthetic	Cesarean Delivery (No. of Cases)	Relapse No.
Epidural	5	1
General	3	1
	Vaginal Delivery	
Epidural	9	4
Local	13	2
General	2	1

From Bader AM, Hunt CO, Datta S, et al: *J Clin Anesth* 1988; 1:21. Used with permission from Elsevier.

Table 13-10. Epidural Local Anesthetics Used for Vaginal Delivery in Patients With Multiple Sclerosis

Drug	No. of Cases	Relapse No.
Bupivacaine, 0.25%	4	0
Bupivacaine, 0.5%	2	2
Bupivacaine, 0.5%, + lidocaine, 2%	1	1
Lidocaine, 2%	1	0
Drugs unknown	1	0

From Bader AM, Hunt CO, Datta S, et al: *J Clin Anesth* 1988; 1:21. Used with permission from Elsevier.

Table 13-11. Local Anesthetics Used for Cesarean Section

Drugs Used	No. of Cases	Relapse No.	Indication
Lidocaine, 2%	2	0	Breech, previa
Lidocaine, 2%, + bupivacaine, 0.5%	1	0	Previa
Bupivacaine, 0.5%, + chloroprocaine, 3%	1	0	Fetal distress
Bupivacaine, 0.5%, + lidocaine, 2%, + chloroprocaine, 3%	1	1	Failure to progress

From Bader AM, Hunt CO, Datta S, et al: *J Clin Anesth* 1988; 1:21. Used with permission from Elsevier.

(3) that lower concentrations of local anesthetics should be used in these individuals to minimize the concentration of anesthetic that reaches the spinal cord.

Space-Occupying Lesions (Brain Tumors)

Labor and Delivery. Spinal anesthesia may be relatively contraindicated in brain tumors because of a sudden reduction in cerebrospinal fluid (CSF) pressure; if it occurs rapidly, it may produce cerebral herniation and death. *On the other hand, painful uterine contractions and bearing-down efforts during labor will increase intracranial pressure; hence epidural or caudal analgesia may be indicated, but one should bear in mind the consequences of accidental dural puncture.* Some authors suggest the use of a bilateral lumbar sympathetic block for the first stage of labor and a pudendal block for the second stage.

Cesarean Section. Most anesthesiologists prefer to use general anesthesia for this purpose. Induction with *large doses of narcotics, hypotensive medication (if necessary), sodium thiopental (Pentothal), and vecuronium* may be used. *Isoflurane is the inhalation anesthetic of choice since it does not increase cerebral blood flow.*[50] *Although hyperventilation can reduce the intracranial pressure, it can affect the uteroplacental circulation, and continuous fetal heart rate monitoring, if possible, may be useful until delivery.* Arterial and CVP lines may be indicated. Depending upon the severity of the increase in intracranial pressure, neurosurgeons may prefer to reduce the intracranial pressure by surgical drainage before cesarean section. *Medical therapy to decrease intracranial pressure includes* steroids and diuretics like furosemide or mannitol, which obviously will be tried before surgical intervention. A close FHR monitoring is necessary while using mannitol because of the possibility of severe maternal and fetal hypovolemia. Reduced uteroplacental circulation is also a possibility. Constant communication is necessary between the neurologist, obstetrician, and anesthesiologist.

In benign intracranial hypertension (pseudotumor cerebri), *the increased intracranial pressure is not related to intracranial mass, infection, or obstruction to CSF outflow and may be related to decreased CSF absorption. Regional anesthesia, spinal or epidural, is preferred for both vaginal delivery and cesarean section.*

Epilepsy

There is no evidence that epileptic group are more susceptible to convulsion from local anesthetics than the normal population. *Spinal or epidural anesthesia is not contraindicated in such cases. For general anesthesia, drugs that have potential convulsive action, e.g., enflurane or ketamine, should be avoided.*

Myasthenia Gravis

The major problems encountered in parturients with myasthenia gravis are as follows:

1. Chance of a prolonged second stage of labor because of muscle weakness
2. Postdelivery pulmonary complications because of respiratory muscle weakness
3. Complications during anesthesia
4. Possibility of neonatal myasthenia gravis

Myasthenic or cholinergic crisis may be evident by progressive generalized bulbar and respiratory weakness. Differential diagnosis occasionally may be difficult:

Myasthenic crisis	Cholinergic crisis
Progressive deteriorization of the disease process evidenced by cranial nerve involvement (ocular symptoms) as well as respiratory muscle weakness	Often associated with high doses of antiacetyl-cholinesterase therapy and accompanied by muscarinic side effects like diarrhea, sweating, abdominal sweating, abdominal muscle cramps, fasciculations, palpitations, increased secretions, and bradycardia

In a controversial situation, parturients may need ventilation and supplemental feeding. Antiacetylcholinesterase should be stopped and then gradually restarted in case of cholinergic crisis. In myasthenic crisis, women may need plasmapheresis followed by immunosuppressive therapy. Although rare, myasthenic parturients may be associated with PIH. Use of magnesium sulfate for PIH is contraindicated in this situation. Phenytoin may be used in these cases.[50a]

Anesthetic Management. ***Labor and Delivery.*** Tranquilizers and narcotics should be used cautiously because of the chance of respiratory depression. *Epidural analgesia will reduce the requirements of systemic analgesics. Amide local anesthetics are preferable to esters because the women are usually receiving anticholinesterase drugs for their treatment and these can prolong ester local anesthetic activity.*[51]

Cesarean Delivery. Because of the need of a higher level of sensory anesthesia for cesarean delivery, there is always a danger of impairment of the respiratory and swallowing muscles following regional anesthesia. Unless contraindicated because of respiratory insufficiency, regional anesthesia should be the technique of choice. If general anesthesia is indicated, succinylcholine should be used to facilitate intubation. However, the effect of depolarizing muscle relaxants has been described as inconsistent.[52] Depolarizing muscle relaxant activity can be prolonged in the presence of anticholinesterase therapy. Myasthenic parturients are overly sensitive to nondepolarizing muscle relaxants. Nondepolarizing muscle relaxants should be used in small doses, and a blockade monitor must be used.

Neonatal Myasthenia Gravis. A transient form of myasthenia gravis happens in 12% of babies born to myasthenic mothers. It develops within the first 4 days of life. Symptoms include lethargy, poor sucking reflex, feeble cry, generalized muscle weakness, or absent or weak Moro's reflex. Diagnosis is confirmed by using edrophonium chloride, 0.05 to 0.1 mL, subcutaneously.

Renal Disorders

Physiological Changes

The major physiological changes are as follows:

1. *The effective renal plasma flow and glomerular filtration rate (GFR) increase by 50% by 16 weeks' gestation.*
2. The high renal plasma flow and GFR result in an increase in creatinine clearance.
3. During normal pregnancy, the blood urea nitrogen (BUN) level averages 8 to 9 mg/dL and creatinine, 0.46 mg/dL. *Therefore, during pregnancy, normal nonpregnant BUN (10 to 20 mg/dL) and creatinine (0.5 to 1.2 mg/dL) levels may represent renal compromise.*
4. One of the most common disorders in pregnancy that involves kidney function is preeclampsia.
5. Acute renal failure in pregnancy can occur in conjunction with hemorrhage, sepsis, or preeclampsia.

Anesthetic Management

Several important factors have to be considered before the anesthetic technique is selected:

I. The parturients should undergo dialysis before surgery if time permits.

II. Arteriovenous fistulas should be carefully protected during surgery.

III. *Because of the presence of severe anemia, hyperventilation should be prevented because this will shift the O_2 dissociation curve to the left.*

IV. Drug interactions:

   A. Abnormal protein binding may cause prolongation of the thiopental effect.

   B. *Nondepolarizing muscle relaxants like gallamine should not be used because they are excreted mainly by the kidney:* vecuronium and pancuronium excretion can also be prolonged in the presence of renal failure.

   C. *Depolarizing muscle relaxants such as succinylcholine can increase serum potassium levels; hence, they should be contraindicated in parturients with hyper-*

kalemia. A low pseudocholinesterase level can prolong the succinylcholine block.

D. *Enflurane and methoxyflurane should not be used.*

Labor and Delivery. *Epidural analgesia should be the technique of choice.*

Cesarean Section. *Epidural technique* is preferred over spinal because of less chance of severe hypotension and less need of volume loading, which might be detrimental in parturients with chronic renal failure. If general anesthesia is essential, succinylcholine may be contraindicated, and halothane or isoflurane should be the inhalation anesthetic of choice.

Hematological Disorders

Besides the hereditary clotting defects, the defects that are of concern in obstetric population are the acquired problems[53]:

1. Drugs that interfere with platelet function (e.g., aspirin, heparin).
2. Massive transfusion of old bank blood.
3. Liver failure.
4. *Disseminated intravascular coagulation, associated with abruptio placentae, amniotic fluid embolism, intrauterine fetal death, and severe preeclampsia. The pathophysiology of disseminated intravascular coagulation consists of simultaneous uncontrolled activation of procoagulants and fibrinolytic enzymes in the microvasculature. The process depletes platelets and procoagulants. Plasma (fibrinolysin) levels are elevated and this leads to further digestion of fibrin clots, which releases fibrin degradation products and inhibits polymerization.*

Anesthetic Management

1. General anesthesia should be the choice because of the clotting problems unless treatment with the medications is stopped beforehand and clotting parameters revert to the normal range (Fig 13-16).
2. Blood volume replacement and circulatory support are necessary.

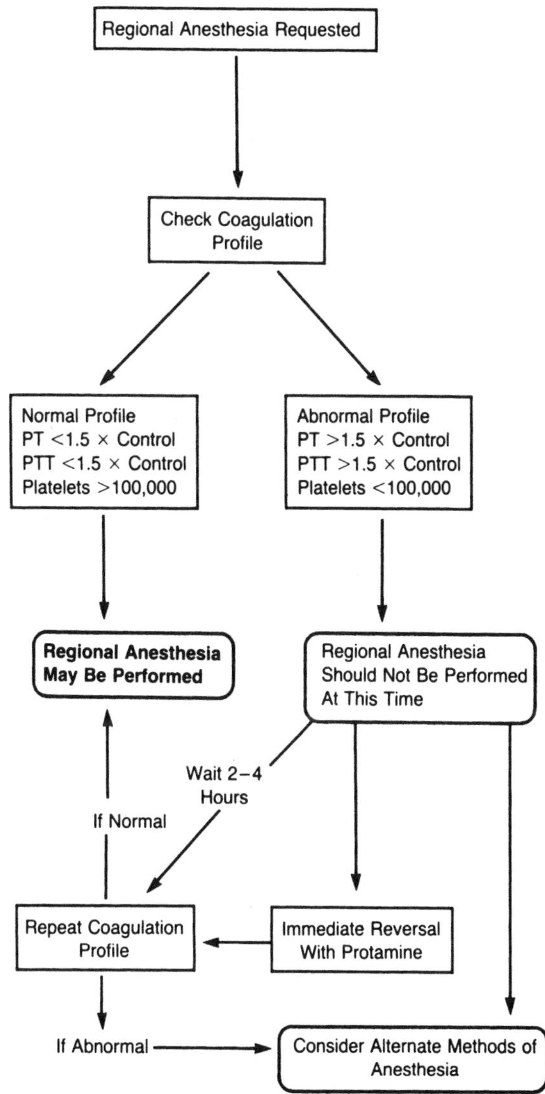

Figure 13–16. Regional anesthesia in the heparinized parturient. (From Sharma SK, Leveno KJ. Anticoagulated Patient. In Datta S (ed): Anesthetic and Obstetric Management of High-Risk Pregnancy 3rd ed. New York, Springer, 2004.)

3. Fresh whole blood or red cells and fresh frozen plasma containing all known clotting factors should be used. A 250-mL unit of fresh frozen plasma contains 200 to 400 mg of fibrinogen and also factors VIII, V, and XIII. Cryoprecipitate is a concentrated preparation of fibrinogen and contains 200 to 400 mg of fibrinogen in 15 to 20 mL.
4. The administration of procoagulants to replace factors that have been consumed is essential.

Sickle Cell Disease

Parturients with sickle cell trait usually have no problems during pregnancy; however, women with S/S or S/C disease are poor obstetric risks. Their anemia becomes more severe during pregnancy, and the incidence of preeclampsia is increased.

Anesthetic Management. Hypoxia and hypotension must be prevented because of the increased chance of sickling.

Labor and Delivery. Epidural analgesia is the technique of choice, and proper volume expansion with warm fluid is important. Oxygen should be administered and aortocaval compression should be avoided. Hypotension should be immediately corrected.

Cesarean Delivery. Epidural anesthesia, if properly performed, will be associated with good maternal and neonatal outcome. It can also be used for postoperative analgesia, which might be necessary in these women because they might be receiving analgesic drugs because of sickle cell crisis. Warm fluid for volume expansion should be used, and treatment of hypotension should be immediate. If general anesthesia is indicated, proper oxygenation and a warm environment are essential.

Idiopathic Thrombocytopenia

Regional anesthesia may be indicated both for labor and delivery and for cesarean section, provided that the clotting parameters are normal. If coagulation parameters are abnormal and clinical features of prolonged bleeding are present, general anesthesia will be necessary for cesarean section.

Gentle intubation with a small-sized endotracheal tube is important for preventing hematoma of the vocal cords.

Classification of Von Willebrand disease (Incidence/1: 10,000)[53a]:

Type 1: Mild to moderate bleeding, mildly decreased vWF (60–70%)

Type 2: Mild to moderate bleeding, normal vWF levels. In type 2a there is a deficiency in the high-molecular-weight forms of vWF, whereas type 2b is due to the inappropriate binding of vWF to platelets.

Type 3: Autosomal recessive (may have severe mucosal bleeding)

Treatment: DDAVP, 0.3 mg/kg, especially in type 1. DDAVP should not be given in type 2a and may worsen type 2b. During therapy, close monitoring of vWF levels is necessary; the patrurient may develop tachyphlaxis when treatment is used for more than 48 hours.

Hypercoaguable States

Protein C is a vitamin K-dependent hepatic protein and is converted to an active protease by thrombin. Activated protein C in conjunction with protein S proteolyses factors Va and VIIIa, which shuts off the fibrin formation. Deficiencies of protein C and S cause recurrent venous thrombosis and pulmonary embolism. *Heparin therapy* may be necessary during pregnancy.[53a]

Factor V Leiden Mutation

Carriers of the factor V Leiden mutation have a high risk of fetal loss because of placental blood vessel thrombosis. Anticoagulant therapy is indicated from the beginning of pregnancy.[53b]

Endocrine Disorders

Hyperthyroidism

Major problems involving parturients with hyperthyroidism include the following:

1. The parturient might be receiving propranolol therapy.
2. If the mother is receiving antithyroid therapy, fetal goiter may occur.
3. The myocardium remains hypersensitive to catecholamines in such cases.
4. There is a possibility of thyroid storm. Thyroid storm, an exaggerated hypermetabolic state of thyrotoxicosis, is rare during pregnancy. Clinical signs include high fever, tachycardia, agitation, and severe dehydration. The important differential diagnosis is malignant hyperthermia.

Anesthetic Management. Regional anesthesia, especially spinal anesthesia, may be avoided, especially for cesarean delivery, if the mother is taking high doses of propranolol.

Pheochromocytoma

During pregnancy this entity carries high maternal and fetal mortality rates. Although epidural anesthesia can be used for labor and delivery, for cesarean section, an epidural or continuous spinal and general anesthesia may be used.[54] Prior treatment with α- followed by β-adrenergic blockers is indicated in elective cesarean section.

Problems Because of Miscellaneous Factors

Prematurity

Major problems connected with prematurity include the following:

1. Respiratory distress syndrome is the major cause of mortality in premature infants. Intrapartum hypoxia and severe maternal stress during labor may increase the severity.
2. Intracranial hemorrhage is usually related to uncontrolled delivery, other causes of birth trauma, or intracranial hemorrhage as a result of neonatal hypertension, which might be associated with asphyxia.
3. Ischemic cerebral damage can occur from intrapartum asphyxia, hypoxia, and hypotension.
4. There is a chance of a prolonged effect of depressant medications because metabolic and excretory systems may be immature in the preterm infant.

5. *Hypoglycemia is more common.*
6. *Hyperbilirubinemia caused by drugs that displace bilirubin from protein-binding sites could be harmful.*
7. *Drug interactions can occur among tocolytic agents, corticosteroids, and anesthetic agents.*

Regarding the etiology of premature labor, recent evidence suggests presence of infection in the reproductive tract. Epidemiologic studies provide information about the association of premature labor with colonization of the genital tract by group B streptococci, *Chlamydia, Neisseria gonorrhoeae* and other organisms that cause bacterial vaginosis.[54a] Fetal fibronectin, a marker of degradation of the extracellular matrix, has been used recently to diagnose preterm labor.[54b]

Tocolytic Agent Therapy. These drugs are used to stop premature contractions. Because of their side effects these agents can expose the mother and fetus to various risks. Various groups of drugs have been used for tocolysis.[55]

Ethanol. This drug inhibits the secretion of antidiuretic hormone and oxytocin. *While the primary mechanism of inhibition of labor by ethanol is related to the inhibition of secretion of oxytocin,* there are several other possible mechanisms. Ethanol may act directly on the myometrium by suppressing intrinsic uterine activity and/or interfering with the action of uterine-stimulating agents such as the prostaglandins. A loading dose of 7.5 mL/kg/hr of 10% ethanol in 5% dextrose is infused over a period of 2 hours. This dose is followed by a maintenance infusion of 10% ethanol at a rate of 1.5 mL/kg/hr for 10 hours. If labor recurs, a second or third course of ethanol is given. However, because of the major side effects and availability of better drugs, this drug has become unpopular. *The possibility of maternal unconsciousness with gastric aspiration remains the major problem.*

Anesthetic Considerations—The following problems should be taken into account with ethanol therapy for prematurity:

1. *Inebriated, uncooperative, and possibly unconscious mother*
2. *Increased acid gastric secretion, nausea, and vomiting*

Magnesium Sulfate. Strips of myometrium excised from gravid human uteri have reduced contractility in the presence of magnesium ions. Magnesium sulfate has been used as the primary tocolytic agent to prevent delivery, as an adjunct to other tocolytic agents, and also in place of other tocolytic agents when they have failed to inhibit preterm labor. The mechanism of action is not fully understood; however, it is possible, by competing with calcium for surface binding sites on smooth muscle membrane, for magnesium to prevent the increase in free intracellular calcium concentration that is necessary for myosin light-chain kinase activity. In addition, there is evidence that an increased magnesium ion concentration activates adenylcyclase and the synthesis of cyclic adenosine monophosphate (cAMP).

Anesthetic Considerations—Parturients receiving magnesium sulfate therapy are more sensitive to both depolarizing and nondepolarizing relaxants. The neuromuscular blockade monitor should be used routinely. The minimum alveolar concentration is decreased in the presence of magnesium.

Calcium Channel Blockers. Although these drugs are primarily used in the treatment of ischemic heart disease and paroxysmal supraventricular tachycardia, these agents remain potentially useful tocolytics. However, the doses necessary to inhibit preterm labor are frequently associated with impairment of atrioventricular conduction and hypotension. Nifedipine, because of its fewer side effects, has been tried as a tocolytic agent. The contractility of myometrium is directly related to the concentration of free calcium with the cytoplasm; a decrease in the cytoplasmic free calcium level decreases contractility. Calcium channel blockers act by altering the net calcium uptake through cellular membranes by blockade of the aqueous voltage-dependent membrane channels selective for calcium or by affecting intracellular uptake and release mechanisms.

Anesthetic Considerations—Parturients receiving calcium channel blockers will be more prone to the cardiovascular depressive effect of inhalational anesthetics. In addition, there may be uterine atony postpartum, which is unresponsive to oxytocin and prostoglandin $F_{2\alpha}$ and which leads to postpartum hemorrhage.

Methylxanthines. These drugs exhibit the action of the phosphodiesterase enzyme responsible for the intracellular catabolism of cAMP. cAMP levels increase, and this results in uterine muscle relaxation. Because of the frequent incidence of side effects and the narrow margin between therapeutic and toxic blood levels, these drugs never became popular.

Prostaglandin Synthetase Inhibitors. Indomethacin has been used in preterm labor with some success. The main disadvantage of this drug is the chance of narrowing of the fetal ductus arteriosus and persistent fetal circulation. Indomethacin has been found to be effective and safe when used for short periods (48 hours) at less than 34 weeks' gestation. This agent can interfere with platelet function and can prolong the bleeding time.

β-Adrenergic Drugs. Currently the most widely used tocolytic agents, these agents act by direct stimulation of the β-adrenergic receptors present in uterine smooth muscle, with resultant increased intracellular cAMP levels and uterine relaxation. Side effects of these drugs can be seen in both mothers and neonates, and these can be classified as follows: (*1*) *CNS: nausea, vomiting, anxiety, and restlessness;* (*2*) *metabolic: hyperglycemia, hyperinsulinemia, hypokalemia, and acidosis; and* (*3*) *cardiovascular system: tachycardia, multiple arrhythmias, decreased diastolic pressure, decreased peripheral vascular resistance, dilutional anemia, low colloidal oncotic pressure, and pulmonary edema.*

Pulmonary Edema—This is one of the most complex problems following β-mimetic therapy, and the incidence has been reported to be 5% in parturients.[56] The exact mechanism is unknown; however, several factors can precipitate this problem (Figs. 13-17, and 13-18):

1. Increased intravenous fluid administration
2. Multiple gestation
3. Tocolysis therapy for more than 24 hours
4. Concomitant $MgSO_4$ therapy
5. Infection
6. Hypokalemia
7. Previously unrecognized heart disease

Signs of left ventricular failure are not always present, and in many instances, pulmonary fluid suggested evidence of

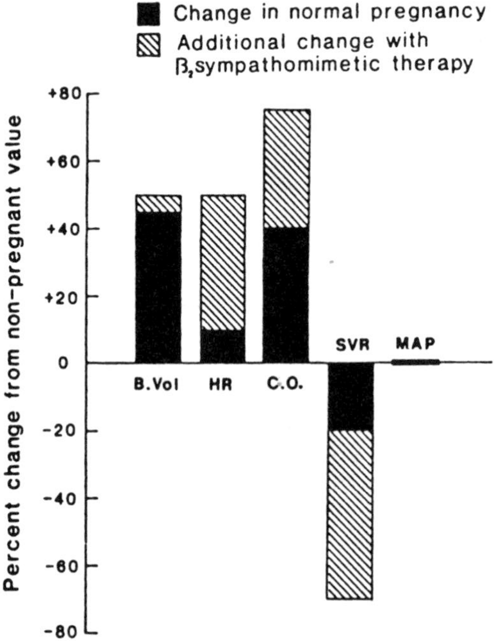

Figure 13–17. Cardiovascular changes of β-sympathomimetic therapy in pregnancy. (From Hawker F: *Anesth Intensive Care* 1984; 12:143. Used by permission.)

increased capillary permeability. Multiple factors may be involved in the pathophysiology of pulmonary edema:

1. *Left Ventricular Dysfunction*—Cardiac output is increased during pregnancy, and this can increase even further in the presence of multiple gestation. The administration of β-mimetic therapy has also been shown to increase the maternal heart rate, cardiac output, and stroke volume.[57] β-Mimetic drugs can increase water retention associated with sodium because of the increased secretion of antidiuretic hormone.[58] This will augment with increased duration of therapy. Acute volume expansion prior to regional anesthesia, especially spinal, can further increase the

cardiac output. All the factors mentioned above can cause left ventricular dysfunction.

2. *Low Colloidal Oncotic Pressure*—In the pregnant woman colloidal oncotic pressure is lower (20 to 25 mm Hg) than in the nonpregnant mother (28 to 32 mm Hg). β-Mimetic therapy, because of sodium and water retention, can further lower colloidal oncotic pressure and thus increase the chance of pulmonary edema.
3. *Infection*—Certain infections can increase pulmonary capillary permeability. Hatjis and Swain surveyed the incidence of pulmonary edema associated with infection following β-mimetic therapy. Out of 527 parturients receiving tocolysis, there was evidence of maternal infection in

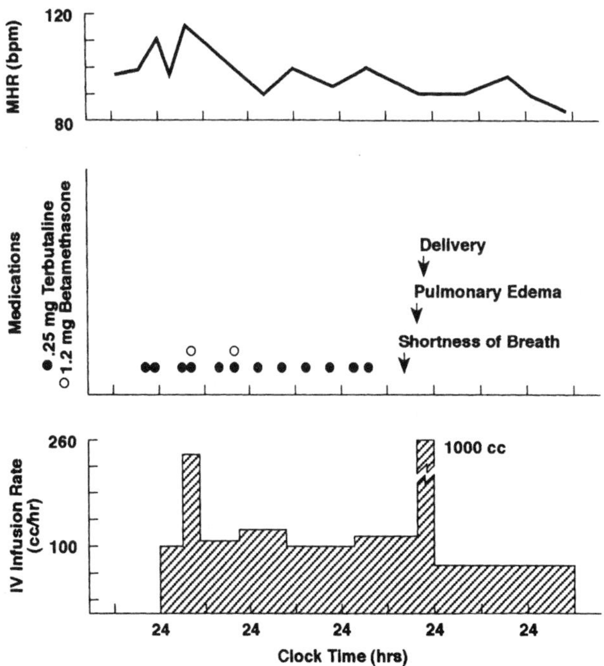

Figure 13–18. Pulmonary edema following long-term β-mimetic therapy. (Reprinted from Benedetti TJ: *Am J Obstet Gynecol* 145:1. © 1983, with permission from Elsevier.)

52 women. The incidence of pulmonary edema was 21% (11/52), whereas it was only 1% (5 of 475) in the absence of infection.[59]

Whatever the mechanism of pulmonary edema, anesthesiologists must take care of these individuals carefully, and the drug interactions that might be associated with tocolytic agents and anesthetics should also be remembered. *Treatment of pulmonary edema usually consists of (1) O_2 by face mask, (2) diuretics such as furosemide, and (3) in cases of refractory pulmonary edema, invasive monitoring with CVP and pulmonary artery lines may be necessary.*

Anesthetic Management of Prematurity. ***Labor and Delivery.*** *Epidural analgesia* has several advantages here: (1) smaller doses of narcotics or tranquilizers may be necessary; (2) there is better placental perfusion in the absence of hypotension, which can reduce the chance of fetal acidosis; and (3) a well-controlled delivery may reduce the chances of intracranial hemorrhage.

Spinal anesthesia may be administered just before delivery.

Cesarean Section. *Regional Anesthesia.* In the presence of unstable cardiovascular system *epidural anesthesia, because of its slower onset, may be associated with less hypotension; thus less fluid for acute volume expansion may be necessary, and less vasopressor will be needed to maintain blood pressure. Spinal anesthesia can also be used in the absence of severe maternal tachycardia. If hypotension occurs, occasionally ephedrine may not be effective in the presence of tachycardia; in this situation small doses of phenylephrine (Neo-Synephrine), 40 μg at a time, may be necessary to maintain the blood pressure. Volume expansion should be carefully regulated; O_2 saturation monitoring and continuous urine output monitoring are absolutely essential. In the presence of pulmonary edema, prior insertion of CVP or pulmonary artery lines may be necessary.* CSE using a smaller amount of local anesthetic with an opiate may be ideal.

General Anesthesia. The following list includes points to keep in mind when using general anesthesia:

1. *Small endotracheal tubes may be necessary in the presence of vocal cord edema* (this can happen if the parturient is kept in a head-down position to stop premature labor).

2. *Inhalation anesthetics should be used carefully in the presence of calcium channel blockers.*
3. *$MgSO_4$ therapy can interact with both depolarizing and nondepolarizing muscle relaxants.*
4. *Parturients receiving β-mimetic tocolytics for more than 24 hours must have their electrolyte levels checked. Hypokalemia can cause cardiac arrhythmias, and hyperventilation can worsen the situation.*
5. *Halothane is contraindicated in the presence of β-mimetic drugs because of the possibility of cardiac arrhythmias.*
6. *Tocolytic drugs are associated with uterine muscle relaxation and atony and can cause severe uterine hemorrhage.*
7. Volume expansion should be restricted.
8. Active neonatal resuscitation may be necessary.
9. Parturients should be monitored closely, especially with the oxygen saturation monitor, in the recovery room because of the possibility of pulmonary edema.

Postmaturity

Major problems encountered in postmaturity include the following:

1. Reduced uteroplacental blood flow causing fetal distress.
2. Umbilical cord compression can occur as a result of oligohydramnios with an increased incidence of fetal distress.
3. Meconium staining of amniotic fluid is common.
4. There is a high frequency of macrosomia and shoulder dystocia.[60]

Anesthetic Management of Postmaturity. ***Labor and Delivery.*** Epidural analgesia is associated with several advantages: (1) relief of labor pain, decreased endogenous catecholamine release, and thus increased uteroplacental perfusion; and (2) it can be used for cesarean section if there is sudden fetal distress. However, continuous close monitoring of the fetal heart rate is mandatory, and hypotension must be prevented.

Cesarean Section. Epidural or spinal anesthesia can be used provided that hypotension is prevented. General anesthesia may be used in the presence of fetal distress if all the precautions mentioned before are observed.

Autoimmune Disease

Rheumatoid Arthritis

Women with severe rheumatoid arthritis may impose multiple problems on the anesthesiology team:

1. Difficult intubation because of severe flexion deformity of the neck along with atlantoaxial instability[61] (Fig. 13-19).
2. Deformity of hip, knee, and intervertebral joints, thus making insertion of an epidural needle difficult and sometimes impossible
3. Restrictive lung disease and occasionally pleural effusion
4. Associated cardiac problems
5. Involvement of peripheral nerves with associated sensory and motor deficits
6. Effect of different medications like high-dose aspirin or nonsteroidal antiinflammatory drugs

Anesthetic Management. *If possible, epidural or continuous spinal analgesia is preferable provided that the clotting parameters are within normal limits. The main advantage of this technique is the avoidance of difficult intubation if emergency cesarean section is indicated.* On the other hand, some anesthesiologists prefer to secure the airway by fiberoptic technique if necessary before proceeding with cesarean delivery.

Systemic Lupus Erythematosus

The major problems of this multiorgan disease include the following:

1. Cardiomyopathy, chronic hypertension, coronary artery disease, nonspecific T-wave changes on the ECG.[62]
2. Higher incidence of pre-eclampsia.
3. Pulmonary vasculitis, pulmonary infarcts.
4. Severe renal problems, evident by the presence of high BUN and creatinine concentrations.

▶

Figure 13-19. Deviated position of the trachea and larynx in association with severe arthritis of the cervical spine. (From Keenan MA, Stiles CM, Kaufman RL, et al: *Anesthesiology* 1983; 58:441–444.)

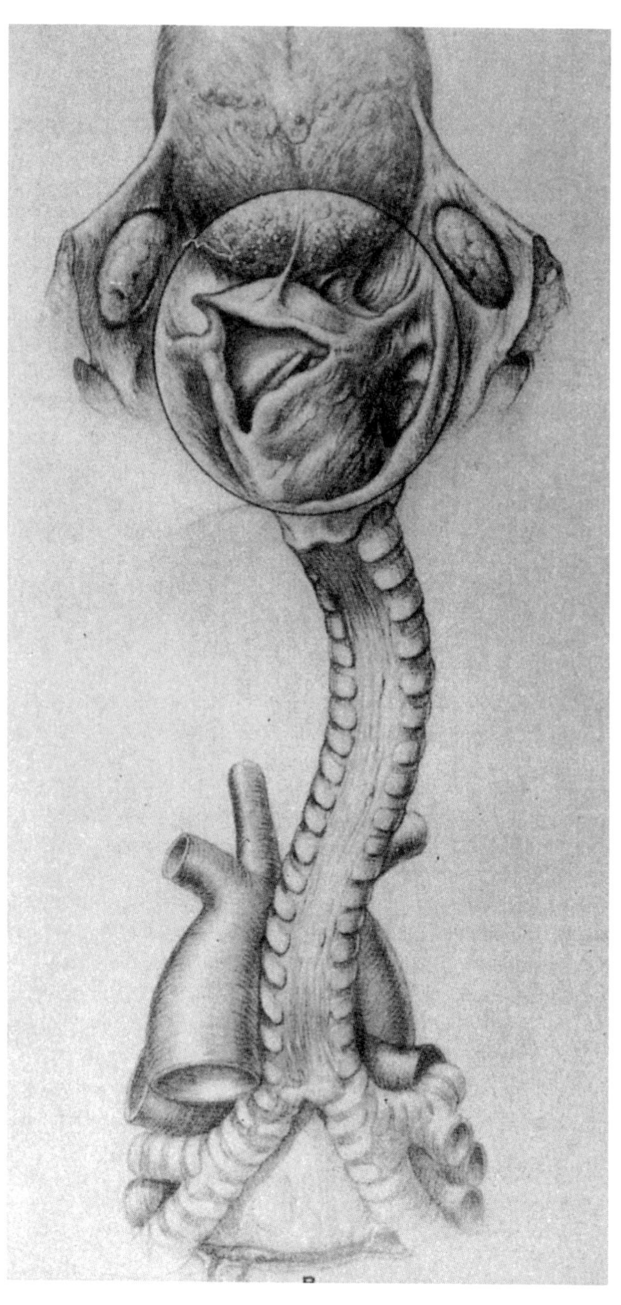

5. CNS as well as peripheral nervous system involvement.
6. Hematologic abnormalities. *The presence of lupus anticoagulant may prolong the PTT and rarely the PT secondary to its reaction with the phospholipids used in the test.*[63] *On the other hand, anticardiolipin antibodies detected in parturients with systemic lupus erythematosus may be associated with thrombocytopenia and women with abnormal PTT or PT.*
7. The increased incidence of thrombosis in parturients with systemic lupus erythematosus may require anticoagulant therapy.
8. Rarely, lupoid hepatitis can complicate the picture.

Anesthetic Management. Anesthetic management either for labor and delivery or for cesarean section will depend on the severity of the disease and organs involved. If clotting parameters are normal, one can use regional anesthesia, but invasive monitoring may be necessary in women with severe respiratory and cardiovascular problems. General anesthesia may be necessary in the presence of clotting abnormalities.

Breech Presentation

Cesarean deliveries for breech presentation are being performed more often in recent years. Unless it is an emergency situation like a prolapsed cord, where general anesthesia may be necessary, spinal or epidural anesthesia can be utilized in elective situations; for labor and delivery, epidural analgesia with a lower concentration of local anesthesia and analgesia may be used with success.

Multiple Gestation

Twins. For labor and delivery, continuous epidural analgesia offers the better approach. This method obviates the use of depressant drugs like narcotics or tranquilizers and also allows a controlled delivery over a relaxed perineum. *Occasionally, however, general anesthesia is needed for version or extraction, especially for the second baby. Inhalation* *anesthetics should be used for proper relaxation of the uterus if necessary.* Nitroglycerin in small doses can also be used for uterine relaxation.

For cesarean delivery, spinal or epidural anesthesia can be used if there is no contraindication. For emergency situations, general anesthesia should be used.

Triplets or Quadruplets. The abdominal route is usually the mode of delivery. Major problems include the following:

1. More profound aortocaval compression and a higher incidence of hypotension are observed.
2. There is an increased tendency toward hypoxemia because of the upward displacement of the diaphragm.
3. In the presence of a grossly enlarged uterus, gastric emptying may be even further compromised, thereby increasing the risk of aspiration in these individuals.
4. Fetuses in multiple gestations are often premature and may have growth retardation.

Anesthetic Management

Epidural anesthesia may be preferred because of a lower incidence of hypotension, less possibility of higher spread, and less time pressure for the termination of surgery.

Spinal anesthesia may be associated with higher incidences of hypotension. Judicial volume replacement and use of vasopressors are mandatory. If there is more than 3 babies one should stay away from spinal anesthesia. CSE using small amounts of local anesthetic for the spinal part will be a viable option.

A well-conducted general anesthesia might also be used. *The induction-delivery and uterine incision—delivery intervals should be minimized because of the chances of partial separation of the placenta.*

Maternal Addiction

The following are among the major problems when faced with maternal narcotic addiction:

1. Withdrawal symptoms occur if parturients do not receive the narcotics.

2. There is an increased likelihood of perinatal mortality from maternal narcotic addiction because of prematurity and low birth weight.
3. Maternal withdrawal may trigger fetal withdrawal and lead to fetal hyperactivity, an increase in oxygen consumption, and fetal hypoxia.
4. An acute drug overdosage may cause hypotension and fetal death.
5. The chance of maternal hypotension during anesthesia is greater because of adrenal insufficiency, associated hypovolemia, or the possibility of maternal overdose from narcotics.
6. Starting an intravenous infusion can be difficult.
7. Cesarean delivery in the presence of cardiovascular, respiratory, or neurological problems secondary to addiction may occasionally make regional anesthesia unsafe. General anesthesia can be given in such situations, but because the majority of these parturients have liver problems, halothane should be avoided, and N_2O, enflurane, sevoflurane or isoflurane may be used instead.

Postoperative pain relief is *always a problem in these cases because of the chance of readdiction. The use of epidural anesthesia for postoperative pain relief might be beneficial in such cases.*

Active resuscitation of the neonate may be necessary.

Alcohol

Major Problems. Medical complications like hemorrhage because of esophageal varices and clotting abnormalities due to abnormal liver function, myocardiopathy, neuropathy, and the possibility of increased gastric volume and gastric acidity will make the administration of anesthesia difficult.

There is also the possibility of fetal alcohol syndrome.

Anesthetic Management. Both for labor and delivery and for cesarean delivery, epidural anesthesia is safe as long as there are no clotting abnormalities. Regional anesthesia will help to minimize the chances of aspiration.

Amphetamines

Anesthetic Management. Since amphetamines are CNS stimulants, they cause depletion of CNS catecholamines and might cause a poor response to indirectly acting sympathomimetic agents like ephedrine.

An increased anesthetic requirement is a possibility if one uses general anesthesia.

Epidural anesthesia might be a better choice in this situation, and hypotension may be treated with small doses of phenylephrine (Neo-Synephrine) if ephedrine is ineffective.

Questions remain about the choice of vasopressors.

Cocaine

Cocaine blocks the presynaptic uptake of norepinephrine, serotonin, and dopamine. In the CNS it increases monoamine neurotransmitter levels and lowers the seizure threshold.[64] "Crack" is commonly smoked at the present time, and pure cocaine is rapidly absorbed across the pulmonary blood vessels and reaches the CNS in high concentration. Severe hypertension and tachycardia can be a problem for the anesthesiologist. Because of its vasoconstriction property, cocaine will reduce uteroplacental blood flow, and abruptio placentae and labor can occur immediately following self-administration of intravenous cocaine.[65] Multiple congenital abnormalities, growth retardation, and decreased weight have been described in neonates of cocaine-addicted mothers.

Anesthetic Management. ***Labor and Delivery.*** Epidural analgesia is the most effective method of pain relief in cocaine-addicted parturients. Chronic cocaine use can cause thrombocytopenia.

Cesarean Section. *Regional anesthesia* should be the anesthetic of choice. Epidural anesthesia is associated with a smaller incidence of hypotension, and it can be used for effective control of postoperative pain. Hypotension has been treated with ephedrine successfully. Neo-Synephrine (50–100 mcg) may be necessary in certain situations. Cocaine may decrease the plasma cholinesterase concentration and may prolong the action of 2-chloroprocaine.

General anesthesia may be necessary in the presence of acute fetal distress associated with abruptio placentae. *Reflex hypertension and tachycardia during intubation can be treated with labetalol. A decreased pseudocholinesterase concentration can prolong the duration of action of succinylcholine. Severe tachyarrhythmias may be associated with general anesthesia.*

Infectious Diseases

Genital Herpes

Caused by herpes simplex virus (HSV) types I and II, the majority of genital herpes lesions are caused by the HSV-2 virus. Most obstetric management issues revolve around possible transmission of the virus to the neonate at the time of birth. Current recommendations for obstetric management include the following[66]:

1. The route of delivery should be determined by assessment of the lesion at the time of delivery.
2. A viral culture is done at the same time.
3. If no evidence of a lesion exists, vaginal delivery is recommended. The viral culture result is delivered to the pediatrician.
4. Any suggestion of a positive lesion will be an indication for cesarean section.

Anesthetic management of a primary lesion is controversial. In the author's institution, regional anesthesia is not used if there is any indication of a primary lesion because primary HSV infections are associated with viremia and the possibility of encephalitis. In the case of secondary infection, we prefer regional anesthesia both for labor and delivery and for cesarean section even during the active phase unless contraindicated for other reasons. Recently, Bader et al reported a 6-year retrospective survey of 169 parturients who underwent cesarean section with a diagnosis of HSV.[67] One hundred sixty-four parturients had secondary infection, whereas 5 had a diagnosis of primary infection. Fifty-nine women had general anesthesia, 75 received spinal anesthesia, and 35 received epidural anesthesia. None of the parturients with secondary infection who received regional anesthesia had any evidence of septic or neurological complications (Fig. 13-20, Table 13-12). Conflicting data exists regarding the use of intraspinal morphine and risk of a recurrent HSV-1 infection. Anesthesiologists should be careful about using the intraspinal morphine for postoperative analgesia in parturients with a history of an HSV-1 infection.

Infection with the Human Immunodeficiency Virus

Acquired immunodeficiency syndrome (AIDS) is the end-stage condition of a disease caused by the human immunodeficiency virus (HIV). The main problems, including the risks involved, are as follows:

1. *Anesthetic Technique*—AIDS is a progressive disease and can ultimately involve the CNS. The CNS manifestations

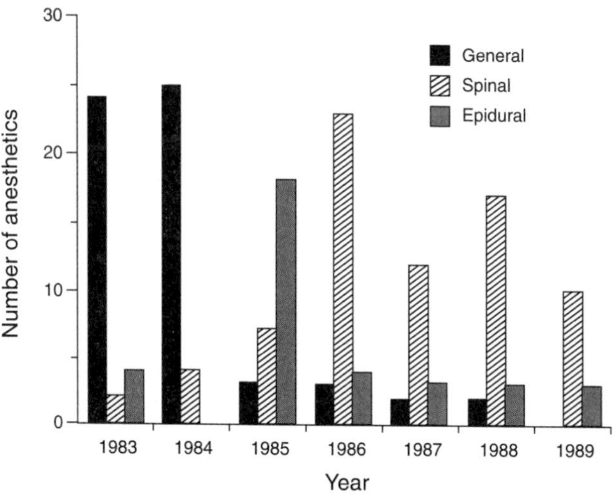

Figure 13–20. Different anesthetic techniques used for cesarean section with a diagnosis of HSV infection between 1983 and 1989. (From Bader AM, Camann WR, Datta S: *Reg Anaesth* 1990; 15:261. Used with permission from Elsevier.)

Table 13-12. Indications for Cesarean Delivery (No. of Cases by Year)

Indication	1983	1984	1985	1986	1987	1988	1989†
Active lesion present at delivery	24	27	27	26	15	20	9
Healing lesion present at delivery	1	1	—	3	—	—	3
No active lesion but positive cultures within 2 wk of delivery	3	1	1	—	1	—	1
Other	2	—	—	1	1	2	—
Total cases	30	29	28	30	17	22	13

Reprinted from Regional Anesthesia & Pain Medicine, 15(5), Bader AM, Camann WR, Datta S, Anesthesia for cesarean delivery in patients with herpes simplex virus type-2 infections, 261-263, Copyright 1990, with permission for American Society of Regional Anesthesia and Pain Medicine.

can include paralysis, ataxia, encephalitis, and coma. The virus has been isolated from the CSF from parturients with HIV.[68] Anesthesiologists should carefully look for any evidence of neurological deficit before the administration of anesthesia, and pregnant women should be told about the possibility of continuation of the neurological problems that might not be related to the anesthetic technique in any way. Regional anesthesia should not be contraindicated in a parturient with AIDS; on the other hand, there is a possibility of difficult endotracheal intubation due to pharyngeal lymphatic hypertrophy.[69] Seroprevalence of HIV during pregnancy has been estimated to be 1.7 per 1000 pregnancies. Knowledge of side effects as well as the drug interactions with the anesthetics of antiretroviral drugs are important.[69a]

2. *Risk to the Anesthesiologist*—Of all cases, 0.5% are estimated to be infected with HIV[70]; hence, care should be taken when contact with bodily fluids is anticipated. Double gloves, mask, gown, eye wear, etc. should be used. Caution is also needed while handling needles and sharp objects.

Emboli in Pregnancy

The leading cause of maternal mortality is emboli,[71] three types of which have been described: thrombotic, amniotic fluid, and air.

Thrombotic Embolism

Pregnancy is a hypercoagulable state, and the incidence of thromboembolism has been reported to be 0.018 to 0.00052 per delivery. Parturients might be receiving low molecular weight or regular heparin for treatment or prophylaxis of deep vein thrombosis. Proper precautions for regional anesthesia is important (Page 355–356).

Amniotic Fluid Embolism

Unique to the pregnant woman, the incidence of amniotic fluid embolism varies from 1 in 8,000 to 1 in 80,000 pregnancies. The mortality rate is very high. Predisposing factors include maternal age, multiple pregnancies, macrosomic fetuses, fast labor, and intense uterine contraction following oxytocin augmentation. Clinical features include the following:

1. Occurrence usually during second stage of labor
2. Sudden chills, shivering, sweating
3. Tachypnea, cyanosis
4. Convulsions and cardiovascular collapse
5. Disseminated intravascular coagulation

A differential diagnosis of amniotic fluid embolism will include the following:

1. Thrombotic pulmonary embolism
2. Air embolism
3. Aspiration of gastric contents
4. Eclamptic convulsions
5. Convulsions from a toxic reaction to local anesthetic drugs
6. Acute left ventricular failure
7. Cerebrovascular accident
8. Hemorrhagic shock associated with pregnancy

Emergency cesarean section under general anesthesia is indicated in the midst of active resuscitation.

Venous Air Embolism

The reported incidence of maternal mortality from venous air embolism is approximately 1 in 100,000 live births. The following are possible causes of venous air embolism:

1. Traumatized vein, open uterine sinuses
2. Negative intrathoracic pressure
3. Uterine manipulation during manual extraction of the placenta and exteriorization of the uterus following cesarean section
4. Douching during pregnancy

Clinical features of venous air embolism include the following:

1. Gasping respiration
2. Chest pain
3. ECG changes
4. Hypotension
5. Changes in heart sounds
6. Cyanosis
7. Cardiac arrest

Immediate treatment, depending on the size of the embolism will include (1) the reverse Trendelenburg position, (2) left lateral position, (3) discontinuation of nitrous oxide and provision of 100% oxygen, (4) immediate cardiopulmonary resuscitation, and (5) a central venous catheter to aspirate air.

Although a major venous air embolism is rare during labor and delivery and cesarean section, careful attention is required, especially during the opening of the uterus for delivery as well as when the uterus is pulled out of the abdominal cavity.

Psychiatric Disorders

Psychiatric disorders of women of childbearing age are as follows:

I. *Schizophrenia*
   A. Paranoid
   B. Schizoaffective
   C. *Medications commonly used:*

    1. Phenothiazenes
    2. Butyrophenones

II. Bipolar disorder
  A. Manic with or without psychotic features
  B. Mixed with or without psychotic features
  C. Depressed with or without psychotic features
  D. *Medications commonly used:*
    1. Lithium
    2. Carbamazepine
    3. Valproic acid (Depakote)

III. *Major depression* with or without suicidal tendency
  A. Medications commonly used:
    1. Tricyclic antidepressants, seratonergic as well as nonadrenergic types
    2. Monoamine oxidase inhibitors

IV. Dysthymia
  A. Medications commonly used: tricyclic antidepressants

V. Miscellaneous diagnostic categories
  A. Panic disorder with or without agoraphobia
  B. Generalized anxiety disorder
  C. Anorexia and/or bulimia
  D. Post-traumatic stress disorder
  E. Obsessive-compulsive disorder
  F. Medications commonly used:
    1. Tricyclic antidepressants
    2. Benzodiazepines
    3. Phenothiazenes
    4. Monoamine oxidase inhibitors

Clinical Implications

Because of recent evidence of the relationship between neurohormonal imbalance and psychiatric disorders, various medications have been used for the treatment of different psychological problems. *Drug interactions between the psychotropic medications and anesthetic techniques and agents are extremely important and have been discussed in Chapter 4.*

Malignant Hyperthermia

Only a few cases of malignant hyperthermia during pregnancy have been reported. The clinical features of malignant hyperthermia under anesthesia include (1) central venous hypercarbia, (2) tachycardia, (3) hypertension, (4) muscle rigidity, (5) tachypnea, (6) lactic acidosis, and (7) rapidly increasing body temperature. Recommended laboratory analyses during malignant hyperthermia are shown in Table 13-13. Figure 13-21 provides a hotline telephone number for the management of malignant hyperthermia.

Anesthetic Management

Regional Anesthesia. It would appear that regional anesthesia is preferable for such cases. *Currently, most anesthesiologists agree with the use of either amide or ester local anesthetics.* The addition of epinephrine to the local anesthetic is felt to be contraindicated because of α-adrenergic agonists precipitate malignant hyperthermia in pigs, but this point is controversial. We have used ephedrine for the treatment of

Table 13-13. Recommended Laboratory Analyses for Malignant Hyperthermia

Central Venous Blood Gas Analysis
Arterial blood gas analysis
Central venous electrolytes (Na^+, K^+ Cl^-, HCO_3^-)
Serum glucose
Central Venous Creatine Phosphokinase
and isoenzymes—immediately and every 12 hr
Hemoglobin or Hematocrit Fibrinogen
and fibrin degradation products
Plasma myoglobin
Urine Myoglobin
Urine pH

From Longmire S, et al: Malignant hyperthermia, in Datta S (ed): *Anesthetic and Obstetric Management of High Risk Pregnancy.* Chicago, Mosby-Year Book, 1991, p 337. Used with permission from Elsevier.

Essential studies shown in boldface type.

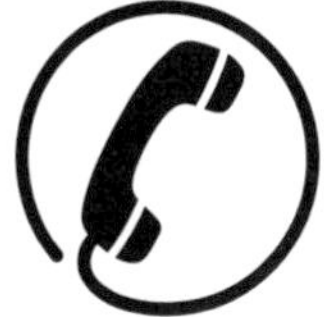
Malignant Hyperthermia Society of North America
MHAUS
(209) 634-4917
Ask for INDEX ZERO.
MHAUS hotline. Call 24 hours a day for information on management of MH crisis.

Figure 13-21. MHAUS hotline. (From Longmire S, Lee W, Pivarnik J: Malignant hyperthermia, in Datta S (ed): *Anesthetic and Obstetric Management of High-Risk Pregnancy.* St Louis, Mosby-Year Book, 1991. Used with permission from Elsevier.)

hypotension without problems, but one might consider using phenylephrine in such cases.

General Anesthesia. If general anesthesia has to be used, then one must avoid depolarizing muscle relaxants and inhalational anesthetics or other triggering agents. The use of prophylactic dantrolene is controversial, but nevertheless it should be always kept handy. Dantrolene crosses the placenta and can cause hypotonia in neonates.

Role of Dantrolene. Dantrolene crosses the placenta, and a fetal blood level of about 60% of that of the mother is reached. There are no reports of adverse neonatal effects. Prophylaxis with dantrolene is a matter of debate. While it seems safe to administer, its use may not be necessary. If used, the prophylactic dose is 2.4 mg/kg intravenously given over a period of about 15 minutes preoperatively. Most of the authors will not use propylactic dantrolene and will avoid the agents that trigger the malignant hyperthermia.

Another potential problem that has been described recently in the literature is the chance of uterine atony following dantrolene treatment.

Obesity

The major problems associated with maternal obesity are as follows:

1. Associated medical problems like hypertension, respiratory insufficiency, diabetes mellitus, etc., are common.
2. The volume of gastric contents with a low pH is large.
3. There can be technical difficulty with regional anesthesia.
4. Obstetric complications are high in this group of parturients.
5. Laryngoscopy may be difficult in such cases.

Recently, in an interesting article authors observed anesthetic and obstetric outcome of 117 morbidly obese parturients. The findings included (1) higher oxytocin use, (2) higher rate of cesarean section (62% compared with 24% in the control group), (3) significantly more initial epidural anesthesia failure (42% compared with 6% in normal parturients), and (4) significantly higher incidence of accidental dural puncture.[72]

Anesthetic Management

Labor and Delivery. Epidural analgesia is preferable and should be used if technically possible. Continuous spinal analgesia has also been used with success.

Elective Cesarean Section. If one considers regional anesthesia, single-shot spinal anesthesia should be used cautiously, if at all, because of the following:

1. Control of the spinal anesthetic level is unpredictable.
2. There is a very high incidence of hypotension.
3. Spinal anesthetic can reach higher levels and cause further compromise of the already abnormal pulmonary function. However, continuous spinal anesthesia can obviate these problems. For epidural anesthesia, the volume of the local anesthetic might have to be reduced. CSE technique using a small amount of local anesthetic for spinal part can be a good option. This will be associated with flexibility of the duration.

General Anesthesia. If general anesthesia is necessary, one should carefully check the airway before the induction of anesthesia. Laryngoscopy may prove difficult in these cases because both the chest and large breasts often impede the use of the

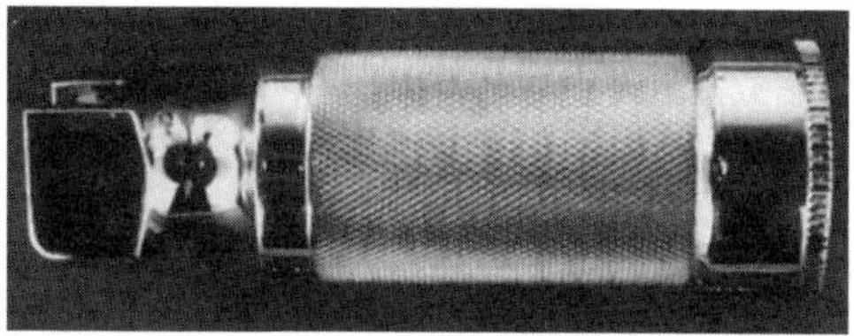

Figure 13-22. Datta-Briwa short-handle laryngoscope.

usual laryngoscope handle. Use of a short-handle laryngoscope (Datta-Briwa) can circumvent this problem (Fig. 13-22).

Fetal Distress

The etiology of fetal distress is associated with maternal causes, placental causes, and fetal problems.[73] Recently, the ACOG has changed the term *fetal distress* to *nonreassuring fetal status.*

Maternal Causes

Maternal factors that may be responsible for fetal distress will include maternal systemic disease, e.g., diabetes, chronic hypertension, drug abuse (cocaine), as well as the physiological problems of supine hypotensive syndrome.

Placental Causes

Decreased placental perfusion because of preeclampsia, diabetes, postmaturity, or separation of the placenta from the uterine bed, e.g., abruptio placentae, can give rise to fetal distress. Umbilical cord problems like a prolapsed cord should also fall into this category.

Fetal Causes

Inherent congenital anatomic as well as other abnormalities will also increase the chances of fetal distress.

Diagnosis

Obstetric diagnostic tools include (1) amniocentesis, (2) ultrasound examination, (3) glucose tolerance test, (4) antepartum testing and intrapartum monitoring, and (5) umbilical cord acid-base values in the postpartum period.

Anesthetic Management

Anesthetic management should include the following points:

1. *Avoidance of aortocaval compression by left uterine displacement should be the first step* in any situation where there is a suspicion of fetal distress.
2. Oxygen supplementation (fetal oxygenation) is necessary. *The fetus normally exists at an almost vertical portion of its oxygen dissociation curve; hence a small change in fetal oxygen tension can result in significant changes in oxygen content and delivery of the oxygen in the fetus* (see Table 13-14).
3. Treatment of hypotension becomes a hallmark in the restoration of placental circulation if there is a drop in blood pressure for any reason. *Ephedrine should be the drug of choice for this purpose because it increases the blood pressure by inotropic and chronotropic means without causing uterine vasoconstriction;* however, if ephedrine use is contraindicated, small doses of phenylephrine (Neo-Synephrine) may be necessary to increase the blood pressure.
4. Oxytocin therapy might be discontinued, but this is decided by the obstetric team.

Table 13-14. Effect of Umbilical Arterial Oxygen Tension with Varying Maternal Inspired Oxygen Concentration

Maternal FIO_2	Maternal PaO_2 (mm Hg)	Umbilical Artery PaO_2 (mm Hg)
0.21	96	15
0.47	232	19
0.74	312	21
1.0	423	25

5. In a few situations, the administration of *tocolytic drugs* like terbutaline can be used to relax the uterus and increase placental circulation. This treatment is also decided by the obstetrician.
6. *Amnioinfusion* has been tried for the treatment of variable deceleration.
7. Epidural anesthesia can increase placental perfusion, especially in parturients in labor, provided that the maternal blood pressure is kept at a normal level. A scalp pH determination may be requested before the initiation of epidural anesthesia if there is any indication of fetal problems. With normal scalp pH (7.25 or higher) an amide local anesthetic can be used. However, in the presence of a borderline fetal heart rate tracing and a low scalp pH, the ester local anesthetic 2-chloroprocaine should be used because of its short maternal and fetal plasma half-life. Hypotension should be prevented by all means.
8. In the case of acute fetal distress, the anesthetic management for cesarean section should include (1) 2-chloroprocaine combined with bicarbonate (1 in 10 mL, 8.4 mEq) if time permits; avoidance of hypotension is extremely important; (2) general anesthesia with proper precautions; and (3) spinal anesthesia, depending on the anesthesiologist.[74] Aggressive neonatal resuscitation may be necessary.

Intrauterine Fetal Death

The major causes of intrauterine fetal death[75] are as follows:

1. Chromosomal causes
2. Congenital malformations, e.g., heart defects, urinary tract anomalies
3. Multiple gestations
4. Infection
5. Placental factors, e.g., abruptio placental hemorrhage, placenta previa, placental insufficiency due to diabetes, pre-eclampsia, postdate pregnancy
6. Cord accidents
7. Maternal immunological diseases
8. Maternal thyroid disease

9. Isoimmunization
10. Maternal trauma

Before making an anesthetic decision, the anesthesiologist must find the associated maternal problems that might have caused the fetal demise. The pain of labor in the case with intrauterine fetal death can be taken care of by epidural analgesia. However, anesthesiologists must examine the clotting parameters before using regional anesthesia in these cases because of the possibility of coagulation problems (abruptio placentae). Pritchard observed disseminated intravascular coagulation in mothers where dead fetuses stayed in the mother for more than 1 month[76] regardless of the etiology; hypofibrinogenemia was a common finding. Pregnant women with abnormal clotting parameters may need general anesthesia if necessary. Large-bore intravenous catheters may be necessary for resuscitation; volume replacement with fluid, blood, cryoprecipitate or fresh frozen plasma that contains high concentrations of factor VIII, and fibrinogen may be indicated.

Composition and Usefulness of Blood Components

1. One unit of platelets (suspended in 20 to 70 mL of plasma) may raise the platelet count by 10,000/mm^3.
2. Fresh frozen plasma (FFP), 1 unit (250 mL), contains 200 to 400 mg of fibrinogen and may raise plasma fibrinogen content by 10 mg/100 mL. FFP also contains various clotting factors excluding platelets.
3. Cryoprecipitate (1 unit = 15 to 20 mL) contains the same fibrinogen as 1 unit (250 mL) of FFP.

Summary

There is a need for further studies on anesthetic needs for high-risk parturients. Successful anesthesia will depend on technical skills and understanding of maternal and fetal physiology, pathophysiology of the disease, and the pharmacology of different drugs and their interactions with the anesthetic techniques.

References

1. Suresh MS, Kinch RA: Antepartum hemorrhage, in Datta S (ed): *Anesthetic and Obstetric Management of High Risk Pregnancy.* Chicago, Mosby-Year Book, 1991.
2. Clark SL, Koonings P, Phelan J, et al: Placenta previa/accreta and prior cesarean section. *Obstet Gynecol* 1985; 66:89.
3. Arcario T, Greene M, Ostheimer GW, et al: Risk of placenta previa/accreta in patients with previous cesarean deliveries (abstract). *Anesthesiology* 1988; 69:659.
4. Chestnut DH, Dewan DM, Redick LF, et al: Anesthetic management for obstetric hysterectomy: A multi-institutional study. *Anesthesiology* 1989; 70:607.

4a. Grange CS, Douglas MJ, Adams TJ, et al: The use of acute hemodilution in parturients undergoing cesarean section. *Am J Obstet Gynecol* 1998; 178:156.

4b. Rebarber A, Lonser R, Jackson S, et al: The safety of intraoperative autologous blood collection and autotransfusion during cesarean section. *Am J Obstet Gynecol* 1998; 179:715.

4c. Hansch E, Chitkara U, McAlpine J, et al: Pelvic arterial embolization for control of obstetric hemorrhage: A five-year experience. *Am J Obstet Gynecol* 1999; 180:1454.

5. Peng AT, Gorman RS, Shulman SM, et al: Intravenous nitroglycerine for uterine relaxation in the postpartum patient with retained placenta. *Anesthesiology* 1989; 71:172.
6. Shah-Hosseini, Evrad JR: Puerperal uterine inversion. *Obstet Gynecol* 1989; 73:567.
7. American College of Obstetricians and Gynecologists: New guidelines to reduce repeat cesareans (news release). Statement by Luella Klein for VBAC News Conference, Washington, DC, January 25, 1985.
8. Brundell M, Chakravarti S: Uterine rupture in labour. *Br Med J* 1975; 2:122.
9. Carlsson C, Nybell-Lindahl G, Ingemarsson I: Extradural block in patients who have previously undergone caesarean section. *Br Anaesth* 1980; 52:827.
10. Crawford JS: The epidural sieve and MBC (minimum blocking concentration): An hypothesis. *Anaesthesia* 1976; 31:1277.
11. Golan A, Sambank O, Rubin A: A rupture of the pregnant uterus. *Obstet Gynecol* 1980; 56:549.
12. Demianczuk N, Hunter D, Taylor D: Trial of labor after previous cesarean section: Prognostic indicators of outcome. *Am J Obstet Gynecol* 1982; 142:640.

12a. Kruskall MS, Leonard S, Klapholz: Autologous blood duration during pregnancy: Analysis of safety and blood use.
12b. Grange CS, Douglas J, Adams TJ, et al: The use of acute hemodilution in parturients undergoing cesarean section. *Am J Obstet Gynecol* 1998; 178:156.
12c. Rainaldi MP, Tazzari PL, Scagliarini G, et al: Blood salvage during cesarean section. *Br J Anesth* 1998; 80:195.
12d. Vedantham S, Goodwin SC, McLucas B, et al: Uterine artery embolization: An under used method of controlling pelvic hemorrhage. *Am J Obstet Gynecol* 1997; 176:938.
13. Friedman SA: Preeclampsia: A review of the role of prostaglandins. *Obstet Gynecol* 1988; 71:122.
14. Gant NF, Daley GL, Chand S: A study of angiotensin II pressor response throughout primigravid pregnancy. *J Clin Invest* 1973; 52:2682.
15. Kambam JR, Handte RE, Brow WU, et al: Effect of normal and preeclamptic pregnancies on the oxyhemoglobin dissociation curve. *Anesthesiology* 1986; 65:426.
15a. Kobayashi T, et al: A new treatment of severe preeclampsia by long-term epidural anesthesia. *J Human Hypertension* 13: 922–926, 1999.
16. Ghoneim MM, Long JP: Interaction between magnesium and other neuromuscular blocking agents. *Anesthesiology* 1970; 32:23.
17. The Eclampsia Trial Collaborative Group: Which anticonvulsion for women with eclampsia? Evidence from the Collaborative Eclampsia trial. *Lancet* 1995; 345:1455.
17a. Jouppila P, Jouppila R, Hollmen A, et al: Lumbar epidural analgesia to improve intervillous blood flow during labor in severe preeclampsia. *Obstet Gynecol* 1982; 59:158.
18. Roberts JM: Magnesium for preeclampsia and eclampsia. *N Engl J Med* 1995; 4:230.
18a. Kelton JG, Hunter DJS, Neamet B: A platelet function defect in preeclampsia. *Obstet Gynecol* 1985; 65:107.
19. DeBoer K, Tencate JW, Sturk A, et al: Enhanced thrombin generation in normal and hypertensive pregnancy. *Am J Obstet Gynecol* 1989; 160:95.
19a. Mallet SV, Cox DJA: Thromboelastography. *Br J Anaesth* 1992; 69:307.
20. Sharma SK, Philip, J, Whitten CN, et al: Assessment of changes in coagulation in parturients with preeclampsia using thromboelastography, *Anesthesiology* 1999; 90:385–90.
20a. Hood DD, Curry R: Spinal versus epidural anesthesia for cesarean section in severely preeclamptic patients. *Anesthesiology* 1999; 90:1276.

20b. Wallace DH, Leveno KJ, Cunningham FG, et al: Randomized comparison of general and regional anesthesia for cesarean delivery in pregnancies complicated by severe preeclampsia. *Obstet Gynecol* 1995; 86:193.
21. Aya GM, Mangin R, Vialles N, et al: Patients with severe preeclampsia experience less hypotension during spinal anesthesia for elective cesarean delivery than healthy parturients: A prospective cohort comparison. *Anesth Analg* 2003; 97:867.
21a. Karinen, J, Räsänen J, Alahuhta S, et al: Maternal and uteroplacental hemodynamic state in preeclamptic patients during spinal anesthesia for caesarean section. *Br J Anaesth* 1996; 76:616.
21b. Fox EJ, Sklar GS, Hill CH, et al: Complications related to the pressor response to endotracheal intubation. *Anesthesiology* 1977;47:524.
22. Joyce TH III, Debnath KS, Baker EA: Preeclampsia: Relationship of CVP and epidural anesthesia. *Anesthesiology* 1979; 51:5297.
23. Benedetti TJ, Kates R, Williams V: Hemodynamic observation in severe preeclampsia complicated by pulmonary edema. *Am J Obstet Gynecol* 1985; 152:330.
24. Clark SI, Greenspoon JS, Aldahn D, et al: Severe preeclampsia with persistent oliguria: Management of hemodynamic subsets. *Am J Obstet Gynecol* 1986; 154:490.
25. Jouppila P, Kirkinen P, Koivula A, et al: Labetalol does not alter the placental and fetal blood flow or maternal prostanoids in preeclampsia. *Br J Obstet Gynaecol* 1986; 93:543.
26. Fenakel K, et al: Nifedipine in the treatment of severe preeclampsia. *Obstet Gynecol* 1991; 77:331.
27. Lawes EG, Downing JW, Duncan PW, et al: Fentanyl-droperidol supplementation of rapid sequence induction in the presence of severe pregnancy induced and pregnancy aggravated hypertension. *Br J Anaesth* 1987; 59:1381.
28. Jouppila R, Jouppila P, Hollmen A: Laryngeal oedema as an obstetric anesthesia complication. *Acta Anaesthesiol Scand* 1980; 24: 97.
29. Moore TR, Key TC, Reisner LS, et al: Evaluation of the use of continuous lumbar epidural anesthesia for hypertensive pregnant women in labor. *Am J Obstet Gynecol* 1985; 152:404.
30. Weinstein L: Syndrome of hemolysis, elevated liver low platelet count: A severe consequence of hypertension in pregnancy. *Am J Obstet Gynecol* 1989; 142:159.
31. Crowther C: Magnesium sulfate versus diazepam in the management of eclampsia: A randomized controlled trial. *Br J Obstet Gynaecol* 1990; 97:110.

32. Dommisse J: Phenytoin sodium and magnesium sulphate in the management of eclampsia. *Br J Obstet Gynaecol* 1990; 97:104.
32a. Frison LM, Dorsey DL: Epidural blood patch and late postpartum eclampsia. *Obgyn* 1996; 82:666.
33. Nylund L, Lunell NO, Lewander R, et al: Uteroplacental blood flow in diabetic pregnancy: Measurements with indium 113m and a computer linked gamma camera. *Am J Obstet Gynecol* 1982; 144:298.
34. Madsen H, Ditzel J: Changes in red blood cell oxygen transport in diabetic pregnancy. *Am J Obstet Gynecol* 1982; 143:421.
35. Pearson JF: The effect of continuous lumbar epidural block on maternal and fetal acid-base balance during labor and at delivery. *Proceedings of the Symposium on Epidural Analgesia in Obstetrics.* London, HK Lewis & Co Ltd, 1972, p 26.
36. Shnider SM, Abboud T, Artal R, et al: Maternal endogenous catecholamine decrease during labor after epidural anesthesia. *Am J Obstet Gynecol* 1983; 147:13.
37. Datta S, Brown WU: Acid-base status in diabetic mothers and their infants following general or spinal anesthesia for cesarean section. *Anesthesiology* 1977; 47:272–276.
38. Datta S, Brown WU, Ostheimer GW, et al: Epidural anesthesia for cesarean section in diabetic parturients: Maternal and neonatal acid-base status and bupivacaine concentration. *Anesth Analg* 1981; 60:574.
39. Milley JR, Rosenberg AA, Philipps AF, et al: The effect of insulin on ovine fetal oxygen extraction. *Am J Obstet Gynecol* 1984; 149:673.
40. Datta S, Kitzmiller JL, Naulty JS, et al: Acid-base status of diabetic mothers and their infants following spinal anesthesia for cesarean section. *Anesth Analg* 1982; 61:662.
41. Datta S, Greene MF: The diabetic parturient, in Datta S (ed): *Anesthetic and Obstetric Management of High Risk Pregnancy.* Chicago, Mosby-Year Book, 1991, pp 407–422.
42. Lev-Ran A: Sharp temporary drop in insulin requirement after cesarean section in diabetic patients. *Am J Obstet Gynecol* 1974; 120:905.
43. Jones TW, Porter P, Sherwin RS, et al: Decreased epinephrine responses to hypoglycemia during sleep. *N Engl J Med* 1998; 338:1657.
43a. Sullivan JM, Rarmanathan KB: Management of medical problems in pregnancy. Severe cardiac disease. *N Engl J Med* 1985; 313: 304.
44. Saltzman DH: Cardiac disease, in Datta S (ed): *Anesthetic and Obstetric Management of High Risk Pregnancy.* Chicago, Mosby-Year Book, 1991, pp 210–259.

45. Freund FG, Bonica JJ, Ward RJ, et al: Ventilatory reserve and level of motor block during high spinal and epidural anesthesia. *Anesthesiology* 1967; 28:824.
46. Mallampati SR: Bronchospasm during spinal anesthesia. *Anesth Analg* 1981; 60:838.
46a. Yun E, Topulos GP, Body SC: Pulmonary function changes during epidural anesthesia for cesarean delivery. *Anesth Analg* 1996; 82:750.
47. Nathan RA, Segall N, Glover GC, et al: The effects of H_1 and H_2 antihistamines on histamine inhalation challenges in asthmatic patients. *Am Rev Respir Dis* 1979; 120:1251.
48. Baraka A: Epidural meperidine for control of autonomic hyperreflexia in a paraplegic parturient. *Anesthesiology* 1985; 62:688.
48a. Confavreux C, Hutchinson M, Hours MM, et al: Rate of pregnancy related relapse in multiple sclerosis. *N Engl J Med* 1998; 339:285.
49. Bader AM, Hunt CO, Datta S, et al: Anesthesia for the obstetric patient with multiple sclerosis. *J Clin Anaesth* 1988; 1:21.
50. Newmann B, Lam AM: Induced hypotension for clipping of cerebral aneurysm during pregnancy. *Anesth Analg* 1986; 65:675.
50a. Repke JT: Myasthenia gravis in pregnancy, in Goldstein PJ, Stern BJ (eds): *Neurological Disorders of Pregnancy,* 2nd ed. Mount Kisco, New York, Futura Publishing Co., 1992, p 225.
51. Rolbin SH, Levinson G, Shnider SM, et al: Anesthetic consideration for myasthenia gravis and pregnancy. *Anesth Analg* 1978; 57:44.
52. Usubiaga JE, Wikinski JA, Morales RL, et al: Interaction of intravenously administered procaine, lidocaine and succinylcholine in anesthetized subjects. *Anesth Analg* 1967; 46:39.
53. Bassel GM, Horbelt DV: Hematologic disease, in Datta S (ed): *Anesthetic and Obstetric Management of High-Risk Pregnancy.* Chicago, Mosby-Year Book, 1991, pp 345–362.
53a. Harrison's Principles of Internal Medicine. New York, McGraw-Hill, p. 1473.
53b. Meinardi JR, Middeldorp S, de Kain J, et al: Increased risk for fetal loss in carriers of the factor V Leiden mutation. *Ann Intern Med* 1999; 130:736.
54. Roizen MF, Horrigan M, Koike EI, et al: A prospective randomized trial of four anesthetic techniques for resection of pheochromocytoma (abstract). *Anesthesiology* 1982; 57:43.
54a. Parry S, Strauss JF: Premature rupture of the fetal membranes. *N Engl Med J* 1998; 338:663.

54b. Jackson GM, Edwin SS, Varner MW, et al: Regulation of fetal fibronectin production in human amnion cells. *J Soc Gynecol Invest* 1996; 3:85.
55. Malinow AM, Gershon RY, Alger LS: Preterm labor and delivery, in Datta S (ed): *Anesthetic and Obstetric Management of High Risk Pregnancy.* Chicago, Mosby-Year Book, 1991, pp 457–486.
56. Eggleston MK: Management of preterm labor and delivery. *Clin Obstet Gynecol* 1986; 29:230.
57. Spielman FJ, Herbert WNP: Maternal cardiovascular effects of drugs that alter uterine activity. *Obstet Gynecol Sur* 1988; 43: 516–522.
58. Jacobs MM, Arias F: Cardiopulmonary complication associated with beta-adrenergic tocolytic therapy, in Berkowitz RL (ed): *Critical Care of the Obstetric Patient.* New York, Churchill Livingstone Inc, 1980, p 505.
59. Hatjis CG, Swain M: Systemic tocolysis for premature labor is associated with an increased incidence of pulmonary edema in the presence of maternal infection. *Am J Obstet Gynecol* 1988; 159:723.
60. Mannino F: Neonatal complications of postterm gestation. *J Reprod Med* 1988; 33:271.
61. Keenan MA, Stiles CM, Kaufman RL: Acquired laryngeal deviation associated with cervical spinal disease in erosive polyarticular arthritis. *Anesthesiology* 1983; 58:44.
62. Steinberg AD: Systemic lupus erythematosus, in Wyngaarden JB, Smith LH, Lloyd H Jr (eds): *Cecil Textbook of Medicine.* Philadelphia, WB Saunders Co, p 2011.
63. Malinow AM, Rickford WJK, Mokriski BLK, et al: Lupus anticoagulant: Implications for obstetric anaesthetists. *Anaesthesia* 1987; 42:1291.
64. Credler L, Mark H: Medical complications of cocaine abuse: *N Engl J Med* 1986; 315:1495.
65. Acker DB, Sachs BP, Tracey KJ, et al: Abruptio placentae associated with cocaine use. *Am J Obstet Gynecol* 1983; 146:220.
66. Camann WR, Tuomala RE: Infectious disease, in Datta S (ed): *Anesthetic and Obstetric Management of High Risk Pregnancy.* Chicago, Mosby-Year Book, 1991, pp 536–563.
67. Bader Am, Camann WR, Datta S: Anesthesia for cesarean delivery in patients with herpes simplex virus type-2 infections. *Reg Anaesth* 1990; 15:261.
68. Ho DM, Rota TR, Schooly RT, et al: Isolation of HTLV-III from cerebrospinal fluid and neural tissues of patients with neurologic syndromes related to the acquired immunodeficiency syndrome. *N Engl J Med* 1985; 313:1493.

69. Barzan L, Carbone A, Saracchini S, et al: Nasopharyngeal lymphatic hypertrophy in HIV-infected patients. *Lancet* 1989; 1:42.

69a. Evron S, Glezerman M, Harow E, et al: Human immunodeficiency virus. Anesthetic and obstetric considerations. *Anesth Analg* 2004; 98:503.

70. Davies JM, Thistlewood JM, Rolbin SH, et al: Infections and the parturient: Anesthetic considerations. *Can J Anaesth* 1988; 35:270.

71. Friedman AM, Kaplan HI, Sadock BJ: *Comprehensive Textbook of Psychiatry,* vol 2. Baltimore, Williams Wilkins, 1976.

72. Hood DD, Dewan DM: Anesthetic and obstetric outcome in morbidly obese parturients. *Anesthesiology* 1993; 79:110.

73. Arcario TJ, Thomas RL: Fetal distress, in Datta S (ed): *Anesthetic and Obstetric Management of High Risk Pregnancy.* Chicago, Mosby-Year Book, 1991, p 613.

74. Marx GF, Luyky W, Cohen S: Fetal-neonatal status following caesarean section for fetal distress. *Br J Anaesth* 1984; 56:1009.

75. Hartwell BL, Reisner DP, Cetrulo CL: Intrauterine fetal death, in Datta S (ed): *Anesthetic and Obstetric Management of High Risk Pregnancy.* Chicago, Mosby-Year Book, 1991, p 657.

76. Pritchard JA: Fetal death in utero. *Obstet Gynecol* 1959; 14:573.

14
Neonatal Resuscitation

▼

Physiology
- Cardiovascular System
- Respiratory System
- Thermoregulation

Maternal Well-Being

Evaluation of the Neonate
- Steps in Neonatal Resuscitation
- Airway
- Breathing
- Circulation
  - *Cardiac massage*
  - *Indications for volume expanders*
  - *Bleeding*

Treatment of Specific Conditions
- Neonates with Apgar Scores of 8 to 10
- Neonates with Apgar Scores of 5 to 7
- Neonates with Apgar Scores of 3 to 4
- Neonates with Apgar Scores of 0 to 2

Equipment and Medications Necessary for Neonatal Resuscitation

Other Specific Causes of Neonatal Respiratory Problems
- Nose: Choanal, Atresia
  - *Clinical findings*
  - *Treatment*
- Upper Airway
  - *Clinical findings*
  - *Treatment*

A discussion of physiological adaptations of neonates at the time of delivery is important before concentrating on specific techniques of neonatal resuscitation.

Physiology

Cardiovascular System

Gas exchange occurs in fetus from the mother via the placenta. Ten percent of maternal cardiac output reaches the placenta. The umbilical vein, which has the highest oxygen saturation, enters the fetal circulation; 50% of the umbilical vein circulation enters the inferior vena cava via the ductus venosus, and the other half enters the hepatoportal system (Fig 14-1). A streaming phenomenon that separates blood with various oxygen saturations as it flows through the blood vessels becomes an extremely important factor for oxygen delivery in the fetal tissue. From the inferior vena cava the blood flow is divided into two distinct streams: oxygenated blood enters the left atrium via the foramen ovale, whereas

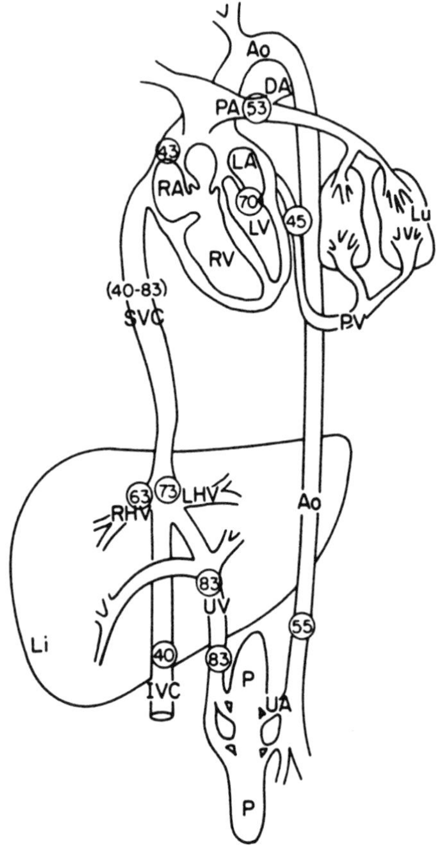

Figure 14–1. Fetal circulation with oxygen saturation in different parts of the fetus (*circled numbers* indicate percent saturation). *P* = placenta; *IVC* = inferior vena cava; *UV* = umbilical vein; *RHV* = right hepatic vein; *LHV* = left hepatic vein; *SVC* = superior vena cava; *RV* = right ventricle; *RA* = right atrium; *LV* = left ventricle; *LA* = left atrium; *PA* = pulmonary artery; *DA* = ductus arteriosus; *AO* = aorta; *PV* = pulmonary vein; *AO* = aorta; *UA* = umbilical artery. (From Martin R. Prepartum and Intrapartum Fetal Monitoring. In Datta S (ed): Anesthetic and Obstetric Management of High-Risk Pregnancy, 3rd ed. New York, Springer, 2004.)

deoxygenated blood enters the right atrium. The left heart blood is responsible for supplying oxygenated blood to the brain, whereas deoxygenated blood from the right atrium returns to the placenta via the umbilical artery and ultimately to the maternal circulation for reoxygenation. The relatively fast fetal heart rate as well as the decreased systemic vascular resistance of the placenta maintains the high fetal cardiac output relative to its total body surface. Forty percent of the fetal cardiac output reaches the placenta. *Obviously oxygen saturation, oxygen and carbon dioxide tension, and pH will be different in the umbilical artery as compared with the umbilical vein* (*Table 14-1*). Another important factor to remember is the higher hemoglobin oxygen saturation in the fetal blood as compared with adult blood at the same oxygen tension. This is due to differences in the oxygen dissociation curve (Fig 14-2) because of the lower affinity of 2,3-diphosphoglycerate (2,3-DPG) to fetal hemoglobin. The *P_{50} of hemoglobin of term infants ranges between 19 and 24 mm Hg as opposed to 26 mm Hg in adult hemoglobin.*

At the time of delivery several changes take place: the onset of respiration increases fetal PO_2 and consequently decreases pulmonary vascular resistance; on the other hand, exclusion of the placental circulation increases systemic vascular resistance. Increased systemic vascular resistance will ultimately cause a closure of the foramen ovale, and the ductus arteriosus will close as a result of an increased fetal arterial PO_2.[1]

Respiratory System

In intrauterine life the fetal tracheobronchial tree is filled with fluid. This fluid represents nearly two thirds of the functional residual capacity.[2] At the time of delivery the fetal lung

Table 14-1. Fetal Blood Gas and Acid-Base Values

	PO_2	PCO_2	Saturation (%)	pH
Umbilical vein	30	40	70	7.3–7.35
Umbilical artery	20	50	28	7.24–7.29

20,30,40,50 formula.

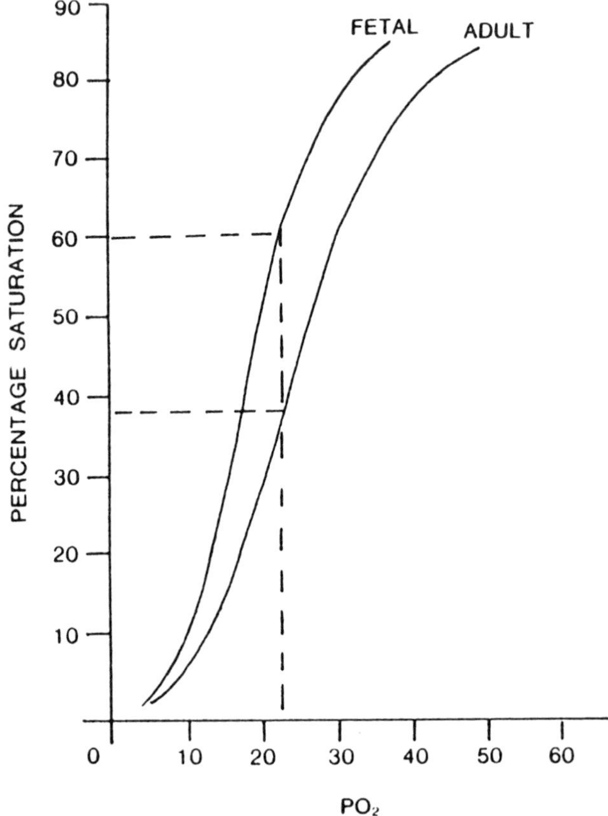

Figure 14-2. Adult and fetal oxyhemoglobin dissociation curves. (From Freeman RK, Gartie TS: *Fetal Heart Rate Monitoring.* Baltimore, Williams & Wilkins, 1981, p 10. Used by permission.)

fluid is cleared by several factors: (1) during vaginal delivery the fluid is squeezed out by compression of the thoracic cage, so babies delivered by cesarean section will have more lung fluid because of the absence of this compression mechanism.

(2) One third of the lung fluid will be absorbed by lymphatics. (3) Some of the fluid will be expelled by the newborns themselves, and finally (4) some of the fluid is deliberately taken out at the time of delivery.

Initiation of respiration is extremely important and takes place within 1 minute after delivery, and regular-rhythm respiration is established within 2 to 10 minutes. The exact stimulus responsible for the establishment of neonatal respiration is unknown; however, several factors may be involved: (1) squeezing of the thoracic cage by the vaginal canal, (2) hypoxia and hypercarbia, (3) tactile stimulation, (4) umbilical cord clamping, and (5) possibly the lower temperature outside the uterus.

The first breath requires an extremely high intrathoracic pressure that can vary from 40 to 100 cm H_2O. The lungs are expanded with 40 to 70 mL of air, and they remain completely inflated after the first few breaths. *Normal term neonates breathe 30 to 60 times per minute with a 10- to 30-mL tidal volume, and the lungs maintain a minute volume of about 500 mL.*

During intrauterine development fetal lung processes two types of epithelial cells (type I and type II). Type II cells are responsible for the production of surfactant (surface-acting material), which is important for counteracting the surface tension and keeping the alveoli open. Surfactant production by type II cells can start by 22 to 24 weeks. Premature babies will obviously have problems in expanding the alveoli because of the absence of surfactant.

Thermoregulation

The most important point to remember regarding thermoregulation is the inability of the neonate to maintain body temperature by shivering, and hence nonshivering thermogenesis becomes an important factor.[3] Breakdown of brown fat is the main source of maintenance of fetal body temperature.[4] The term fetus stores abundant brown fat in the neck, interscapular area, back, and axillary area as well as around different abdominal viscera, especially the kidney and adrenals. Brown fat is extremely vascular and receives as much as

25% of the cardiac output in hypothermic conditions. Cold stress will liberate norepinephrine, which is important for the metabolism of brown fat; this complex process involves an exothermic reaction that liberates heat with the utilization of a significant amount of oxygen (Fig 14-3).[5] Warm blood from different sources reaches the vertebral venous plexus surrounding the spinal cord and ultimately reaches the heart via the jugular and azygos vein. Maintenance of body temperature is extremely important for the neonates because cold temperature will cause pulmonary vasoconstriction, increased

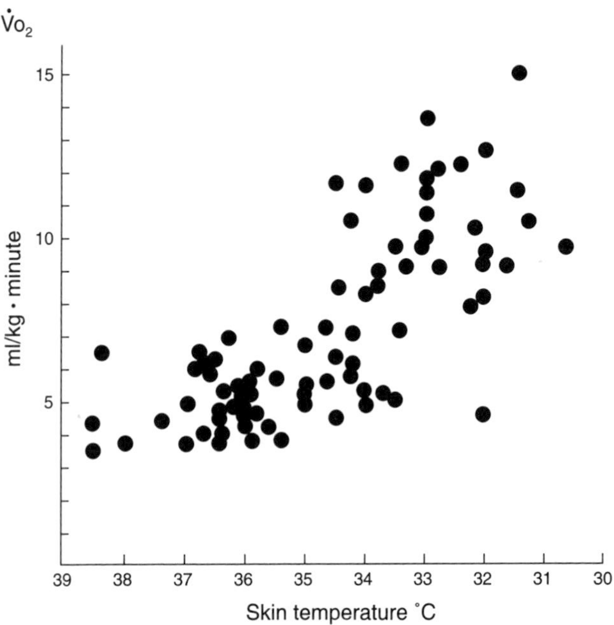

Figure 14-3. The relationship between oxygen consumption and skin temperature of neonates. (From Levinson G, Shnider SM: *Anesthesia for Obstetrics.* Baltimore, Williams & Wilkins, 1987, p 512. Used by permission.)

right-to-left shunt, hypoxemia, and metabolic acidosis, which will further increase the right-to-left shunt.

All of the above are important factors in a proper approach to neonatal resuscitation.

Maternal Well-Being

Anesthesiologists should be primarily responsible for maternal well-being; hence when active neonatal resuscitation becomes necessary, a person other than the anesthesiologist should be responsible for this task. This will vary from one institution to another. A prior knowledge of a difficult delivery or delivery of a high-risk fetus will help the resuscitation process. Factors can be classified in the following manner:

I. Maternal factors
   A. Uteroplacental insufficiency
      1. Diabetes mellitus
      2. Preeclampsia
      3. Postmaturity
      4. Intrauterine growth retardation
      5. Cocaine addiction
      6. Autoimmune disease
   B. Infection from any source
   C. Hemorrhage
      1. Placenta previa
      2. Abruptio placentae
      3. Ruptured uterus
      4. Vasa previa
   D. Endocrine problems
      1. Hypothyroidism or hyperthyroidism
      2. Hypoadrenalism or hyperadrenalism
      3. Pheochromocytoma
   E. Maternally administered drugs (high doses)
      1. Narcotics
      2. Sedatives and tranquilizers
      3. Muscle relaxants
      4. Magnesium sulfate
      5. Local anesthetics
      6. Calcium channel blockers
      7. β-Blockers

II. Difficult deliveries
    A. Traumatic
    B. Intrauterine manipulation
    C. Breech extraction
    D. Forceps delivery
III. Fetal factors
    A. Premature neonates
    B. Abnormal presentation, e.g., breech
    C. Multiple births
    D. Congenital anomalies for any reason
    E. Acute fetal distress for any reason
    F. Presence of meconium

Evaluation of the Neonate

Dr. Virginia Apgar devised a scoring system for quick evaluation of the neonate immediately after delivery[6] (Table 14-2). Scores are evaluated by observing the following criteria and are recorded at 1 and 5 minutes.

Steps in Neonatal Resuscitation

Neonatal resuscitation should be divided into three major steps[7] (Fig. 14-4).

1. Taking care of the *airway*
2. Taking care of the *breathing*
3. Taking care of the *circulation*

Airway

The first important step is clearing and establishing an open airway. Suction should begin immediately after the delivery by the obstetric team. The neonate should be placed immediately under a radiant heat source, and the drying-up process should begin as soon as possible. The neonate should be placed in a slight head-down position with the neck slightly extended. Turning the head to the side will allow better drainage and

Table 14-2. Apgar Scoring System

Sign	Score 0	1	2
Appearance	Blue, pale	Pink body, blue extremity	Pink all over
Pulse	Absent	> 100/min	> 100/min
Grimace	No response	Some response	Cry, cough
Activity	Limp	Some flexion	Active motion
Respiration	Absent	Slow	Strong cry

removal of the secretion. Suction with a bulb syringe will be satisfactory in most cases, but *caution should be used to prevent stimulation of the posterior portion of the pharynx during the first few minutes after delivery to prevent vagally mediated bradycardia.* In the presence of meconium stained fluid, thin or thick, the resuscitation will depend upon the condition of the neonate. If the infant has absent or depressed respiration, decreased muscle tone and heart rate below 100, direct laryngoscopy should be done for suction of meconium from hypopharynx as well as from trachea. If the infant is vigorous regardless of the consistency of meconium laryngoscopy and tracheal suction should not be performed.[8] (Fig 14-5) *Gastric suction is also important in these cases.*

Continuous suction can be used by the wall suction de-vice via an adaptor, but *if mechanical suction is used, one should make sure that the negative pressure does not exceed 100 mm Hg.*

Breathing

Once the oral cavity is cleared, the majority of neonates will start breathing spontaneously, but in a few cases tactile stimulation may be necessary to initiate respiration. In the absence of respiratory effort and movement, positive-pressure

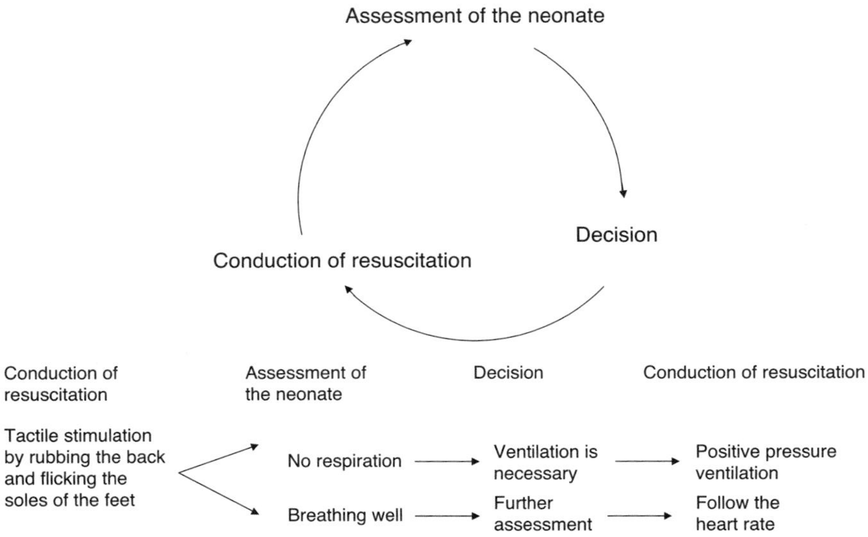

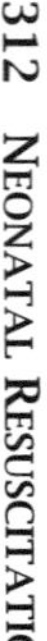

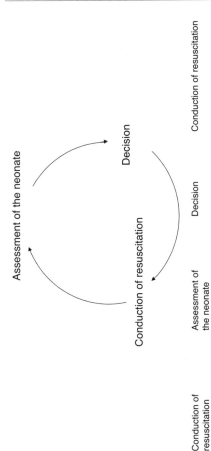

Figure 14–4. Decision making in neonatal resuscitation. (Modified from Text of Neonatal resuscitation of American Heart Association 1987, 1990, 1994.)

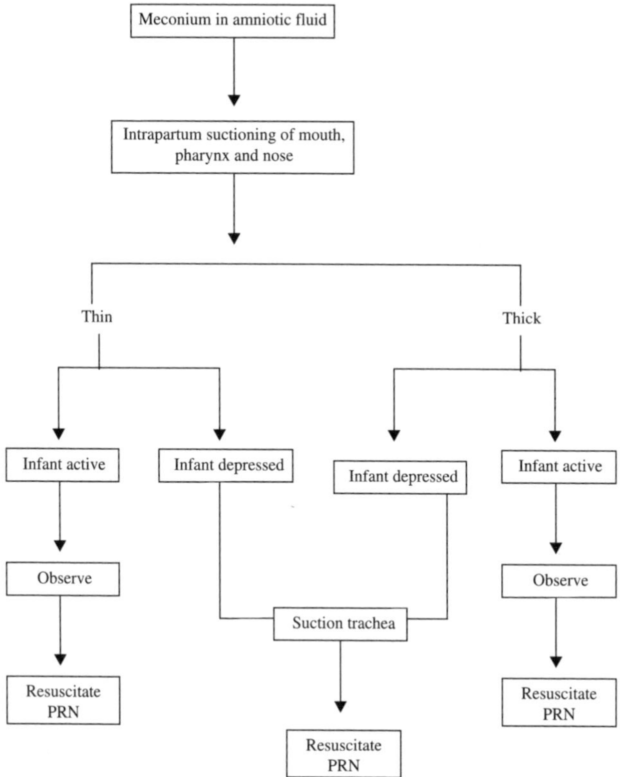

Figure 14–5. Treatment for meconium aspiration. (From *Textbook of Neonatal Resuscitation,* Dallas, American Heart.)

ventilation using a bag and mask should be initiated. The heart rate should also be checked at the same time; adequate oxygenation with proper ventilation will improve the heart rate as well as the color. *Most neonatal resuscitation bags have a built-in pressure-release valve that is set to release at 30 to 35 cm H_2O.* Neonates should be ventilated at a rate of 40 per minute. The adequacy of chest movement should be observed and also be confirmed by listening for bilateral breath sounds. If the heart rate and color do not improve after adequate ventilation or if there is any difficulty in ventilation (diaphragmatic hernia), endotracheal intubation may be necessary. Laryngeal mask airway can be used for ventilation if bag and mask ventilation is inadequate or endotracheal intubation is not successful.

Circulation

If the heart rate drops or stays below 80 beats per minute, external cardiac compression should be started. Chest compression will compress the heart against the spinal column, and this will help to maintain circulation in the vital organs. There are two techniques for external cardiac massage. Epinephrine should be used if heart rate remains below 60, despite 60 seconds of assisted ventilation and circulation.

Cardiac Massage

Thumb Technique. In this technique the fingers encircle the chest, with the thumbs lying over the midsternum. The sternum is compressed 1 to 2 cm 120 times per minute. This technique might have an advantage that it generates better peak systolic and coronary perfusion pressure compared to the two-finger technique.

Two-finger Technique. In this technique the tips of the middle finger and either the index finger or ring finger of the same hand are used to compress the sternum; the other hand can support the back of the neonate in the absence of a rigid surface. The sternum is again compressed 1 to 2 cm 120 times per minute. Ventilation should be continued at 30 to 60 breaths per minute. In the absence of improvement one should think about using medications and volume expanders to stimulate the heart rate, increase tissue perfusion, and normalize acid-base values. *The umbilical vein should be the preferred route:* a catheter is introduced through the umbilical stump until the tip of the catheter is just below the skin level because *threading the catheter too far will entail the risk of infusion of the solutions into the liver and cause liver damage.*

Indications for Volume Expanders

Volume expanders should be used in the following situations:

1. Persistence of pallor after adequate oxygenation
2. Presence of weak pulses
3. Inadequate response to resuscitative measures
4. Low blood pressure

Bleeding

If there is acute bleeding with associated hypovolemia, one of the following volume expanders can be used: (1) whole blood (O-negative blood crossmatched with the mother's blood), (2) albumin is not usually used, other plasma expanders, (3) normal saline, and (4) Ringer's lactate. It is usually administered at 10 mL/kg over a period of 5 to 10 minutes. Epinephrine at 1:10,000 (0.1 to 0.3 ml/kg) can be used intravenously or intra tracheally if necessary. Use of bicarbonate is discouraged for a short period of cardiopulmonary resuscitation. If it is used following prolonged arrests unresponsive to other medications, it should be used only after establishment of adequate ventilation and circulation. Later use of bicarbonate should be associated with persistent fetal metabolic acidosis or hyperkalemia. A 4.2% solution at a dose of 2 m Eq/kg is used, and it is given slowly at a rate of 1 m Eq/kg/min. The risk of intraventricular hemorrhage following bicarbonate infusion can be minimized by using dilute solution (4.2%) and injecting slowly. Naloxone hydrochloride can be used in the presence of neonatal respiratory depression following maternal narcotic administration within 4 hours of delivery. It is given in a dose of 0.1 mg/kg either intravenously, intramuscularly, or intratracheally. *Naloxone should not be administered to a newborn infant whose mother is a narcotic addict and suspected of having recently abused narcotic because of possibility of acute withdrawal.*

Treatment of Specific Conditions

Neonates With Apgar Scores of 8 to 10

The majority of neonates will fall into this category, and they do not need any special treatment. They should be kept warm and dried immediately.

Neonates With Apgar Scores of 5 to 7

These newborns may need tactile stimulation and oxygen to breathe. With the onset of spontaneous rhythmic respiration, the heart rate and color should improve rapidly. If improvement is delayed, positive-pressure ventilation with oxygen may be necessary.

Neonates With Apgar Scores of 3 to 4

These babies are more hypoxic and acidotic and need a longer time for resuscitation. Positive-pressure ventilation using oxygen and a mask will be absolutely necessary. Unless there is hypovolemia or other congenital anomalies, the color and heart rate will rapidly improve.

Neonates With Apgar Scores of 0 to 2

These newborns should be immediately ventilated with mask and 100% oxygen. This should be followed by immediate intubation, ventilation with 100% oxygen, and external cardiac massage. Umbilical vein catheter introduction might be indicated since volume expansion and the use of medications such as epinephrine, sodium bicarbonate, or naloxone hydrochloride may be necessary.

Equipment and Medications Necessary for Neonatal Resuscitation

The following outline lists items that the neonatal team should have on hand.

I. Radiant warmer
II. Equipment for suction
  A. Bulb syringe
  B. De Lee mucus trap with a 10-F catheter or mechanical suction
  C. Suction catheters, 5, 6, 8, and 10 F
  D. An 8-F feeding tube and a 20-mL syringe
III. Bag and mask
  A. Resuscitation bag with a pressure-release valve
  B. Face masks of different sizes
  C. Laryngeal mask airway.
  D. Oral airways of different sizes
  E. Oxygen with a flow meter and tubing
IV. Equipment for intubation
  A. Laryngoscope with straight blades (nos. 0 and 1)
  B. Endotracheal tubes (2.5, 3.0, 3.5, and 4.0 mm)
  C. Stylet
  D. Scissors
  E. Gloves
V. Medication and intravenous fluid
  A. Epinephrine, 1: 10,000 (3- or 10-mL ampules)
  B. Naloxone hydrochloride (0.02 mg/ml in 2-mL ampules)
  C. Albumin, 5% solution
  D. Normal saline
  E. Ringer's lactate
  F. Sodium bicarbonate (4.2% in 10-mL ampules)
  G. Dextrose, 10% (250 mL)
  H. Sterile water (30 mL)
  I. Normal saline (30 mL)

Other Specific Causes of Neonatal Respiratory Problems

These are classified by parts of the respiratory system.

Nose: Choanal Atresia

This condition is associated with anatomic obstruction of the nasal passage.

Clinical Findings

Breathing via the nose will demonstrate an absence of breath sounds, and the newborn will be cyanotic. Breathing via the mouth or crying will make the baby pink, and breath sounds will be present.

Choanal atresia is characterized by an inability to pass a soft rubber or plastic catheter through the nose. A small amount of contrast media through the nose will confirm the anatomic obstruction.

Treatment

Choanal atresia is treated by insertion of a rubber or plastic oral airway and, if necessary, an endotracheal tube.

Upper Airway

The Pierre Robin syndrome can cause neonatal respiratory problems and is a congenital malformation associated with glossoptosis, micrognathia, and possibly a cleft palate.

Clinical Findings

Clinical findings include sternal retraction, cyanosis, and specific congenital anomalies.

Treatment

Treatment of upper airway causes of neonatal respiratory problems include the following:

1. Anterior pulling of the tongue
2. Oral airway insertion
3. Small nasal tube positioned in the posterior portion of the pharynx
4. Orotracheal tube if possible
5. Blind nasal intubation
6. Placement of the neonate in the prone position

Anomalies of the Larynx

This can include webs, fusions, atresia, and vocal cord paralysis.

Clinical Findings

Clinical findings include stridor, cyanosis, and prolonged inspiration and expiration.

Treatment

Placement of an endotracheal tube distal to the obstruction will alleviate the clinical problems.

Anomalies of the Trachea

These include subglottic stenosis, tracheal rings, hemangiomas and webs, vascular rings, and tumors.

Clinical Findings

Clinically, anomalies of the trachea can be detected by the following:

1. Inspiratory stridor
2. Retraction
3. Decreased breath sounds
4. Collapse of the trachea during inspiration in the presence of incomplete tracheal rings
5. Tracheal bleeding in the presence of hemangiomas

Treatment

An endotracheal tube should be inserted beyond the site of obstruction. If there is pulmonary hemorrhage because of trauma to the hemangioma, the situation can be life-threatening. Ventilation with 100% oxygen via an endotracheal tube becomes less essential. Positive end-expiratory pressure (5 to 10 cm H_2O) may be used for producing a tamponade to ease the bleeding.

Esophageal Atresia and Tracheoesophageal Fistula

This is a congenital anomaly in which there is esophageal atresia with an associated tracheoesophageal fistula. Several different varieties have been described[9]: (1) atresia of the upper portion of the esophagus and a fistula connection between the lower part of the esophagus and trachea (85%), (2) atresia of the proximal aspect of the esophagus as well as a fistula connection with the trachea (1%), (3) atresia of both the proximal and distal portions of the esophagus without a tracheal connection (8%), (4) atresia of both the proximal and distal aspects of the esophagus with two separate esophagotracheal fistula connections (1%), (5) a tracheoesophageal fistula without esophageal atresia (4%), and (6) constriction of the esophagus without any fistula connection.

Clinical findings include the following:

1. Presence of polyhydramnios.
2. Excessive oropharyngeal secretions.
3. Inability to pass a catheter via the esophagus to the stomach. X-ray films will confirm the diagnosis.
4. Coughing, cyanosis while feeding.
5. Possibility of respiratory distress following aspiration.
6. Distension of the stomach from swallowing air.

Treatment involves surgical correction following proper preparation of the neonate.

Congenital Bronchial Stenosis

Clinical findings are difficult expiration following easy inspiration as well as hyperinflation of the lungs.

Aspiration Syndrome

Meconium aspiration is one of the important causes of neonatal morbidity and mortality. Intrauterine meconium aspiration is common after 42 weeks of gestation. Meconium is a combined product of amniotic fluid, gastrointestinal cells, and intestinal secretions; aspiration occurs in about 9% of cases, mainly because of peripartum asphyxia. Peripartum asphyxia will increase intestinal motility and relax the anal sphincter and will cause fetal gasping and ultimately meconium aspiration. Inhalation of meconium can produce chemical pneumonitis, plugging and obstruction of the airways with air trapping, and consequent ventilation-perfusion mismatch.

Clinical Findings

Clinical findings include the following:

1. Presence of meconium at birth
2. Cyanosis
3. Retractions
4. Tachypnea
5. Grunting
6. Hypoxia and acidosis

Treatment

Treatment is summarized in Figure 14-6.[10]

Blood aspiration should be treated the same way as meconium aspiration. The medications that can be administered endotracheally are lidocaine, atropine, naloxone, and epinephrine (LANE).

Diaphragmatic Hernia

Diaphragmatic hernia is a congenital defect in the diaphragm with entrance of the gut into the thoracic cavity.[11]

Clinical Findings

Clinical findings at examination include the following:

1. Scaphoid abdomen at birth
2. Cyanosis
3. Intercostal retractions
4. Grunting
5. Confirmation by x-ray studies

Treatment

Intubation of the trachea and the use of 100% oxygen should be started immediately. Careful ventilation is necessary

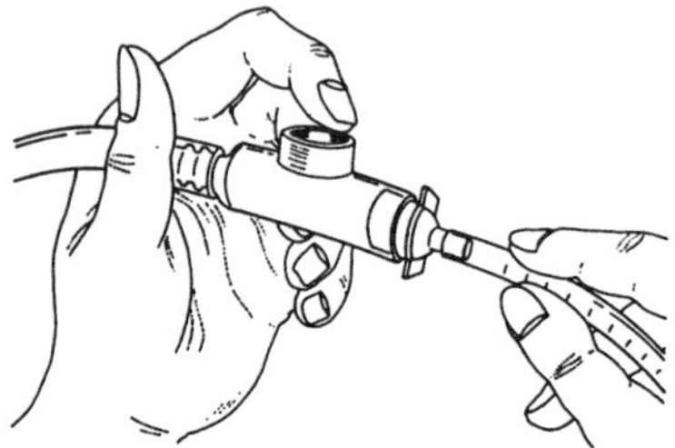

Figure 14-6. Meconium aspirator attached to wall suction (Modified from *Textbook of Neonatal Resuscitation*, Dallas, American Heart Association, 1994).

because excessive pressure may cause pneumothorax. Surgical intervention will be needed in these cases.

Pneumothorax

A collection of air in the pleural cavity (pneumothorax) can occur spontaneously or during ventilation with high pressure in situations like respiratory distress syndrome or meconium aspiration syndrome.

Clinical Findings

Examination reveals the following findings:

1. Tachypnea
2. Cyanosis
3. Reduced breath sounds at the site of the lesion
4. Displacement of the heart
5. Hypotension

The diagnosis is confirmed by a chest x-ray transillumination test or insertion of a needle or chest tube.

Treatment

Removal of air by a chest tube or intravenous catheter will be necessary in symptomatic cases.

Table 14–3. Medications for Neonatal Resuscitation

Medication	Concentration	Dosage route	Rate/ Precautions
Epinephrine	1:10,000	0.1-0.3 ml/kg IV or ET	Give rapidly May dilute with normal saline to 1-2 ml (ET)
Volume expanders	Whole blood 5% Albumin-saline Normal saline Ringer's lactate	10 ml/kg IV	Give over 5-10 minutes
Sodium bicar-bonate	0.5 mEq/ml (4.2% solution)	2 mEq/kg IV	Give slowly, over at least 2 minutes. Give only if infant is being effectively ventilated
Naloxone hydro-chloride	0.4 mg or 1 mg/ml	0.1 mg/kg IV, ET, IM, SQ	Give rapidly IV, ET preferred IM, SQ acceptable
Dopamine	Desired concen-tration	5 mcg/kg/min may increase to 20 mcg/kg/min if necessary	Give as a continuous infusion using an infusion pump, monitor heart rate and blood pressure closely, seek consultation

IV = intravenous, ET = endotracheal, IM = intramuscular, SQ = subcutaneous.

Conclusion

The majority of the deliveries remain uncomplicated; however, a proper knowledge of neonatal resuscitation, which may become necessary, is important in taking care of high-risk neonates.

References

1. Clayman RI, Heymann EH, Rudolph AM: Ductus arteriosus response to prostaglandin E_1 at high and low oxygen concentrations. *Prostaglandins* 1977; 13:219.
2. Avery ME, Cook CD: Volume-pressure relationships of lungs and thorax in fetal, newborn, and adult goats. *J Appl Physiol* 1961; 16:1034.
3. Deham LS, James LS: Newborn temperature and calculated heat loss in the delivery room. *Pediatrics* 1972; 49:504.
4. Avery GB: *Neonatology: Pathophysiology and Management of the Newborn,* ed 2. Philadelphia, JB Lippincott, 1981.
5. Adamsons K Jr, Gandy GM, James LS: The influence of thermal factors upon oxygen consumption of the newborn infant. *J Pediatr* 1965; 66:495.
6. Apgar V: A proposal for a new method of evaluation of the newborn infant. *Curr Res Anesth* 1953; 32:260.
7. Bloom RS, Croppley C: *Textbook of Neonatal Resuscitation.* Dallas, American Heart Association, 1987.
8. Niermeyer S, Kattiwinkel J, Reempts PV, et al. International guidelines for neonatal resuscitation: An excerpt from the guidelines 2000 for cardiopulmonary resuscitation and emergency cardiovascular care: International consensus on science. Pediatrics 2000;106:29.
9. Avery ME, Fletcher BD: *The Lung and Its Disorders in the Newborn Infant,* ed 3. Philadelphia, WB Saunders Co, 1974, p 134.
10. Shnider SM, Levinson G: *Anesthesia for Obstetrics,* ed 2. Baltimore, William & Wilkins, 1987, p 526.
11. deLorimier AA, Tierney DF, Parker HR: Hypoplastic lungs in fetal lambs with surgically produced congenital diaphragmatic hernia. *Surgery* 1967; 62:12.

15
Postpartum Tubal Ligation

Gastric Emptying in the Postpartum Period
Anesthetic Technique
Epidural Anesthesia
Spinal Anesthesia
General Anesthesia

Many obstetricians prefer to perform postpartum tubal ligation immediately after the delivery or before the women are discharged from the hospital. This procedure has a few *distinct advantages:*

1. Immediately after delivery, the uterine fundus lies between the umbilicus and symphysis pubis, so the fallopian tubes remain easily accessible.
2. Uncomplicated postpartum sterilization does not increase the hospital stay.
3. There is less medical cost.

On the other hand, one can find a *few disadvantages* in performing this procedure immediately after delivery:

1. The physiological changes of pregnancy do not revert back to the normal stage for at least 6 weeks.
2. One should not anesthetize any women with a full stomach for elective surgery like tubal ligation.

The possibility of a full stomach and increased gastric acidity remains the major problem in parturients. Gastric motility can be further decreased in the presence of labor pain as well as because of the use of narcotics. These factors will place parturients at high risk for gastric aspiration even after delivery, and controversy exists regarding the time for gastric emptying after delivery.

Gastric Emptying in the Postpartum Period

A gastric volume of more than 25 mL and a pH of less 2.5 will put the parturient at risk.[1]

Blouw and colleagues performed an interesting study to observe the differences in gastric volume and pH between parturients undergoing tubal ligation 8 hours postpartum vs. nonpregnant women having laparoscopic tubal ligation.[2] Thirty-three percent of the postpartum women and 64% of the control women were found to be at risk. The next study regarding this issue was done by Uram and colleagues.[3] They measured gastric volume and pH in 40 postpartum women in whom tubal ligations were performed between 2 and 48 hours after delivery and found that 28% of these women were at risk (Figs 15-1 and 15-2). Finally, James et al, in a more extensive and well-controlled study, observed three groups of postpartum women undergoing tubal ligation.[4] They were divided

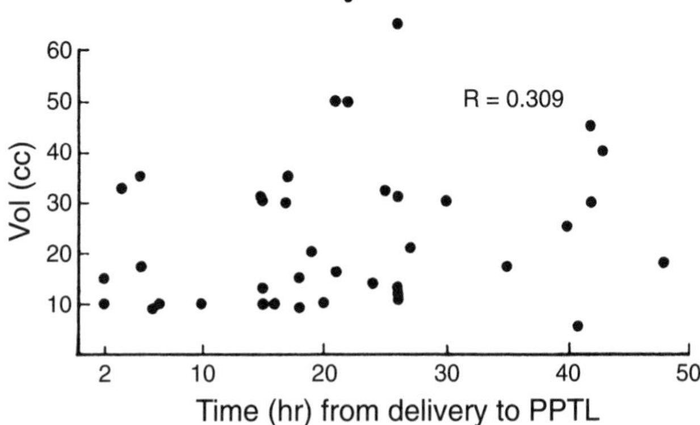

Figure 15-1. Correlation between time to postpartum tubal ligation (*PPTL*) and gastric volume. (Adapted from Uram M, Abouleish E, McKenzie R, et al: The risk of aspiration pneumonitis with postpartum tubal ligation (abstract). Presented at the Society for Obstetric Anesthesia and Perinatology, Jackson Hole, WY, 1982.

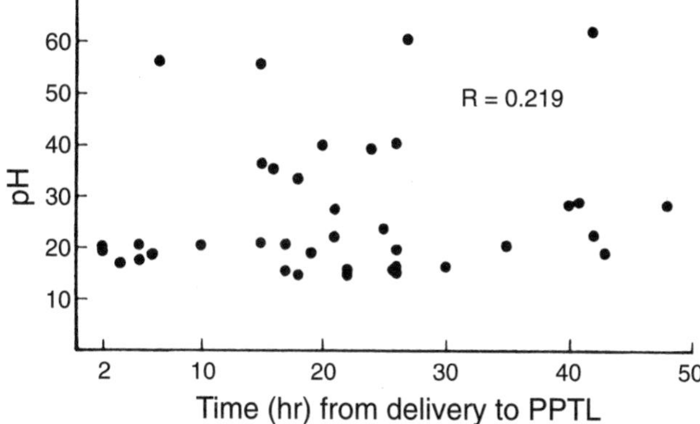

Figure 15–2. Correlation between the time to postpartum tubal ligation (*PPTL*) and gastric pH. (Adapted from Uram M, Abouleish E, McKenzie R, et al: The risk of aspiration pneumonitis with postpartum tubal ligation (abstract). Presented at the Society for Obstetric Anesthesia and Perinatology, Jackson Hole, WY, 1982, p 2. Used by permission.)

into groups by the time of their surgery following delivery: (1) 1 to 8 hours, (2) 9 to 23 hours, and (3) 24 to 25 hours; the control group was composed of surgical cases of the same age and weight. There were no differences in the number of women who were at risk among the groups, and the results in the control group were no different from those in the experimental groups. Sixty percent of their women were at risk, which was higher than two previous studies. So it is obvious from these studies that one cannot be sure about the gastric volume and pH up to 48 hours postpartum and that at least 33% of women will be at risk.

There is controversy among anesthesiologists regarding the optimum time for performing postpartum tubal ligation as well as the choice of anesthetic. At Brigham and Women's Hospital we encourage the obstetric team to inform the women to have epidural anesthesia for their labor and delivery if they are contemplating postpartum tubal ligation. These women are also consulted by the anesthetic team as soon as they arrive on the labor floor. If women desire postpartum tubal ligation after natural childbirth and induction of epidural anesthesia is not possible because of time restriction, most of the anesthesiologists in our institution will use a subarachnoid block for surgical intervention. *However, the ultimate decision is made by the individual anesthesiologist.* The following guidelines are followed by most of the anesthesiologists at Brigham and Women's Hospital.

1. A consent form should be appropriate and ready.
2. Women are encouraged to have epidural anesthesia for labor and delivery if they desire to have postpartum tubal ligation.
3. Women contemplating natural childbirth and postpartum tubal ligation are consulted by the anesthesiologist and are advised against food intake. Spinal anesthesia is used in these cases unless contraindicated.
4. Postpartum tubal ligation will be canceled if the parturient remains unstable.

Anesthetic Technique

Epidural Anesthesia

Pregnant women need less local anesthetic as compared with their nonpregnant counterparts. Although the mechanism is not exactly known, increased neuronal sensitivity has been suggested.[5] However, there is controversy regarding the duration of this increased sensitivity after delivery. In an elegant study, *Brooks and colleagues observed an increased spread of sensory anesthesia up to 36 hours postpartum, and following this period, the dose requirements were not significantly different from those of nonpregnant population.*[6] A sensory level encompassing T5–6 is necessary when performing postpartum tubal ligation to prevent discomfort. I personally prefer 2% plain lidocaine with 50 μg of fentanyl for this procedure because of its relatively short duration of action, less intense motor block, as well as absence of interference with μ-receptor agonist drugs (e.g., fentanyl, morphine). One can also use other local anesthetics like 2% lidocaine with epinephrine, 0.5% bupivacaine, or 3% 2-chloroprocaine. I prefer to use 10 mg of metoclopramide intravenously and nonparticulate antacid at least 30 minutes prior to the operative procedure. This will decrease gastric volume and increase gastric pH.[7]

Spinal Anesthesia

Like epidural anesthesia, less local anesthetic is required in parturients than in nonpregnant women when a subarachnoid block is performed. This decreased requirement does not reach prepregnant values for at least 24 hours (Fig 15-3).[8] The techniques for spinal anesthesia are summarized below:

1. Metoclopramide, 10 mg intravenously (unless contraindicated), plus nonparticulate antacid.
2. Volume expansion with 1,500 mL Ringer's lactate or dextrose Ringer's lactate.
3. Routine monitoring (blood pressure, electrocardiogram, pulse oximeter).
4. Hyperbaric bupivacaine or lidocaine. Doses should be similar to those used for cesarean section. Because of the

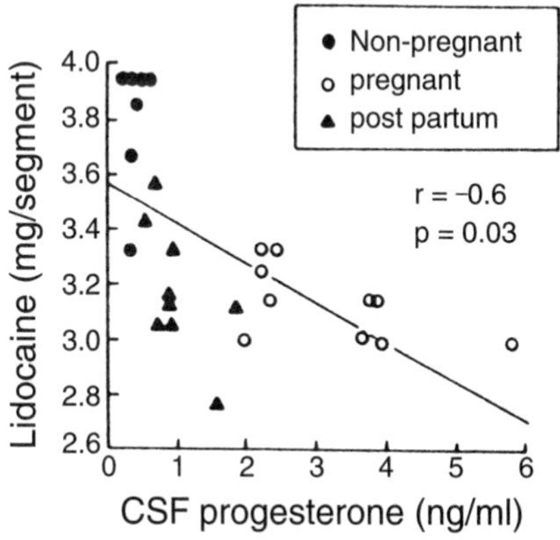

Figure 15-3. Correlation between cerebrospinal fluid (*CSF*) progesterone (ng/mL) and lidocaine (milligrams per segment) in nonpregnant patients, parturients having cesarean section, and patients 24 hours after delivery. (Adapted from Datta S, Hurley RJ, Naulty JS: *Anesth Analg* 1986; 65:950.)

possibility of transient radicular symptoms (TRS), use of lidocaine has been controversial. However, incidences of TRS in supine position have been observed to be low. Some centers have used intrathecal meperidine (1 mg/kg) for postpartum tubal ligation. The duration was observed to be 30–60 minutes and the duration analgesia was 6–7 hours.[9] Tubal ligation is usually a painful procedure. Hence, adequate postoperative pain relief is important. Small doses of intrathecal or epidural morphine have been used in a few centers. Others have used infiltration of bupivacaine of the mesosalpinx or topical application of local anesthetic over the fallopian tubes with success.[10] Intravenous meperidine may be used for postoperative pain relief.

5. Ten micrograms of fentanyl mixed with local anesthetic can intensify the sensory anesthesia.
6. Vital signs should be maintained throughout the procedure.
7. A small amount of narcotics and tranquilizers can be used.

General Anesthesia

At Brigham and Women's Hospital we try to avoid general anesthesia for postpartum tubal ligation. If general anesthesia is necessary, one should be aware of the reduction in the minimum alveolar concentration in parturients; again it is not known how long this reduction in the minimum alveolar concentration lasts following delivery. The use of a small amount of nondepolarizing muscle relaxants before administering depolarizing relaxants is controversial, and we at Brigham and Women's Hospital do not routinely use nondepolarizing muscle relaxants before induction of anesthesia. The techniques for general anesthesia for postpartum tubal ligation are as follows:

1. Intravenous line
2. Metoclopramide, 10 mg intravenously (unless contraindicated), plus nonparticulate antacid
3. Rapid-sequence induction: preoxygenation, cricoid pressure, and a cuffed endotracheal tube 7 to 7.5 F in size
4. Sodium thiopental (Pentothal), 4 mg/kg, or ketamine, 1 to 1.5 mg/kg, plus succinylcholine, 1 to 1.5 mg/kg

5. Routine monitoring (blood pressure, electrocardiogram, pulse oximeter, capnometer, temperature, block aid monitor)
6. Ventilation with O_2 and N_2O and a low concentration of inhalation anesthetics (to prevent uterine relaxation and bleeding) like enflurane, isoflurane, desflurane and sevoflurane
7. Continuous infusion of 0.1% succinylcholine or nondepolarizing muscle relaxants to ease ventilation
8. Narcotics like fentanyl, sufentanil, or alfentanil
9. Deflation of the stomach by a nasogastric tube inserted via the mouth
10. Extubation after the women is awake

Postpartum tubal ligation is an elective procedure; hence there is controversy regarding the optimum time for performing this surgery.[11] This will obviously vary from one hospital to another, depending upon personnel, expertise, and local policy.

References

1. Roberts RB, Shirley MA: Reducing the risk of acid aspiration during cesarean section. *Anesth Analg* 1974; 53:859.
2. Blouw R, Scatliff J, Craig DB: Gastric volume and pH in postpartum patients. *Anesthesiology* 1976; 45:456.
3. Uram M, Abouleish E, McKenzie R, et al: The risk of aspiration pneumonitis with postpartum tubal ligation (abstract). Presented at the Society for Obstetric Anesthesia and Perinatology, Jackson Hole, WY, 1982. p 2.
4. James CF, Gibbs CP, Banner T: Postpartum perioperative risk of aspiration pneumonia. *Anesthesiology* 1984; 61:756.
5. Datta S, Lambert DH, Gregus J, et al: Differential sensitivities of mammalian nerve fibers during pregnancy. *Anesth Analg* 1983; 61:1070.
6. Brooks GZ, Mandel ALZ: The early postpartum dermatomal spread of epidural 2-chloroprocaine, in *Abstracts of Scientific Papers.* Annual meeting of the Society for Obstetric Anesthesia and Perinatology, San Antonio, 1984, p 25.
7. Murphy D, Nally B, Gardiner J, et al: Effect of metoclopramide on gastric emptying before elective and emergency caesarean section. *Br J Anaesth* 1984; 56:1113.

8. Datta S, Hurley RJ, Naulty JS: Plasma and cerebrospinal fluid progesterone concentrations in pregnant and nonpregnant women. *Anesth Analg* 1986; 65:950.
9. Norris MC, Honet JE, Leighton BL, et al: A comparison of meperidine and lidocaine for spinal anesthesia for postpartum tubal ligation. *Reg Anesth* 1996; 21:84.
10. Alexander, Wetchler BV, Thompson RE: Bupivacaine infiltration of the mesosalpinx in ambulatory surgical laparoscopic tubal sterilization. *Can J Anaesth* 1987; 34:362.
11. Bucklin BA, Smith CV: Postpartum tubal ligation safety, timing and other implications for anesthesia. Anesth Analg 1999; 89:1269.

16
Anesthesia for Surgery During Pregnancy

▼

It has been estimated that every year in the United States about 50,000 pregnant women (0.5% to 2.2%) will receive anesthesia for various surgical indications during their pregnancy. The purpose of this surgery may be (1) to prolong gestation, (2) unrelated to the pregnancy, or (3) to correct fetal anomalies. Hence, an appreciation of the effects of different anesthetic drugs and techniques in such situations is essential in the care of these women. Recently, a question of preoperative pregnancy testing in adolescents has been raised. The authors observed retrospectively 412 adolescent women undergoing surgery. The overall incidence of positive testing was 1.2%. The authors concluded that mandatory pregnancy testing is advisable in all adolescent, surgical candidates aged 15 years and older.[1] However, compulsory pregnancy testing is not practiced in all hospitals; a hospital policy should be established after a discussion with the obstetric as well as anesthesia divisions.

Ideal anesthetic consideration for these women should include maternal safety, fetal well-being, and continuation of pregnancy.

Maternal Safety

A thorough knowledge of physiological changes during pregnancy is very important. This has been discussed in Chapter 1. However, the most important points will be mentioned here in a nutshell.

I. Respiratory system changes
   A. Capillary engorgement of respiratory mucous membrane
   B. Increased minute ventilation due mainly to an increase in tidal volume and to a lesser extent to an increase in respiratory rate
   C. Decreased end tidal CO_2
   D. Decreased functional residual capacity
   E. Increased oxygen demand

II. Cardiovascular system changes
   A. Increased cardiac output
   B. Increased blood volume
   C. Aortocaval compression from the gravid uterus

III. Gastrointestinal system changes
   A. Increased gastric volume and acidity because of decreased gastric motility; decreased lower gastroesophageal sphincter pressure

IV. Central and peripheral nervous system changes
   A. Decreased anesthetic requirement both for general, epidural, and spinal anesthesia

Fetal Well-Being

Avoidance of the teratogenic effects of anesthetics on the neonate is paramount in caring for this population. One should also try to avoid derangement of neonatal homeostasis, which can be affected directly and indirectly by anesthetic drugs and techniques.

The teratogenic effect of anesthetic drugs is a very controversial issue that has no clear-cut answer. Exposure to anesthetic agents may be either acute during surgery—sedatives, hypnotics, narcotics, muscle relaxants, local anesthetics, oxygen and carbon dioxide, or inhalational anesthetics—or chronic because of occupational exposure to inhalational anesthetics.

Acute Exposure

Even though human studies of the effect of acute exposure of anesthetics demonstrated an increased incidence of spontaneous abortion, they failed to show any teratogenic effects on the fetus.[1–4] In 1986 Duncan and colleagues retrospectively reviewed the incidence of congenital anomalies and spontaneous abortions in 2,565 pregnant women who underwent surgery.[5] These women were matched with a control group consisting of a similar number of pregnant women with similar maternal ages as well as areas of residence. *No significant differences in the rate of congenital anomalies were observed between the study and control groups. However, there was a significant increase in spontaneous abortions in women who underwent surgery during their first and second trimesters. One of the drawbacks of this study was that the vast majority of surgeries were performed with the woman under general anesthesia, so one could not differentiate the effect of regional or general anesthesia on the incidence of spontaneous abortion.* Mazze and Kallen retrospectively analyzed pregnant women from Swedish health care registries (1973 to 1981).[6] Out of 720,000 cases, 5,405 underwent surgery. *The incidence of congenital malformation was not different between the group that underwent surgery and the one that did not; however, there was a high incidence of prematurity and intrauterine growth retardation in the group that had surgery. The authors did not observe any association of this adverse outcome with the anesthetic used or the operation the woman underwent.*

Chronic Exposure

Several reports of increased congenital anomalies as well as spontaneous abortions among anesthesiologists and other operating room personnel have been published.[7,8] An important report regarding this issue was published by an ad hoc committee of the American Society of Anesthesiologists.[9] They found an increased risk of congenital anomalies and spontaneous abortions in women working in operating room areas when compared with non–operating room female hospital employees. In a separate study, an increased rate of spontaneous abortions was reported among female dentists and assistants who used inhalational anesthetics as compared with those who used local anesthetics in their practice.[10] On the other hand, in a different study, Ericson and Kallen were unable to demonstrate an increased risk of adverse fetal outcome in operating room or anesthesia nurses as compared with a control group of medical floor nurses.[11]

Until now, no causal relationship has been proved between the chronic exposure to inhalational anesthetics and spontaneous anomalies. However, the importance of the scavenging system has been stressed in the operating room environment. Rowland et al. observed the effect of nitrous oxide on pregnancy in 459 dental assistants and divided them into five groups 1) unexposed 2) low scavenged 3) high scavenged 4) low unscavenged 5) high unscavenged. The mean time to conception was significantly higher in the high unscavenged group.[11a]

Teratogenic studies of different anesthetic agents have been studied mainly in animals. It is very difficult as well as impractical to extrapolate these results to humans. However, a comprehensive knowledge of the effect of anesthetic agents on teratogenicity is important.

Sedative and Hypnotic Agents

Barbiturates have been used in humans as induction agents for a long time. Although there is a conflicting report in animals regarding the teratogenic effect of barbiturates, in pregnant women these agents have been found to be safe.[12] Phenothiazines have also been observed to be without any adverse effect in humans.[13] The association of minor tranquilizers with teratogenicity is controversial, although retrospective studies have shown diazepam and chlordiazepoxide to be associated with congenital malformations.[14,15] One the other hand, more recent studies did not find any increased risk of congenital anomalies following use of diazepam.[16] Midazolam has not been observed with any teratogenecity.

Narcotics

Geber and Schramm observed the teratogenicity of a wide variety of narcotics administered to pregnant hamsters at critical periods of fetal central nervous system development.[17] Comparative studies using single or multiple doses showed increased fetal anomalies with diacetylmorphine, thebaine, pentazocine, morphine, hydromorphone, as well as meperidine.

On the other hand, other authors observed that the chronic administration of morphine, fentanyl, sufentanil, or alfentanil in pregnant rats was not associated with any teratogenic effect.[18,19] There is also no evidence that these opioids are associated with teratogenicity in humans.

Muscle Relaxants

There is no evidence of an adverse effect in fetal development following the use of muscle relaxants.

Local Anesthetics

In a very large study by the Collaborative Perinatal Project, no evidence of teratogenicity was found in pregnant rats following the administration of benzocaine, procaine, tetracaine, or lidocaine.[20] *In contrast, the use of cocaine is associated with fetal congenital malformations both in humans and animals.[21] This may be explained by cocaine-mediated vasoconstriction and, hence, fetal tissue hypoxia.*

Oxygen and Carbon Dioxide

Hypoxia as well as hypercarbia have been associated with teratogenicity in animal species.[22,23] Although a high concentration of inspired oxygen at atmospheric pressure does not produce any adverse effects,[24] hyperbaric oxygen exposure is associated with fetal anomalies in animals.[25]

Inhalation Anesthetics

The addition of inhalational anesthetics such as nitrous oxide or halogenated agents to oxygen has become a routine practice when administering general anesthesia. Some of these agents have been implicated in the development of fetal anomalies as well as in premature births.

Nitrous Oxide. Interest in the teratogenic effect of nitrous oxide has grown significantly among anesthesiologists since Nunn and colleagues observed the effect of the short-term nitrous oxide anesthetic administration on plasma concentrations of methionine, tryptophan, phenylalanine, and *S*-adenosylmethionine in humans.[26] The authors observed a 15% reduction in tryptophan concentration after exposure to 60% to 70% nitrous oxide for a mean duration of 88 minutes. *The plasma methionine concentration decreased significantly following exposure to 50% nitrous oxide for up to 11 days in rats.*[27] Using nitrous oxide during surgery and up to 24 hours postoperatively, Skacel and colleagues observed a significant decrease in the plasma methionine concentration following major vascular surgery in humans.[28] Recovery took place following discontinuation of nitrous oxide administration. *The main reason for the decreased plasma methionine concentration is related to inhibition of enzyme methionine synthetase.*[26] *Thus the teratogenic effect of nitrous oxide may be related to the interference with DNA synthesis by altering folate metabolism*[26] (Fig 16-1). *Keeling and colleagues observed the effect of pretreatment with folinic acid on the teratogenic effect of nitrous oxide in rats.*[29] *Major skeletal abnormalities in the group receiving nitrous oxide without pretreatment increased five times as compared with the control group, whereas the group that was pretreated with folinic acid was not significantly different from controls.* Mazze et al also observed teratogenicity in rats after exposure to 50% or more of nitrous oxide for 24 hours on day 8 of pregnancy.[30] *Interestingly, the teratogenic effect was prevented by the addition of fentanyl or halogenated anesthetics with nitrous oxide.*[31,32] *Hence the authors concluded that the mechanism of teratogenicity following nitrous oxide exposure may not be related to interference in DNA synthesis but rather*

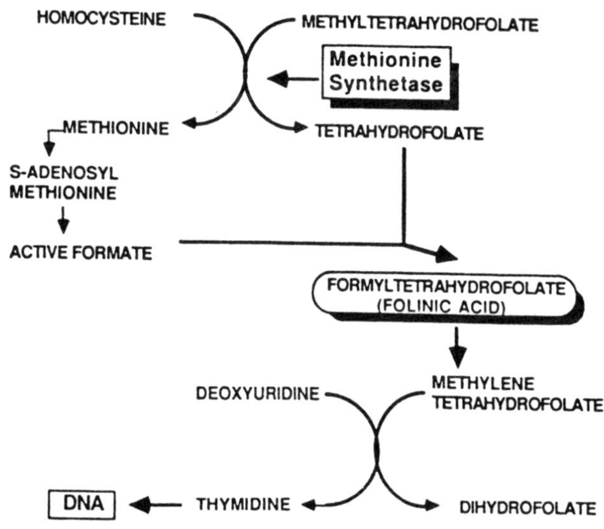

Figure 16-1. Mechanisms of the interference of nitrous oxide in DNA synthesis. Nitrous oxide directly blocks the transmethylation reaction by which methionine is synthesized from homocysteine and methyltetrahydrofolate. Nitrous oxide oxidizes vitamin B_{12}, the cofactor of the enzyme methionine synthetase. (From Levinson G, Shnider SM: *Anesthesia for Obstetrics.* Baltimore, Williams & Wilkins, 1987, p 188. Used by permission.)

to a physiological effect of nitrous oxide, such as reduction in uterine blood flow due to increased sympathetic activity.[32] However, when an α-antagonist like phenoxybenzamine was used, the investigators could not completely abolish the teratogenic effect of nitrous oxide.[33] In summary, although in rats there is a relationship between the use of nitrous oxide and teratogenicity, the exact mechanism is not clear at the present time. In humans, short exposures to nitrous oxide during the second trimester were not associated with any adverse effect.[34]

Halogenated Anesthetics. Halothane, enflurane, and isoflurane at physiological minimum alveolar concentrations are not associated with any teratogenicity in rats.[32] Nor has evidence of teratogenicity been seen in humans with these agents. Recently a review article has been published related to drugs in pregnancy.[35a]

The newer inhalation anesthetics sevoflurane and desflurane are not associated with any teratogenecity.

Continuation of the Pregnancy

Surgery during pregnancy is associated with a higher incidence of premature labor and spontaneous abortion. *The incidence is higher in lower abdominal, pelvic, and cervical surgery.* Tocolytic drugs, both for prophylactic and ther apeutic reasons, are used quite often to prevent premature delivery.

General and Specific Recommendations

Elective surgery should be postponed until delivery. In semielective cases, it is best if surgery can be postponed until after the first trimester. In emergency cases, the anesthetic of choice should depend on the site and extent of the surgery to be performed. If possible, regional anesthesia, e.g., spinal, epidural, or nerve block, is advisable. However, general anesthesia can be administered if necessary.

Preoperative medications, if necessary, may include barbiturates and morphine. Routine, nonparticulate antacid should be used, and rapid-sequence induction is recommended. *Although there is no general consensus, it is reasonable to use an endotracheal tube from the 12th week of gestation onward.* Depending on the duration of surgery, one can use either depolarizing or nondepolarizing muscle relaxants. Anesthesia can be maintained with nitrous oxide, oxygen, and halogenated anesthetics. Morphine, fentanyl, sufentanil, or alfentanil can be used as analgesics. *Hyperventilation should always be avoided because it can reduce uteroplacental perfusion as well as shift the maternal hemoglobin dissociation curve to the left.*

For regional anesthesia, maintenance of normal blood pressure is absolutely necessary, and the routine use of oxygen by face mask is recommended. *Whether general or regional anes-*

thesia has been chosen, left uterine displacement from the second trimester onward is mandatory.

Routine monitoring should include blood pressure, electrocardiogram, oxygen saturation, capnograph, and temperature. In addition, fetal heart rate monitoring, if possible, should be performed from 16 weeks onward. Close communication between the anesthesiologist and obstetrician regarding fetal heart rate monitoring is necessary as well as interpretation of the tracings. Because most of the medications used for general anesthesia can abolish the fetal heart rate variability, the baseline fetal heart rate should be the main indicator of fetal well-being during general anesthesia. Depending upon the location of surgery, tocodynamometry can be used to monitor uterine contractions. This obviously becomes routine in the postoperative period when treating pregnant women with preterm contractions with tocolytics. Recently, laparoscopic surgery during pregnancy has been used with success. One must have a basic knowledge of physiological changes during pregnancy. During laparoscopic cholecystectomy, the women is placed in a head-up position during dissection and in a head-down position for irrigation. In parturients, these positions may have significant cardiovascular and respiratory effects. Peritoneal insufflation pressure should be kept low because of the possibility of aortocaval compression. Ventilation should be optimal to maintain end-tidal PCO_2 at 32–35 mmHg.[35]

Intrauterine Surgery

Intrauterine surgery is becoming popular for treating fetal congenital anomalies. In the majority of cases the pregnancy is continued, whereas for the ex-utero intrapartum treatment (EXIT) procedure surgery is performed on the fetus on placental support followed by delivery. Maternal and fetal considerations for anesthetic implications have already been discussed. The minimum alveolar concentration for halothane has been observed to be 50% lower in the fetal lamb as compared with the pregnant ewe (0.33% vol. vs 0.69% vol.)[36] (Fig 16-2). Invasive fetal therapy may be associated with preterm labor. Hence avoidance of preterm labor remains the major issue. High concentrations of inhalation anesthetics are used for uterine relax-

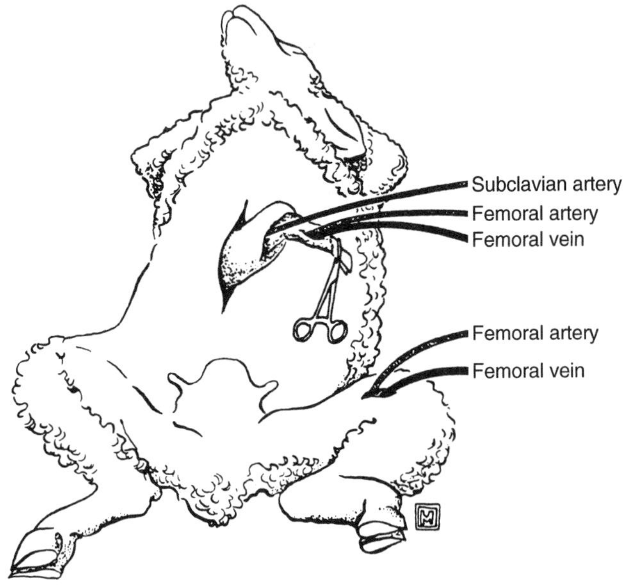

Figure 16–2. The foot of the fetus is withdrawn through a hysterotomy and stimulated with a Kocher clamp for evaluation of the minimum alveolar concentration. (From Gregory GA, Wade JG, Biehl DR, et al: *Anesth Analg* 1983; 62:9. Used by permission.)

ation, as well as to prevent uterine contractions, nitroglycerin can also be used if necessary. Tocolytic drugs like magnesium sulfate is used for the prevention of preterm labor following discontinuation of the inhalation anesthetic at the conclusion of the surgery. Ephedrine or phenylephrine is used for maintenance of baseline blood pressure to prevent uteroplacental insufficiency. In case of EXIT procedure, uterine relaxation is also important to prevent uterine contraction and separation of placenta. Following delivery of the infant, inhalation anesthetic should be discontinued and use of uterotonic drugs are mandatory. The other indication for the use of anesthetics is to prevent fetal movements. This can be accomplished by administering anesthetics, narcotics, or muscle relaxants to the mother, which will ultimately reach the fetus via the placenta. Epidural or combined spinal epidural can also be used for the surgery. Uterine relaxation can be achieved with nitroglycerin. Muscle relaxants and narcotics can directly be administered to the fetus. Pancuronium maintained better fetal cardiovascular stability than did curare, vecuronium can also be used.[37,38] To prevent hypothermia of the fetus the operating room should be kept as warm as possible and the uterus should be irrigated with a warm solution. Fetal monitoring will depend on the surgery and will vary from continuous fetal heart rate monitoring to pulse oximetry and transcutaneous electrode measurement of blood pH and PO_2 if a body part is accessible. Following surgery, monitoring of the fetal heart rate and uterine contractions should be routine because of the possibility of the onset of premature labor. For post operative pain relief patient controlled intravenous analgesia can be used, if an epidural catheter is present use of Duramorph will be ideal.

References

1. Azzam FJ, Padda GS, DeBoard JW, et al: Preoperative pregnancy testing in adolescents. *Anesth Analg* 1996; 82:4.

1a. Shnider SM, Webster GM: Maternal and fetal hazards of surgery. *Am J Obstet Gynecol* 1965; 92:891.

2. Brodsky JB, Cohen EN, Brown BW: Surgery during pregnancy and fetal outcome. *Am J Obstet Gynecol* 1980; 138:1165.

3. Keneddy RL, Miller RP, Bell JU, et al: Uptake and distribution of bupivacaine in fetal lambs. *Anesthesiology* 1986; 65:247.

4. Smith BE: Fetal prognosis after anesthesia during gestation. *Anesth Analg* 1963; 42:521.

5. Duncan PB, Pope WDB, Cohen MM, et al: Fetal risk of anesthesia and surgery during pregnancy. *Anesthesiology* 1986; 64:790.

6. Mazze RI, Kallen B: Reproductive outcome after anesthesia and operation during pregnancy: A registry study of 5405 cases. *Am J Obstet Gynecol* 1989; 161:1178.

7. Vaisman AI: Working conditions in surgery and their effect on the health of anesthesiologists. *Eksp Khir Anesth* 1967; 3:44.

8. Knill-Jones RP, Rodrigues LV, Moir DD, et al: Anesthetic practice and pregnancy-controlled survey of women anaesthetists in the United Kingdom. *Lancet* 1972; 1:1326.
9. Ad Hoc Committee on the Effect of Trace Anesthetics on the Health of Operating Room Personnel, American Society of Anesthesiologists: Occupational disease among operating room personnel—a national study. *Anesthesiology* 1974; 41:321.
10. Cohen EN, Brown BW, Wu ML, et al: Occupational disease in dentistry and chronic exposure to trace anesthetic gases. *J Am Dent Assoc* 1980; 101:21.
11. Ericson HA, Kallen AJB: Hospitalization and miscarriage and delivery outcome among Swedish nurses working in operating rooms. 1973–1978. *Anesth Analg* 1985; 64:981.
11a. Rowland AS, Baird DD, Weinberg CR, et al: Reduced fertility among women employed as dental assistants exposed to high levels of nitrous oxide. *N Eng J Med* 1992; 327:993.
12. Heinonen OP, Slone D, Shapiro D: *Birth Defects and Drugs in Pregnancy.* Littleton, MA, Publishing Sciences Group, 1977, p 337.
13. Slone D, Siskind V, Heinonon O, et al: Antenatal exposure to the phenothiazines in relation to congenital malformations, perinatal mortality rate, birth weight and intelligence quotient score. *Am J Obstet Gynecol* 1977; 128:486.
14. Safra M, Oakley GP: Association between the cleft lip with or without cleft palate and prenatal exposure to diazepam. *Lancet* 1975; 2:478.
15. Milkovich L, VandenBerg BJ: Effects of prenatal meprobamate and chlordiazepoxide hydrochloride on human embryonic and fetal development. *N Engl J Med* 1974; 291:1268.
16. Koren G, Pastuszak A, Ito S: Drugs in pregnancy. *N Eng J Med* 1998; 338:1128.
17. Geber WF, Schramm LC: Congenital malformations of the central nervous system produced by narcotic analgesics in the hamster. *Am J Obstet Gynecol* 1975; 123:705.
18. Zagon IS, McLaughlin PJ: Effects of chronic morphine administration on pregnant rats and their offspring. *Pharmacology* 1977; 15:302.
19. Fujinaga M, Stevenson JB, Mazze RJ: Reproductive and teratogenic effects of fentanyl in Sprague-Dawley rats. *Teratology* 1986; 34:51.
20. Fujinaga M, Mazze RI, Jackson EC: Reproductive and teratogenic effects or sufentanil and alfentanil in Sprague-Dawley rats. *Anesth Analg* 1988; 67:166.

21. Bingol N, Fuchs M, Diaz V, et al: Teratogenicity of cocaine in humans. *J Pediatr* 1987; 110:93.
22. Haring OM: The effects of prenatal hypoxia on the CV system in the rat. *Arch Pathol* 1965; 80:351.
23. Haring OM: Cardiac malformations in rats induced by exposure of the mother to CO_2 during pregnancy. *Circ Res* 1960; 8:1218.
24. Fujikura T: Retrolental fibroplasia and prematurity in newborn rabbits induced by maternal hyperoxia. *Am J Obstet Gynecol* 1964; 90:854.
25. Fern BH: Teratogenic effects of hyperbaric O_2. *Proc Soc Exp Biol Med* 1964; 116:975.
26. Nunn JF, Sharer NM, Bottiglieri T, et al: Effect of short-term administration of nitrous oxide on plasma concentrations of methionine, tryptophan, phenylalanine and *S*-adenosylmethionine in man. *Br J Anaesth* 1986; 58:1.
27. Lumb M, Shater N, Deacon R: Effects of nitrous oxide-induced inactivation of cobalamin on methionine and *S*-adenosylmethionine metabolism in the rat. *Biochim Biophys Acta* 1983; 756:354.
28. Skacel PO, Hewlett AM, Lewis JD: Studies on the haemopoietic toxicity of nitrous oxide in man. *Br J Haematol* 1983; 53:189.
29. Keeling PA, Rocke DA, Nunn JF: Folinic acid protection against nitrous oxide teratogenicity in the rat. *Br J Anaesth* 1986; 58:528.
30. Mazze RI, Wilson AI, Rice SA: Reproductive and fetal development in rats exposed to nitrous oxide. *Teratology* 1984; 30:259.
31. Mazze RI, Fujinaga M, Baden JM: Reproductive and teratogenic effects of nitrous oxide, fentanyl and their combination in Sprague-Dawley rats. *Br J Anaesth* 1987; 59:1291.
32. Mazze RI, Fujinaga M, Rice SA, et al: Reproduction and teratogenic effects of nitrous oxide, halothane, isoflurane and enflurane in Sprague-Dawley rats. *Anesthesiology* 1986; 64: 339.
33. Fujinaga M, Baden JM, Suto A, et al: Preventive effects of phenoxybenzamine on N_2O induced reproductive toxicity in Sprague-Dawley rats (abstract). *Anesthesiology* 1990; 73:920.
34. Aldridge LM, Tunstall ME: Nitrous oxide and the fetus. A review and the results of a retrospective study of 175 cases of anaesthesia for insertion of Shirodker suture. *Br J Anaesth* 1986; 50:134.
35. Steinbrook RA, Brooks DC, Datta S: Laparoscopic cholecystectomy during pregnancy. *Surg Endosc* 1996; 10:511.

35a. Koren G, Pastuszak A, Ito S: Drugs in pregnancy. *N Engl J Med* 1998; 338:1128.
36. Gregory GA, Wade JG, Biehl DR, et al: Fetal anesthetic requirement (MAC) for halothane. *Anesth Analg* 1983; 62:9.
37. Moise KJ, Carpenter RJ, Deter RL, et al: The use of fetal neuromuscular blockade during intrauterine procedures. *Am J Obstet Gynecol* 1987; 157:874.
38. Chestnut DH, Weiner CP, Thompson CS: Intravenous administration of *d*-tuborcurarine and pancuronium in fetal lambs (abstract). *Anesthesiology* 1988; 69:652.

17
In Vitro Fertilization

▼

Recent improvement in scientific knowledge and biochemical technology has increased the success rate of in vitro fertilization.

Since Edwards and associates of England performed the first successful in vitro fertilization,[1] gamete transfer has become very popular worldwide.

The technique involves obtaining mature oocytes from ovarian follicles and incubating them with sperm. The embryos are then transferred into the uterine cavity.

Preparation of the Embryo

Hormonal manipulation are done to achieve a number of oocytes for retrieval. To start with ovarian down regulation is achieved with the administration of gonadotropin-releasing hormone agonist like Lupron. The ovarian down regulation is done to minimize the formation of single dominant follicle or the onset of premature ovulation. Following down regulation ovarian hyperstimulation is achieved with human menopausal gonadotropin and the result is followed by ultrasonographic confirmation of follicular growth and a progressive increase in serum estrogen levels. Once follicular maturity is reached, ovulation is induced by human chorionic gonadotropin hormone. Multiple oocytes are collected as close as possible to the time of expected ovulation. The oocytes are placed in an organ culture dish containing the sperm, insemination medium, and fetal serum. The transfer is made when the embryo reaches the four to eight-cell stage via a transfer catheter into the uterine cavity. Occasionally in the presence of normal fallopian tubes the mixture of oocytes and liquefied semen is directly introduced into the tubes by laparoscopy. Gamete intrafallopian transfer (GIFT).

Anesthetic Requirement

At the present time, most oocyte retrievals are done through the ultrasonographic transvaginal approach and rarely by the laparoscopic technique. Oocyte collection requires anesthetics, whereas embryo transfer to the uterus is a painless procedure and does not usually require anesthesia. *The GIFT procedure (Fig. 17-1) is a combined technique usually involving transvaginal oocyte retrieval followed by deposit of the mixture of oocytes and semen in the fallopian tube by laparoscopy,* and it requires anesthetics. At present, there is no consensus regarding the anesthetic techniques or anesthetic agents of choice for this procedure. There are only a few reports addressing the effect of anesthetics on the cleavage rate of the embryo. Shatford and colleagues assessed pain associated with transvaginal ultrasonography-guided oocyte recovery in 164 women.[2] The intensity of pain was assessed from the McGill pain questionnaire. Seventy-eight percent of women assessed visual analogue scale (VAS) to be 5 or less (reasonably tolerable level of discomfort), and 6% of the participants scored the pain 7 or more (relatively intense pain) immediately after the procedure; however the pain intensity decreased significantly after 1 hour of the procedure. All women in the study of Shallord et al received narcotics 1 hour before the procedure and a paracervical block with 14 mL of 0.5% lidocaine (Xylocaine) at the time of surgery. Lewin and colleagues compared the oocyte recovery rate and

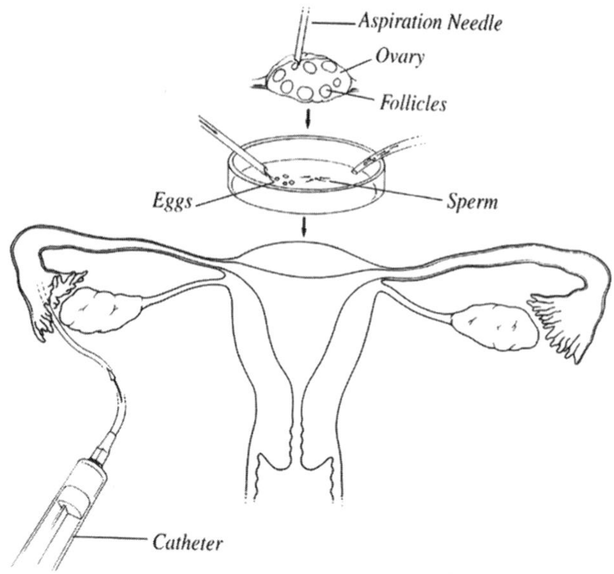

Figure 17-1. In GIFT, eggs are retriered from the ovaries and Mixed with sperm. The sperm–egg mixture is loaded into a catheter and injected directly into the fallopian tube(s). (From The American Society for Reproductive Medicine: IVF and GIFT: A Guide to Assisted Reproductive Technologies; A Guide for Patients, 1995. Used with permission of the publisher, the American Society for Reproductive Medicine. ASRM revised this booklet in 2003 as Assisted Reproductive Technologies: A Guide for Patients. It may be found on the ASRM web site at www.asrm.org.)

the fertilization rate in two groups of women[3]: ten women who had follicular aspiration during laparoscopy under general anesthesia vs. ten women who had ultrasonically guided follicular aspiration with local anesthetic. Ten to 15 mL of 0.5% bupivacaine hydrochloride was used for local infiltration and intravenous infusion of meperidine, 1.5 mg/kg, and diazepam, 10 mg, with saline administered during the procedure. They did not observe any difference in the oocyte recovery and the fertilization rate. On the other hand, they concluded that ultrasonically guided oocyte retrieval may be associated with fewer complications.

Finally, in a recent study Palot and colleagues observed deleterious effects of N_2O on the cleavage rate of the embryo. However, when halothane was combined with O_2 alone or with O_2 and N_2O, it did not affect the cleavage rate.[4] The authors could not explain the exact mechanism for these findings. Some of the conclusions one can derive from the above studies are as follows:

1. Ultrasonographic transvaginal oocyte retrieval is preferred over laparoscopic technique.
2. The transvaginal approach can be done under local anesthesia.
3. Although the mechanism is not known, N_2O can affect the cleavage rate.

Propofol was found to be an adequate induction agent for GIFT procedure. Recently, ultrasound and fiberoptic techniques have been used for approaching fallopian tubes; these techniques avoid the laparoscopic procedures.

Specific Anesthetic Techniques for Ultrasound-Guided Transvaginal Oocyte Retrieval

General anesthesia-In a busy service like ours, general anesthesia is preferred as the procedure is short and the women can be discharged faster compared to spinal anesthesia. Intravenous general anesthesia is provided by propofol either by intermittent injection or continuous infusion. Fentanyl and midazolam are also used routinely by a few. Women are allowed to breath spontaneously via high flow oxygen mask and the use of a capnograph. Spinal-anesthesia – this technique has some distinct advantages

1. It requires a small amount of local anesthetic
2. One can avoid large narcotic doses and tranquilizers
3. N2O can be avoided
4. There is a smaller incidence of postoperative nausea and/or vomiting compared to general anesthesia. Lidocaine 45mg (1.5%) mixed with 10mcg of fentanyl or lidocaine 30mg (1.5%) mixed with 25mcg of fentanyl is commonly used. One can avoid intravenous narcotics or tranquilizers.

Comparing 3mg of hyperbaric bupivacaine with an equipotent dose of lidocaine 30mg (1.5%) mixed with 25mcg of fentanyl, a longer duration for voiding was observed in the bupivacaine group.

Epidural Anesthesia – It is rarely done for this procedure. 2-chloroprocaine is avoided because of possible back pain.[4a]

General anesthesia is used for GIFT and ZIFT techniques, in which laparoscopic procedure is used to inject the gametes in the fallopian tube. This consists of the following steps:

1. A small amount of nondepolarizing muscle relaxant is used to prevent fasciculation from succinylcholine
2. Induction of anesthesia can be initiated with propofol
3. Intubation is performed following succinylcholine administration
4. The stomach is deflated with a gastric tube to prevent possible stomach perforation
5. Relaxation is maintained by using either a succinylcholine drip (0.1%) or nondepolarizing muscle relaxants
6. N2O plus O2 plus inhalation anesthetic or O2 plus inhalation anesthetic is used
7. Small amount of narcotics are administered
8. Neuromuscular block is reversed if nondepolarizing muscle relaxant is used.

The use of N2O is controversial, and no major study exists at this time regarding the detrimental effect of N2O on the clevage rate. The majority of the anesthesiologists use a combination of N2O and O2 and inhalation anesthetics like isoflurane, desflurane or enflurane.

Ovarian hyperstimulation syndrome (OHSS)—It is well understood that *during OHSS cycles the concentrations of thrombin-antithrombin III and plasma X2 antiplasmin complexes in plasma may rise within a few days after hCG administration.* There were also other characteristic changes in OHSS cycles in other hemostatic markers, such as a *decrease in the levels of antithrombin III and prekallikrein and shortened activated partial thromboplastin time.*[5] Three categories of OHSS has been described by their clinical and sonographic findings. In mild form women may complain of mild abdominal discomfort. The severe OHSS is characterized by the presence of intraperitoneal fluid, pleural effusion, hypotension and oliguria. Clinical findings may consist of fluid and electrolyte imbalance, torsion of the ovarian cyst as well as thromboembolic phenomenon.

Major Complications of In Vitro Fertilization

The success rate of in vitro fertilization at the present time varies from 25% to 30%, and the major problems connected with this procedure are as follows[6]:

1. Premature labor with fetal loss
2. Ectopic pregnancies
3. Multiple pregnancies
4. Vaginal bleeding
5. Congenital abnormalities
6. Pregnancy-induced hypertension

References

1. Edwards RG, Steptoe PC, Purely JM: Establishing full term human pregnancies using cleaving embryos grown in vitro. *Br J Obstet Gynaecol* 1980; 87:737.
2. Shatford LA, Brown SE, Yuzpe AA: Assessment of experienced pain associated with transvaginal ultrasonography-guided percutaneous aspiration of follicles in an in vitro fertilization program. *Am J Obstet Gynecol* 1985; 151:621.
3. Lewin A, Margakoth EJ, Rabinowitz R, et al: Comparative study of ultrasonically guided percutaneous aspiration of follicles in an in vitro fertilization program. *Am J Obstet Gynecol* 1985; 151:621.
4. Palot M, Visseaux MD, Harika G, et al: Effects of nitrous oxide and/or halothane on cleavage rate during general anesthesia for oocyte retrieval (abstract). *Anesthesiology* 1990; 73:930.

4a. Fibuch EE, Opper SE: Back pain following epidurally administered nesacaine-MPF. *Anesth Analg* 1989; 69:113.

5. Kodama H, Fukuda J, Karube H, et al: Status of the coagulation and fibrinolytic system in ovarian hyperstimulation syndrome. *Fertil Steril* 1996; 66:417.
6. Andrews MC, Muasher SJ, Levy DL, et al: An analysis of the obstetric outcome of 125 consecutive pregnancies conceived in vitro and resulting in 100 deliveries. *Am J Obstet Gynecol* 1986; 154:848.

18
Maternal Mortality and Morbidity

Maternal mortality and morbidity have always been important matters for discussion in obstetric anesthesia. Confidential inquires into maternal mortality in England and Wales have been used for international comparison because of strict record keeping.[1] However, in recent past several important statistics regarding maternal mortality and morbidity have been published in the American literature.[2–5]

The latest report of confidential inquires from England and Wales was published in 2001. The first report with anesthesia as an entity was published in 1952. Since that time anesthetic agents as well as techniques have changed dramatically. Regional anesthesia has become the technique of choice for labor and delivery as well as cesarean section. Between 1997 and 1999, three deaths were directly associated with anesthesia. In addition to the three deaths, there were a number of deaths that contain messages for anesthesia services. In a recent report the direct maternal mortality rate was 5.0 deaths per 100,000 maternities, this was lower than in any of other four preceding triennia for which the UK data have been collected. The indirect maternal mortality rate, 6.4 deaths per 100,000 maternities, was higher than in any of the preceding four triennia. For the first time, the number of indirect maternal deaths was greater than direct maternal deaths. Like the last report, the recent report also observed an increased incidence of cesarean section, there was also an increase in maternal age. Thrombosis and thromboembolism was the number one cause for maternal mortality followed by hypertensive disease of pregnancy and hemorrhage. Recognized instances of substandard care is shown in Table 18-1.

Table 18-1. Direct Deaths Assessed as Having Substandard Care; United Kingdom 1997-1999

Category	Chapter # in report	% category of deaths due to substandard care
Thrombosis	35	20 (57%)
Hypertension	15	12 (80%)
Hemorrhage	7	5 (71%)
Amniotic Fluid Embolism	8	2 (25%)
Early Pregnancy	17	11 (65%)
Sepsis	14	7 (50%)
Other Direct	7	4 (57%)
Anesthetic	3	3 (100%)

One important problem of general anesthesia for cesarean section is maternal awareness. This problem was found to have an incidence of 0.4%. Awareness claims were further subdivided into awake paralysis (0.4% of all claims) and recall rate (1.5% of all claims). Payments were made to 78% of awake paralysis claims compared with 55% of all other claims (55%).

Some of the key recommendations of anesthesia related maternal mortality were: (1) Dedicated obstetric anesthesia services should be available in all consultant obstetric unit. (2) Adequate advance notice of elective high risk cases must be given to the obstetric anesthetic service. (3) Care of women at high risk of maternal hemorrhage must involve consultant obstetric anesthetists at the earliest possible time.

Maternal mortality figures from the U.S. were reported in 1997 Table 18-2. This report observed that although the incidence of general anesthesia dropped dramatically from 79–84 to 85–90 maternal deaths remained the same; whereas the incidence of maternal mortality dropped even with significant increase in numbers of regional anesthesia.[2] It has been well recognized that regional anesthesia is safer than general anesthesia for cesarean section. Difficulty and inability to intubate remain the major problems with general anesthesia.

Besides mortality, the maternal morbidity rate also should be recognized. A closed claim study of 1991 showed the inci-

Table 18-2. Delivery by Type of Anesthesia, United States, 1979-1984 and 1985-1990

Anesthesia	Number of deaths		Case fatality rate		Risk ratio	
	79-84	85-90	79-84	85-90	79-84	85-90
General	33	32	20.0*	32.3*	2.3	16.7
Regional	19	9	8.6†	1.9†	Referent	Referent

*Per million general anesthetics for cesarean section
†Per million regional anesthetics for cesarean section

dences of malpractice claim in nonobstetric and obstetric population.[6] (Table 18-3)

More frequent nerve injuries were related to lumbo sacral plexus and spinal cord damage. Ninety-three percent of lumbosacral nerve root injuries were associated with difficult spinal and epidural needle placement with paraesthesia. Spinal cord injuries were related to epidural hematoma which occurred in anticoagulated patients. The major problem is the popularity of low-molecular weight heparin. The American Society of Regional Anesthesia published consensus statements regarding the use of neuraxial anesthesia in anticoagu-

Table 18-3. Injuries in the Obstetric Anesthesia Claims

	% Non obstetric n = 1351	% Obstetric n = 190	% Obstetric Regional anesthesia n = 124	% Obstetric General anesthesia n = 62
Headache	1 (10)	12 (23)	19 (23)	0
Pain during anesthesia	<0.5 (5)	8 (16)	13 (16)	0
Nerve injury	16 (209)	8 (16)	10 (12)	7 (4)
Emotional distress	2 (30)	6 (12)	7 (9)	5 (3)
Back pain	1 (8)	5 (9)	7 (9)	0 (0)

Percentages are based on the total claims (in parenthesis) in each group. Some claims had more than one injury and represented more than once. Chadwick HS, et al. Anesthesiology 1991;74:242.

lated patients. Patients on preoperative low molecular weight heparin (LMWH) can be assumed to have altered coagulation. In these patients, needle placement should occur at least 10–12 hours after the LMWH dose. Whereas patients receiving higher doses of LMWH (e.g. enoxaparin 1 mg/kg twice daily) will require longer delays (24 hours). First dose of LMWH should be administered two hours after catheter removal.[6]

Appendix A

American Society of Anesthesiologists Guidelines for Regional Anesthesia in Obstetrics*

These guidelines apply to the use of regional anesthesia or analgesia in which local anesthetics are administered to the parturient during labor and delivery. They are intended to encourage quality patient care but cannot guarantee any specific patient outcome. Because the availability of anesthesia resources may vary, members are responsible for interpreting and establishing the guidelines for their own institutions and practices. These guidelines are subject to revision from time to time as warranted by the evolution of technology and practice.

GUIDELINE I

Regional anesthesia should be initiated and maintained only in locations in which appropriate resuscitation equipment and drugs are immediately available to manage procedurally related problems.

---

*Approved by House of Delegates on October 12, 1988 and last amended on October 18, 2000.

Resuscitation equipment should include, but is not limited to: sources of oxygen and suction, equipment to maintain an airway and perform endotracheal intubation, a means to provide positive pressure ventilation, and drugs and equipment for cardiopulmonary resuscitation.

GUIDELINE II

Regional anesthesia should be initiated by a physician with appropriate privileges and maintained by or under the medical direction[7] of such an individual.

Physicians should be approved through the institutional credentialing process to initiate and direct the maintenance of obstetric anesthesia and to manage procedurally related complications.

GUIDELINE III

Regional anesthesia should not be administered until: (1) the patient has been examined by a qualified individual[8]; and (2) a physician with obstetrical privileges to perform operative vaginal or cesarean delivery, who has knowledge of the maternal and fetal status and the progress of labor and who approves the initiation of labor anesthesia, is readily available to supervise the labor and manage any obstetric complications that may arise.

Under circumstances defined by department protocol, qualified personnel may perform the initial pelvic examination. The physician responsible for the patient's obstetrical care should be informed of her status so that a decision can be made regarding present risk and further management.[8]

GUIDELINE IV

An intravenous infusion should be established before the initiation of regional anesthesia and maintained throughout the duration of the regional anesthetic.

GUIDELINE V

Regional anesthesia for labor and/or vaginal delivery requires that the parturient's vital signs and the fetal heart rate be monitored and documented by a qualified individual. Additional monitoring appropriate to the clinical condition of the parturient and the fetus should be employed when indicated. When extensive regional blockade is administered for complicated vaginal delivery, the standards for basic anesthetic monitoring[9] should be applied.

GUIDELINE VI

Regional anesthesia for cesarean delivery requires that the standards for basic anesthetic monitoring[9] be applied and that a physician with privileges in obstetrics be immediately available.

GUIDELINE VII

Qualified personnel, other than the anesthesiologist attending the mother, should be immediately available to assume responsibility for resuscitation of the newborn.[9]

The primary responsibility of the anesthesiologist is to provide care to the mother. If the anesthesiologist is also requested to provide brief assistance in the care of the newborn, the benefit to the child must be compared to the risk to the mother.

GUIDELINE VIII

A physician with appropriate privileges should remain readily available during the regional anesthetic to manage anesthetic complications until the patient's postanesthesia condition is satisfactory and stable.

GUIDELINE IX

All patients recovering from regional anesthesia should receive appropriate postanesthesia care. Following cesarean delivery and/or extensive regional blockade, the standards for postanesthesia care[10] should be applied.

1. A postanesthesia care unit (PACU) should be available to receive patients. The design, equipment and staffing should meet requirements of the facility's accrediting and licensing bodies.
2. When a site other than the PACU is used, equivalent postanesthesia care should be provided.

GUIDELINE X

There should be a policy to assure the availability in the facility of a physician to manage complications and to provide cardiopulmonary resuscitation for patients receiving postanesthesia care.

Appendix B

Practice Guidelines for Obstetrical Anesthesia*

*A Report by the American Society of Anesthesiologists Task Force on Obstetrical Anesthesia**

Practice guidelines are systematically developed recommendations that assist the practitioner and patient in making deci-

---

Developed by the Task Force on Obstetrical Anesthesia: Joy L. Hawkins, M.D. (Chair), Denver, Colorado; James F. Arens, M.D., Galveston, Texas; Brenda A. Bucklin, M.D., Omaha, Nebraska; Robert A. Caplan, M.D., Seattle, Washington; David H. Chestnut, M.D., Birmingham, Alabama; Richard T. Connis, Ph.D., Woodinville, Washington; Patricia A. Dailey, M.D., Hillsborough, California; Larry C. Gilstrap, M.D., Houston, Texas; Stephen C. Grice, M.D., Alpharetta, Georgia; Nancy E. Oriol, M.D., Boston, Massachusetts; Kathryn J. Zuspan, M.D., Edina, Minnesota.

From Practice Guidelines for Obstetrical Anesthesia: A report by the American Society of Anesthesiologists Task Force on Obstetrical Anesthesia. *Anesthesiology* 1999: 90:600–611. Reprinted by permission.

sions about health care. These recommendations may be adopted, modified, or rejected according to clinical needs and constraints.

Practice guidelines are not intended as standards or absolute requirements. The use of practice guidelines cannot guarantee any specific outcome. Practice guidelines are subject to periodic revision as warranted by the evolution of medical knowledge, technology, and practice. The guidelines provide basic recommendations that are supported by analysis of the current literature and by a synthesis of expert opinion, open forum commentary, and clinical feasibility data (Appendix).

A. Purposes of the Guidelines for Obstetrical Anesthesia

The purposes of these Guidelines are to enhance the quality of anesthesia care for obstetric patients, reduce the incidence and severity of anesthesia-related complications, and increase patient satisfaction.

B. Focus

The Guidelines focus on the anesthetic management of pregnant patients during labor, nonoperative delivery, operative delivery, and selected aspects of postpartum care. The intended patient population includes, but is not limited to intrapartum and postpartum patients with uncomplicated pregnancies or with common obstetric problems. The Guidelines do not apply to patients undergoing surgery during pregnancy, gynecological patients or parturients with chronic medical disease (e.g., severe heart, renal or neurological disease).

C. Application

The Guidelines are intended for use by anesthesiologists. They also may serve as a resource for other anesthesia providers and health care professionals who advise or care for patients who will receive anesthesia care during labor, delivery and the immediate postpartum period.

D. Task Force Members and Consultants

The ASA appointed a Task Force of 11 members to review the published evidence and obtain consultant opinion from a representative body of anesthesiologists and obstetricians. The Task Force members consisted of anesthesiologists in both private and academic practices from various geographic areas of the United States.

The Task Force met its objective in a five-step process. First, original published research studies relevant to these issues were reviewed and analyzed. Second, Consultants from various geographic areas of the United States who practice or work in various settings (e.g., academic and private practice) were asked to participate in opinion surveys and review and comment on drafts of the Guidelines. Third, the Task Force held two open forums at major national meetings to solicit input from attendees on its draft recommendations. Fourth, all available information was used by the Task Force in developing the Guideline recommendations. Finally, the Consultants were surveyed to assess their opinions on the feasibility of implementing the Guidelines.

E. Availability and Strength of Evidence

Evidence-based guidelines are developed by a rigorous analytic process. To assist the reader, the Guidelines make use of several descriptive terms that are easier to understand than the technical terms and data that are used in the actual analyses. These descriptive terms are defined below:

The following terms describe the availability of scientific evidence in the literature.

Insufficient: There are too few published studies to investigate a relationship between a clinical intervention and clinical outcome.

Inconclusive: Published studies are available, but they cannot be used to assess the relationship between a clinical intervention and a clinical outcome because the studies either do not meet predefined criteria for content as defined in the "Focus of the Guidelines," or do not meet research design or analytic standards.

Silent: There are no available studies in the literature that address a relationship of interest.

The following terms describe the strength of scientific data.

Supportive: There is sufficient quantitative information from adequately designed studies to describe a statistically significant relationship ($p < 0.01$) between a clinical intervention and a clinical outcome, using the technique of meta-analysis.

Suggestive: There is enough information from case reports and descriptive studies to provide a directional assessment of the relationship between a clinical intervention and a clinical outcome. This type of qualitative information does not permit a statistical assessment of significance.

Equivocal: Qualitative data have not provided a clear direction for clinical outcomes related to a clinical intervention and (1) there is insufficient quantitative information or (2) aggregated comparative studies have found no quantitatively significant differences among groups or conditions.

The following terms describe survey responses from Consultants for any specified issue. Responses are weighted as agree = +1, undecided = 0, or disagree = –1.

Agree: The average weighted responses must be equal to or greater than +0.30 (on a scale of –1 to 1) to indicate agreement.

Equivocal: The average weighted responses must be between –0.30 and +0.30 (on a scale of –1 to 1) to indicate an equivocal response.

Disagree: The average weighted responses must be equal to or less than –0.30 (on a scale of –1 to 1) to indicate disagreement.

Guidelines

I. Perianesthetic Evaluation

1. History and Physical Examination. The literature is silent regarding the relationship between anesthesia-related obstetric outcomes and the performance of a focused history and physical examination. However, there is suggestive data that a patient's medical history and/or findings from a physical exam may be related to anesthetic outcomes. The Consultants and Task Force agree that a focused history and physical examination may be associated with reduced maternal, fetal and neonatal complications. The Task Force agrees that the obstetric patient benefits from communication between the anesthesiologist and the obstetrician.

Recommendations: The anesthesiologist should do a focused history and physical examination when consulted to deliver anesthesia care. This should include a maternal health history, an anesthesia-related obstetric history, an airway examination, and a baseline blood pressure measurement. When a regional anesthetic is planned, the back should be examined. Recognition of significant anesthetic risk factors should encourage consultation with the obstetrician.

2. Intrapartum Platelet Count. A platelet count may indicate the severity of a patient's pregnancy-induced hypertension. However, the literature is insufficient to assess the predictive value of a platelet count for anesthesia-related complications in either uncomplicated parturients or those with pregnancy-induced hypertension. The Consultants and Task Force both agree that a routine platelet count in the healthy parturient is not necessary. However, in the patient with pregnancy-induced hypertension, the Consultants and Task Force both agree that the use of a platelet count may reduce the risk of anesthesia-related complications.

Recommendations: A specific platelet count predictive of regional anesthetic complications has not been determined. The anesthesiologist's decision to order or require a platelet count should be individualized and based upon a patient's history, physical examination and clinical signs of a coagulopathy.

3. Blood Type and Screen. The literature is silent regarding whether obtaining a blood type and screen is associated with fewer maternal anesthetic complications. The Consultants and Task Force are equivocal regarding the routine use of a blood type and screen to reduce the risk of anesthesia-related complications.

Recommendations: The anesthesiologist's decision to order or require a blood type and screen or crossmatch should be individualized and based on anticipated hemorrhagic complications (e.g., placenta previa in a patient with previous uterine surgery).

4. Perianesthetic Recording of the Fetal Heart Rate. The literature suggests that analgesic/anesthetic agents may influence the fetal heart rate pattern. There is insufficient literature to demonstrate that perianesthetic recording of the fetal heart rate prevents fetal complications. However, both the Task Force and Consultants agree that perianesthetic recording of the fetal heart rate reduces fetal and neonatal complications.

Recommendations: The fetal heart rate should be monitored by a qualified individual before and after administration of regional analgesia for labor. The Task Force recognizes that *continuous* electronic recording of the fetal heart rate may not be necessary in every clinical setting[12] and may not be possible during placement of a regional anesthetic.

II. Fasting in the Obstetric Patient

1. Clear Liquids. Published evidence is insufficient regarding the relationship between fasting times for clear liquids and the risk of emesis/reflux or pulmonary aspiration during labor. The Task Force and Consultants agree that oral intake of clear liquids during labor improves maternal comfort and satisfaction. The Task Force and Consultants are equivocal whether oral intake of clear liquids increases maternal risk of pulmonary aspiration.

Recommendations: The oral intake of modest amounts of clear liquids may be allowed for uncomplicated laboring patients. Examples of clear liquids include, but are not limited to, water, fruit juices without pulp, carbonated beverages, clear tea, and black coffee. The volume of liquid ingested is less important than the type of liquid ingested. However, patients with additional risk factors of aspiration (e.g., morbid obesity, diabetes, difficult airway), or patients at increased risk for operative delivery (e.g., nonreassuring fetal heart rate pattern) may have further restrictions of oral intake, determined on a case-by-case basis.

2. Solids. A specific fasting time for solids that is predictive of maternal anesthetic complications has not been determined. There is insufficient published evidence to address the safety of *any* particular fasting period for solids for obstetric patients. The Consultants agree that a fasting period for solids of 8 hours or more is preferable for uncomplicated parturients undergoing *elective* cesarean delivery. The Task Force recognizes that in laboring patients the timing of delivery is uncertain; therefore compliance with a predetermined fasting period is not always possible. The Task Force supports a fasting period of at least 6 hours before elective cesarean delivery.

Recommendations: Solid foods should be avoided in laboring patients. The patient undergoing elective cesarean delivery should undergo a fasting period for solids consistent with the hospital's policy for nonobstetric patients undergoing elective surgery. Both the amount and type of food ingested must be considered when determining the timing of surgery.

III. Anesthesia Care for Labor and Vaginal Delivery

A. Overview of Recommendations. Anesthesia care is not necessary for all women for labor and/or delivery. For women who request pain relief for labor and/or delivery, there are many effective analgesic techniques available. Maternal request represents sufficient justification for pain relief, but the selected analgesia technique depends on the medical status of the patient, the progress of the labor, and the resources of the facility. When sufficient resources (e.g., anesthesia and nursing staff) are available, epidural catheter techniques should be one of the analgesic options offered. The primary goal is to provide adequate maternal analgesia with as little motor block as possible when regional analgesia is used for uncomplicated labor and/or vaginal delivery. This can be achieved by the administration of local anesthetic at low concentrations. The concentration of the local anesthetic may be further reduced by the addition of narcotics and still provide adequate analgesia.

B. Specific Recommendations

1. Epidural Anesthetics:

a. Epidural Local Anesthetics. The literature supports the use of single-bolus epidural local anesthetics for providing greater quality of analgesia compared to *parenteral opioids.* However, the literature indicates a reduced incidence of spontaneous vaginal delivery associated with single-bolus epidural local anesthetics. The literature is insufficient to indicate causation. Compared to *single-injection spinal opioids* the literature is equivocal regarding the analgesic efficacy of single-bolus epidural local anesthetics. The literature suggests that epidural local anesthetics compared to spinal opioids are associated with a lower incidence of pruritus. The literature is insufficient to compare the incidence of other side-effects.

b. Addition of Opioids to Epidural Local Anesthetics. The literature supports the use of epidural local anesthetics with opioids, when compared with *equal* concentrations of epidural local anesthetics without opioids for providing greater quality and duration of analgesia. The former is associated with reduced motor block and an increased likelihood of spontaneous delivery, possibly as a result of a reduced total dose of local anesthetic administered over time.[†]

The literature is equivocal regarding the analgesic efficacy of *low* concentrations of epidural local anesthetics with opioids compared to *higher* concentrations of epidural local anesthetics without opioids. The literature indicates that low concentrations of epidural local anesthetics with opioids compared to higher concentrations of epidural local anesthetics are associated with reduced motor block.

No differences in the incidence of nausea, hypotension, duration of labor, or neonatal outcomes are found when epidural local anesthetics with opioids were compared to epidural local anesthetics without opioids. However, the literature indicates that the addition of opioids to epidural local anesthetics results in a higher incidence of pruritus. The liter-

---

[†]No meta-analytic differences in the likelihood of spontaneous delivery were found when studies using morphine or meperidine were added to studies using only fentanyl or sufentanil.

ature is insufficient to determine the effects of epidural local anesthetics with opioids on other maternal outcomes (e.g., respiratory depression, urinary retention).

The Task Force and majority of Consultants are supportive of the case-by-case selection of an analgesic technique for labor. The subgroup of Consultants reporting a preferred technique, when all choices are available, selected an epidural local anesthetic technique. When a low concentration of epidural local anesthetic is used, the Consultants and Task Force agree that the addition of an opioid(s) improves analgesia and maternal satisfaction without increasing maternal, fetal, or neonatal complications.

Recommendations: The selected analgesic/anesthetic technique should reflect patient needs and preferences, practitioner preferences or skills, and available resources. When an epidural local anesthetic is selected for labor and delivery, the addition of an opioid may allow the use of a lower concentration of local anesthetic and prolong the duration of analgesia. Appropriate resources for the treatment of complications related to epidural local anesthetics (e.g., hypotension, systemic toxicity, high spinal anesthesia) should be available. If opioids are added, treatments for related complications (e.g., pruritus, nausea, respiratory depression) should be available.

c. Continuous Infusion Epidural (CIE) Techniques. The literature indicates that effective analgesia can be maintained with a low concentration of local anesthetic with an epidural infusion technique. In addition, when an opioid is added to a local anesthetic infusion, an even lower concentration of local anesthetic provides effective analgesia. For example, comparable analgesia is found, with a reduced incidence of motor block, using bupivacaine infusion concentrations of *less than* 0.125% with an opioid compared to bupivacaine concentrations *equal to* 0.125% without an opioid.[‡] No comparative differences are noted for incidence of instrumental delivery.

[‡]References to bupivacaine are included for illustrative purposes only, and because bupivacaine is the most extensively studied local anesthetic for CIE. The Task Force recognizes that other local anesthetic agents are equally appropriate for CIE.

The literature is equivocal regarding the relationship between different local anesthetic infusion regimens and the incidence of nausea or neonatal outcome. However, the literature suggests that local anesthetic infusions with opioids are associated with a higher incidence of pruritus.

The Task Force and Consultants agree that infusions using low concentrations of local anesthetics with or without opioids provide equivalent analgesia, reduced motor block, and improved maternal satisfaction when compared to higher concentrations of local anesthetic.

Recommendations. Adequate analgesia for uncomplicated labor and delivery should be provided with the secondary goal of producing as little motor block as possible. The lowest concentration of local anesthetic infusion that provides adequate maternal analgesia and satisfaction should be used. For example, an infusion concentration of bupivacaine equal to or greater than 0.25% is unnecessary for labor analgesia for most patients. The addition of an opioid(s) to a low concentration of local anesthetic may improve analgesia and minimize motor block. Resources for the treatment of potential complications should be available.

2. Spinal Opioids with or Without Local Anesthetics. The literature suggests that spinal opioids with or without local anesthetics provide effective labor analgesia without significantly altering the incidence of neonatal complications. There is insufficient literature to compare spinal opioids with parenteral opioids. However, the Consultants and Task Force agree that spinal opioids provide improved maternal analgesia compared to parenteral opioids.

The literature is equivocal regarding analgesic efficacy of spinal opioids compared to epidural local anesthetics. The Consultants and Task Force agree that spinal opioids provide equivalent analgesia compared to epidural local anesthetics. The Task Force agrees that the rapid onset of analgesia provided by single-injection spinal techniques may be advantageous for selected patients (e.g., those in advanced labor).

Recommendations: Spinal opioids, with or without local anesthetics, may be used to provide effective, although time-limited, analgesia for labor. Resources for the treatment of potential complications (e.g., pruritus, nausea, hypotension, respiratory depression) should be available.

3. Combined Spinal-Epidural Techniques. Although the literature suggests that combined spinal-epidural techniques (CSE) provide effective analgesia, the literature is insufficient to evaluate the analgesic efficacy of CSE compared to epidural local anesthetics. The literature indicates that use of CSE techniques with opioids when compared to epidural local anesthetics with or without opioids results in a higher incidence of pruritus and nausea. The Task Force and Consultants are equivocal regarding improved analgesia or maternal benefit of CSE versus epidural techniques. Although the literature is insufficient to evaluate fetal and neonatal outcomes of CSE techniques, the Task Force and Consultants agree that CSE does not increase the risk of fetal or neonatal complications.

Recommendations: Combined spinal-epidural techniques may be used to provide rapid and effective analgesia for labor. Resources for the treatment of potential complications (e.g., pruritus, nausea, hypotension, respiratory depression) should be available.

4. Regional Analgesia and Progress of Labor. There is insufficient literature to indicate whether timing of analgesia related to cervical dilation affects labor and delivery outcomes. Both the Task Force and Consultants agree that cervical dilation at the time of epidural analgesia administration does not impact the outcome of labor.

The literature indicates that epidural analgesia may be used in a trial of labor for previous cesarean section patients without adversely affecting the incidence of vaginal delivery. However, randomized comparisons of epidural versus other specific anesthetic techniques were not found, and comparison groups were often confounded.

Recommendations: Cervical dilation is not a reliable means of determining when regional analgesia should be initiated. Regional analgesia should be administered on an individualized basis.

5. Monitored or Stand-By Anesthesia Care for Complicated Vaginal Delivery. Monitored anesthesia care refers to instances in which an anesthesiologist has been called upon to provide specific anesthesia services to a particular patient undergoing a planned procedure.[13] For these Guidelines, stand-by anesthesia care refers to availability of the anesthesiologist in the facility, in the event of obstetric complications. The literature is silent regarding the subject of monitored or stand-by anesthesia care in obstetrics. However, the Task Force and Consultants agree that monitored or stand-by anesthesia care for complicated vaginal delivery reduces maternal, fetal, and neonatal complications.

Recommendations. Either monitored or stand-by anesthesia care, determined on a case-by-case basis for complicated vaginal delivery (e.g., breech presentation, twins, and trial of instrumental delivery), should be made available when requested by the obstetrician.

IV. Removal of Retained Placenta

1. Anesthetic Choices. The literature is insufficient to indicate whether a particular type of anesthetic is more effective than another for removal of retained placenta. The literature is also insufficient to assess the relationship between a particular type of anesthetic and maternal complication. The Task Force and Consultants agree that spinal or epidural anesthesia (i.e., regional anesthesia) is associated with reduced maternal complication and improved satisfaction when compared to general anesthesia or sedation/analgesia. The Task Force recognizes that circumstances may occur when general anesthesia or sedation/analgesia may be the more appropriate anesthetic choice (e.g., significant hemorrhage).

Recommendations: Regional anesthesia, general endotracheal anesthesia, or sedation/analgesia may be used for removal of retained placenta. Hemodynamic status should be assessed before giving regional anesthesia to a parturient who has experienced significant bleeding. In cases involving significant maternal hemorrhage, a general anesthetic may be preferable to initiating regional anesthesia. Sedation/analgesia should be titrated carefully due to the potential risk of pulmonary aspiration in the recently delivered parturient with an unprotected airway.

2. Nitroglycerin for Uterine Relaxation. The literature suggests and the Task Force and Consultants agree that the administration of nitroglycerin is effective for uterine relaxation during removal of retained placental tissue.

Recommendations: Nitroglycerin is an alternative to terbutaline sulfate or general endotracheal anesthesia with halogenated agents for uterine relaxation during removal of retained placental tissue. Initiating treatment with a low dose of nitroglycerin may relax the uterus sufficiently while minimizing potential complications (e.g., hypotension).

V. Anesthetic Choice for Cesarean Delivery

The literature suggests that spinal, epidural or CSE anesthetic techniques can be used effectively for cesarean delivery. When compared to regional techniques, the literature indicates that general anesthetics can be administered with shorter induction-to-delivery times. The literature is insufficient to determine the relative risk of maternal death associated with general anesthesia compared to other anesthetic techniques. However, the literature suggests that a greater number of maternal deaths occur when general anesthesia is administered. The literature indicates that a larger proportion of neonates in the general anesthesia groups, compared to those in the regional anesthesia groups, are assigned Apgar scores of less than 7 at one and five minutes. However, few studies have utilized randomized comparisons of general versus regional anesthesia, resulting in potential selection bias in the reporting of outcomes.

The literature suggests that maternal side effects associated with regional techniques may include hypotension, nausea, vomiting, pruritus and postdural puncture headache. The literature is insufficient to examine the comparative merits of various regional anesthetic techniques.

The Consultants agree that regional anesthesia can be administered with fewer maternal and neonatal complications and improved maternal satisfaction when compared to general anesthesia. The consultants are equivocal about the possibility of increased maternal complications when comparing spinal or epidural anesthesia with CSE techniques. They agree that neonatal complications are not increased with CSE techniques.

Recommendations: The decision to use a particular anesthetic technique should be individualized based on several factors. These include anesthetic, obstetric and/or fetal risk factors (e.g., elective versus emergency) and the preferences of the patient and anesthesiologist. Resources for the treatment of potential complications (e.g., airway management, inadequate analgesia, hypotension, pruritus, nausea) should be available.

VI. Postpartum Tubal Ligation

There is insufficient literature to evaluate the comparative benefits of local, spinal, epidural or general anesthesia for postpartum tubal ligation. Both the Task Force and Consultants agree that epidural, spinal and general anesthesia can be effectively provided without affecting maternal complications. Neither the Task Force nor the Consultants agree that local anesthetic techniques provide effective anesthesia, and they are equivocal regarding the impact of local anesthesia on maternal complications. Although the literature is insufficient, the Task Force and Consultants agree that a postpartum tubal ligation can be performed safely within eight hours of delivery in many patients.

Recommendations: Evaluation of the patient for postpartum tubal ligation should include assessment of hemodynamic status (e.g., blood loss) and consideration of anesthetic risks. The patient planning to have an elective postpartum tubal ligation within 8 hours of delivery should have no oral intake of solid foods during labor, and postpartum until the time of surgery. Both the timing of the procedure and the decision to use a particular anesthetic technique (i.e., regional versus general) should be individualized, based on anesthetic and/or obstetric risk factors and patient preferences. The anesthesiologist should be aware that an epidural catheter placed for labor may be more likely to fail with longer postdelivery time intervals. If a postpartum tubal ligation is to be done before the patient is discharged from the hospital, the procedure should not be attempted at a time when it might compromise other aspects of patient care in the labor and delivery area.

VII. Management of Complications

1. Resources for Management of Hemorrhagic Emergencies. The literature suggests that the availability of resources for hemorrhagic emergencies is associated with reduced maternal complications. The Task Force and Consultants agree that the availability of resources for managing hemorrhagic emergencies is associated with reduced maternal, fetal and neonatal complications.

Recommendations: Institutions providing obstetric care should have resources available to manage hemorrhagic emergencies (Table 18-4). In an emergency, the use of type-specific or O-negative blood is acceptable in the parturient.

2. Equipment for Management of Airway Emergencies. The literature suggests, and the Task Force and Consultants agree, that the availability of equipment for the management of airway emergencies is associated with reduced maternal complications.

Recommendations: Labor and delivery units should have equipment and personnel readily available to manage airway emergencies. Basic airway management equipment should be immediately available during the initial provision of regional analgesia (Table 18-5). In addition, portable equipment for difficult airway management should be readily available in the operative area of labor and delivery units (Table 18-6).

Table 18-4. Suggested Resources for Obstetric Hemorrhagic Emergencies*

1. Large bore iv catheters
2. Fluid warmer
3. Forced air body warmer
4. Availability of blood bank resources
5. Equipment for infusing iv fluids and/or blood products rapidly. Examples include (but are not limited to) hand squeezed fluid chambers, hand inflated pressure bags, and automatic infusion devices.

*The items listed represent suggestions. The items should be customized to meet the specific needs, preferences, and skills of the practitioner and healthcare facility.

Table 18–5. Suggested Resources for Airway Management During Initial Provision of Regional Anesthesia*

1. Laryngoscope and assorted blades
2. Endotracheal tubes, with stylets
3. Oxygen source
4. Suction source with tubing and catheters
5. Self-inflating bag and mask for positive pressure ventilation
6. Medications for blood pressure support, muscle relaxation, and hypnosis

*The items listed represent suggestions. The items should be customized to meet the specific needs, preferences, and skills of the practitioner and health care facility.

Table 18–6. Suggested Contents of a Portable Unit for Difficult Airway Management for Cesarean Section Rooms*

1. Rigid laryngoscope blades and handles of alternate design and size from those routinely used†
2. Endotracheal tubes of assorted size
3. Laryngeal mask airways of assorted sizes
4. At least one device suitable for emergency nonsurgical airway ventilation. Examples include (but are not limited to) retrograde intubation equipment, a hollow jet ventilation stylet or cricothyrotomy kit with or without a transtracheal jet ventilator, and the esophageal–tracheal combitube.
5. Endotracheal tube guides. Examples include (but are not limited to) semirigid stylets with or without a hollow core for jet ventilation, light wands, and forceps designed to manipulate the distal portion of the endotracheal tube.
6. Equipment suitable for emergency surgical airway access
7. Topical anesthetics and vasoconstrictors

*The items listed represent suggestions. The items should be customized to meet the specific needs, preferences, and skills of the practitioner and health-care facility.

†The Task Force believes fiberoptic intubation equipment should be readily available.

Adapted from Practice guidelines for management of the difficult airway: A report by the American Society of Anesthesiologists Task Force on Management of the Difficult Airway. *Anesthesiology* 1993; 78:599–602.

3. Central Invasive Hemodynamic Monitoring. There is insufficient literature to indicate whether pulmonary artery catheterization is associated with improved maternal, fetal or neonatal outcomes in patients with pregnancy-related hypertensive disorders. The literature is silent regarding the management of obstetric patients with central venous catheterization alone. The literature suggests that pulmonary artery catheterization has been used safely in obstetric patients; however, the literature is insufficient to examine specific obstetric outcomes. The Task Force and Consultants agree that it is not necessary to use central invasive hemodynamic monitoring routinely for parturients with severe preeclampsia.

Recommendations: The decision to perform invasive hemodynamic monitoring should be individualized and based on clinical indications that include the patient's medical history and cardiovascular risk factors. The Task Force recognizes that not all practitioners have access to resources for utilization of central venous or pulmonary artery catheters in obstetric units.

4. Cardiopulmonary Resuscitation. The literature is insufficient to evaluate the efficacy of CPR in the obstetric patient during labor and delivery. The Task Force is supportive of the immediate availability of basic and advanced life-support equipment in the operative area of labor and delivery units.

Recommendations: Basic and advanced life-support equipment should be immediately available in the operative area of labor and delivery units. If cardiac arrest occurs during labor and delivery, standard resuscitative measures and procedures, including left uterine displacement, should be taken. In cases of cardiac arrest, the American Heart Association has stated the following: "Several authors now recommend that the decision to perform a perimortem cesarean section should be made rapidly, with delivery effected within 4 to 5 minutes of the arrest."[14]

Appendix C

American Society of Anesthesiologists Optimal Goals for Anesthesia Care in Obstetrics*

This joint statement from the American Society of Anesthesiologists (ASA) and the American College of Obstetricians and Gynecologists (ACOG) has been designed to address issues of concern to both specialties. Good obstetric care requires the availability of qualified personnel and equipment to administer general or regional anesthesia both electively and emergently.[15] The extent and degree to which anesthesia services are available varies widely among hospitals. However, for any hospital providing obstetric care, certain optimal anesthesia goals should be sought. These include:

I. Availability of a licensed practitioner who is credentialed to administer an appropriate anesthetic whenever necessary. For many women, regional anesthesia (epidural, spinal or combined spinal-epidural) will be the most appropriate anesthetic.

II. Availability of a licensed practitioner who is credentialed to maintain support of vital functions in any obstetric emergency.

III. Availability of anesthesia and surgical personnel to permit the start of a cesarean delivery within 30 minutes of the decision to perform the procedure; in cases of VBAC, appropriate facilities and personnel, including obstetric anesthesia, nursing personnel, and a physician capable of monitoring labor and performing cesarean delivery, immediately available during active labor to perform emergency cesarean delivery (ACOG 1999). The definition of immediate availability of personnel and facilities remains a local

*Approved by House of Delegates on October 28, 2000.

decision, based on each institution's available resources and geographic location.

IV. Appointment of a qualified anesthesiologist to be responsible for all anesthetics administered. There are obstetric units where obstetricians or obstetrician-supervised nurse anesthetists administer anesthetics. The administration of general or regional anesthesia requires both medical judgment and technical skills. Thus, a physician with privileges in anesthesiology should be readily available.

Persons administering or supervising obstetric anesthesia should be qualified to manage the infrequent but occasionally life-threatening complications of major regional anesthesia such as respiratory and cardiovascular failure, toxic local anesthetic convulsions, or vomiting and aspiration. Mastering and retaining the skills and knowledge necessary to manage these complications require adequate training and frequent application.

To ensure the safest and most effective anesthesia for obstetric patients, the director of anesthesia services, with the approval of the medical staff, should develop and enforce written policies regarding provision of obstetric anesthesia. These include:

I. Availability of a qualified physician with obstetrical privileges to perform operative vaginal or cesarean delivery during administration of anesthesia. Regional and/or general anesthesia should not be administered until the patient has been examined and the fetal status and progress of labor evaluated by a qualified individual. A physician with obstetrical privileges who has knowledge of the maternal and fetal status and the progress of labor, and who approves the initiation of labor anesthesia, should be readily available to deal with any obstetric complications that may arise.

II. Availability of equipment, facilities, and support personnel equal to that provided in the surgical suite. This should include the availability of a properly equipped and staffed recovery room capable of receiving and caring for all patients recovering from major regional or general anesthesia. Birthing facilities, when used for analgesia or anesthesia, must be appropriately equipped to provide safe anesthetic care during labor and delivery or post-anesthesia recovery care.

Personnel other than the surgical team should be immediately available to assume responsibility for resuscitation of the depressed newborn. The surgeon and anesthesiologist are responsible for the mother and may not be able to leave her care for the newborn even when a regional anesthetic is functioning adequately. Individuals qualified to perform neonatal resuscitation should demonstrate:

A. Proficiency in rapid and accurate evaluation of the newborn condition including Apgar scoring.
B. Knowledge of the pathogenesis of a depressed newborn (acidosis, drugs, hypovolemia, trauma, anomalies and infection), as well as specific indications for resuscitation.
C. Proficiency in newborn airway management, laryngoscopy, endotracheal intubations, suctioning of airways, artificial ventilation, cardiac massage and maintenance of thermal stability.

In larger maternity units and those functioning as high-risk centers, 24-hour in-house anesthesia, obstetric and neonatal specialists are usually necessary. Preferably, the obstetric anesthesia services should be directed by an anesthesiologist with special training or experience in obstetric anesthesia. These units will also frequently require the availability of more sophisticated monitoring equipment and specially trained nursing personnel.

A survey jointly sponsored by the ASA and ACOG found that many hospitals in the United States have not yet achieved the above goals. Deficiencies were most evident in smaller delivery units. Some small delivery units are necessary because of geographic considerations. Currently, approximately 50 percent of hospital providing obstetric care have fewer than 500 deliveries per year. Providing comprehensive care for obstetric patients in these small units is extremely inefficient, not cost-effective and frequently impossible. Thus, the following recommendations are made:

1. Whenever possible, small units should consolidate.
2. When geographic factors require the existence of smaller units, these units should be part of a well-established regional perinatal system.

The availability of the appropriate personnel to assist in the management of a variety of obstetric problems is a necessary feature of good obstetric care. The presence of a pediatrician or other trained physician at a high-risk cesarcan delivery to care for the newborn or the availability of an anesthesiologist during active labor and delivery when vaginal birth after cesarcan delivery (VBAC) is attempted, and at a breech or twin delivery are examples. Frequently, these professionals spend a considerable amount of time standing by for the possibility that their services may be needed emergently but may ultimately not be required to perform the tasks for which they are present. Reasonable compensation for these standby services is justifiable and necessary.

A variety of other mechanisms have been suggested to increase the availability and quality of anesthesia services in obstetrics. Improved hospital design to place labor and delivery suites closer to the operating rooms would allow for more efficient supervision of nurse anesthetists. Anesthesia equipment in the labor and delivery area must be comparable to that in the operating room.

Finally, good interpersonal relations between obstetricians and anesthesiologists are important. Joint meetings between the two departments should be encouraged. Anesthesiologists should recognize the special needs and concerns of the obstetrician and obstetricians should recognize the anesthesiologist as a consultant in the management of pain and life-support measures. Both should recognize the need to provide high quality care for all patients.

References

1. Confidential enquiry into maternal deaths 2003, Why mothers die 97/99 report.
2. Hawkin JL, Koonin LM, Palmer SK, et al. Anesthesia related deaths during obstetric delivery in the United States 1979–1990. Anesthesiology 1997;86:227.
3. Chadwick HS, Posner K, Caplan RA, et al. A comparison of obstetric and nonobstetric anesthesia malpractice claims. Anesthesiology 1991;74:242.

4. Cheney FW, Domino KB, Caplan RA, et al. Nerve injury associated with anesthesia: A closed claim analysis. Anesthesiology 1999;90:1062.
5. Domino KB, Posner KL, Caplan RA. Awareness during anesthesia: A closed claim analysis. Anesthesiology 1999;90:1053.
6. Horlocker TT, Wedel DJ. Neuraxial block and low-molecular weight heparin: Balancing perioperative analgesia and thromboprophylaxis. Reg Anesth 1998;23:164.
7. The Anesthesia Care Team (Approved by ASA House of Delegates 10/26/82 and last amended 10/25/95).
8. Guidelines for Perinatal Care (American Academy of Pediatrics and American College of Obstetricians and Gynecologists, 1988).
9. Standards for Bask Anesthetic Monitoring (Approved by ASA House of Delegates 10/21/85 and last amended 10/21/98).
10. Standards for Postanesthesia Care (Approved by ASA House of Delegate 10/12/88 and last amended 10/19/94).
11. Practice guidelines for obstetrical anesthesia: A report by the American Society of Anesthesiologists Task Force on Obstetrical Anesthesia. *Anesthesiology* 1999; 90:600.
12. Guidelines for Perinatal Care, 4th ed. American Academy of Pediatrics and American College of Obstetricians and Gynecologists, 1997, p 100–102.
13. American Society of Anesthesiologists: Position on monitored anesthesia care, ASA Standards, Guidelines and Statements. Park Ridge, IL, American Society of Anesthesiologists, October 1997, pp 20–21.
14. Guidelines for cardiopulmonary resuscitation and emergency cardiac care: Recommendations of the 1992 national conference. JAMA 1992; 268:2249.
15. American College of Obstetricians and Gynecologists. Vaginal birth after previous cesarean delivery. ACOG Practice Bulletin. Washington, DC: ACOG, 1999.
16. Committee on Perinatal Health. Toward Improving the Outcome of Pregnancy. The 90s and Beyond. White Plains. New York: March of Dimes Birth Defects Foundation, 1993.

Index